DISCARDED

T5-BQC-921

FATHERS AND MOTHERS: DILEMMAS OF THE WORK-LIFE BALANCE

Social Indicators Research Series
Volume 21

General Editor:

ALEX C. MICHALOS
*University of Northern British Columbia,
Prince George, Canada*

Editors:

ED DIENER
University of Illinois, Champaign, U.S.A.

WOLFGANG GLATZER
J.W. Goethe University, Frankfurt am Main, Germany

TORBJORN MOUM
University of Oslo, Norway

MIRJAM A.G. SPRANGERS
University of Amsterdam, The Netherlands

JOACHIM VOGEL
Central Bureau of Statistics, Stockholm, Sweden

RUUT VEENHOVEN
Erasmus University, Rotterdam, The Netherlands

This new series aims to provide a public forum for single treatises and collections of papers on social indicators research that are too long to be published in our journal *Social Indicators Research*. Like the journal, the book series deals with statistical assessments of the quality of life from a broad perspective. It welcomes the research on a wide variety of substantive areas, including health, crime, housing, education, family life, leisure activities, transportation, mobility, economics, work, religion and environmental issues. These areas of research will focus on the impact of key issues such as health on the overall quality of life and vice versa. An international review board, consisting of Ruut Veenhoven, Joachim Vogel, Ed Diener, Torbjorn Moum, Mirjam A.G. Sprangers and Wolfgang Glatzer, will ensure the high quality of the series as a whole.

The titles published in this series are listed at the end of this volume.

FATHERS AND MOTHERS: DILEMMAS OF THE WORK-LIFE BALANCE

A Comparative Study in Four European Countries

by

MARGRET FINE-DAVIS
*Centre for Gender and Women's Studies,
Trinity College, Dublin, Ireland*

JEANNE FAGNANI
*Centre National de la Recherche Scientifique,
MATISSE, University of Paris-1, France*

DINO GIOVANNINI
*Department of Social, Cognitive and Quantitative Sciences,
University of Modena & Reggio Emilia, Italy*

LIS HØJGAARD
*Institute of Political Science,
University of Copenhagen, Denmark*

and

HILARY CLARKE
*Centre for Gender and Women's Studies,
Trinity College, Dublin, Ireland*

KLUWER ACADEMIC PUBLISHERS
DORDRECHT / BOSTON / LONDON

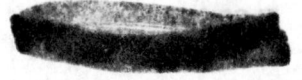

A C.I.P. Catalogue record for this book is available from the Library of Congress.

ISBN 1-4020-1807-X

Published by Kluwer Academic Publishers,
P.O. Box 17, 3300 AA Dordrecht, The Netherlands.

Sold and distributed in North, Central and South America
by Kluwer Academic Publishers,
101 Philip Drive, Norwell, MA 02061, U.S.A.

In all other countries, sold and distributed
by Kluwer Academic Publishers,
P.O. Box 322, 3300 AH Dordrecht, The Netherlands.

Printed on acid-free paper

All Rights Reserved
© 2004 Kluwer Academic Publishers
No part of this work may be reproduced, stored in a retrieval system, or transmitted
in any form or by any means, electronic, mechanical, photocopying, microfilming,
recording or otherwise, without written permission from the Publisher, with the exception
of any material supplied specifically for the purpose of being entered
and executed on a computer system, for exclusive use by the purchaser of the work.

Printed in the Netherlands.

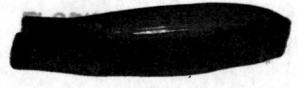

PREFACE

At the risk of sounding frivolous, there is a good case to be made for the argument that women constitute the revolutionary force behind contemporary social and economic transformation. It is in large part the changing role of women that explains the new household structure, our altered demographic behaviour, the growth of the service economy and, as a consequence, the new dilemmas that the advanced societies face.

Most European countries have failed to adapt adequately to the novel challenges and the result is an increasingly serious disequilibrium. Women explicitly desire economic independence and the societal collective, too, needs to maximise female employment. And yet, this runs up against severe incompatibility problems that then result in very low birth rates. Our aging societies need more kids, yet fertility levels are often only half of what citizens define as their desired number of children. No matter what happens in the next decade, we are doomed to have exceedingly small cohorts that, in turn, must shoulder the massive burden of supporting a retired baby-boom generation. Hence it is tantamount that tomorrow's adults be maximally productive and, yet, the typical EU member state invests very little in its children and families.

Our politicians have come to recognize, more or less seriously, the need for a recast welfare state. Indeed, the new clarion call is for mother-friendly policies, usually defined as a basic package of maternity/parental leave plus access to day care. Some governments, like the Spanish, prefer that the package be delivered via tax-deductions – an approach that does little to help lower income families. Others, like the Dutch, attempt to persuade employers to furnish the package – a strategy that may run up against the hardening international competitive pressures that firms face. And, still others – Scandinavia *par excellence* favour public guarantees – putting their faith in the citizenry's willingness to pay taxes.

The great contribution of *Fathers and Mothers* is that it forces us to reconsider the merits of the basic mother-friendly policy package. This excellent cross-national study unambiguously shows that a truly workable and positive social equilibrium needs more than public support for mothers. It needs, somehow or other, to equalize the employment *and* caring roles of men and women alike. The conclusion I draw from this book is that policies that help reconcile women's dual role are, perhaps, necessary but they are not sufficient. To be also sufficient, we need policies that will make it more attractive and possible for men to dedicate themselves to their families.

The societal revolution that latter-day women are bringing about is mainly spurred by radical change in women's own life course behaviour. When one studies the life course behaviour of Europeans over the past 30-40 years, one is struck by an amazing asymmetry: beginning with educated women and eventually extending to most, we detect a clear masculinisation of female biographies. Women are converging with men in educational attainment, in participation rates and, especially, in life-long employment. The amazing thing is that women have done all the changing while men stubbornly cling to a life course model that closely resembles that of their fathers and grandfathers.

What *Fathers and Mothers* helps us realize is that no workable social equilibrium can materialise unless we somehow begin to also reconstruct the male life course. True, the data show that there are distinct national differences in the way men and women jointly distribute their energies, time, and responsibilities. As a Dane, I am of course happy to see that Danish men are somewhat more advanced along the 'feminisation' project than are their Italian, Irish or French brethren. But anything that would look like democratic sharing is nowhere to be seen. So the question we must ask ourselves is: what are the true obstacles to more equality between the sexes?

The empirical work that underpins *Fathers and Mothers* provides the reader with some valuable clues. The samples of citizens that the team of researchers study are quite small, but they opted for a design that is quite clever: interviewing people in both public and private sector jobs, and people from both high and low socio-economic status backgrounds. The need to improve upon productivity in the public sector will probably harden conditions for its workforce, but it is still evident that being employed in the 'soft economy' makes it far more easy for a parent to reconcile career and family. In contrast, there is little doubt that being employed in highly competitive, hard-economy firms implies levels of work and career commitment that leave less time and energy for children, cooking or cleaning. The huge public sector in Denmark is no doubt one reason why Danes appear somewhat more gender egalitarian. But only up to a point. Public sector employment is in large part a female ghetto, whereas Danish men tend to be highly concentrated in the hard economy. Why? Perhaps because of Denmark's gender equality policies. With only small gender wage differentials and a very generous package of mother-friendly policy, the median Danish employer will rationally discriminate against female candidates, simply because it is statistically highly probable that the woman will take full advantage of the opportunities for leave and absenteeism that are offered to her. The paradox here is that policies aimed to strengthen women's capabilities may, inadvertently, reproduce gender segregation in the labour market.

We should, of course, be careful not to place the entire blame on 'structure'. As Katherine Hakim and others have taught us, contemporary women remain exceedingly heterogeneous with regard to their life preferences. The full-blown career woman remains a fairly small minority. And, no doubt, a substantial proportion remain principally dedicated to motherhood and, hence, select educational and employment trajectories that are inherently mother friendly. We also know that marital homogamy remains as powerful as always, meaning that pressure on the male partner to share household and caring work will depend very much on the female partner's preference set. Much of the variation that *Fathers and Mothers* identifies among couples – and between nations – may be explained by factors related to working life or welfare state programs. But I think it is a safe guess that much of the variation is also caused by differences in preferences and how these, in turn, shape the bargaining process that unfolds between mothers and fathers.

Existing obstacles to equal sharing may be formidable and preferences are surely deeply rooted in our cultures. The good news that emanates from this book is that neither one or the other is immune to change. Fathers and mothers in Denmark fare substantially better than in other countries, in part because the welfare state diminished incompatabilities and, I believe, also because there are stronger incentives for men to embrace a more feminine life course. In Denmark – and even more in Sweden – a growing proportion of fathers now interupt their careers in order to dedicate more time to their family. The best news on this front is that the duration of these interruptions is increasing.

Existing dilemmas of the work-life balance will clearly not evaporate soon, probably not during my life-time. Indeed, when we consider the current status of the policy debate across the European Union, there is clearly a very long way to go. But we can accelerate good policy making and this is what this important book should help accomplish. A far greater equality between the sexes in the family-work nexus is now, more than ever before, a precondition for the welfare of individual citizens and, simultaneously, also for the collective good.

Gosta Esping-Andersen

Barcelona, 15th September 2003.

ACKNOWLEDGEMENTS

The authors wish to gratefully acknowledge the support given to the study by the European Commission, Directorate General, Employment and Social Affairs; and the Irish Department of Justice, Equality and Law Reform, who provided national co-funding through the National Development Plan (NDP) 2000-2006.

The authors also wish to express their great appreciation to all of the individuals who contributed to the study in various ways:

In France, Jeanne Galinié, Research Assistant to Dr. Jeanne Fagnani, assisted in the French literature review and data collection.

In Italy, Eloisia Goriup and Serena Pattaro assisted Prof. Dino Giovannini with the Italian literature review. Adriano De Blasi, Elisabetta Trippa and Silvia Zoboli assisted with the Italian data collection.

In Denmark, Malou Juelskjaer collaborated with Prof. Lis Hojgaard in carrying out the Danish literature review and data collection, and she organised the Danish Interviews. Maria Dohlmann, Gitte Henchel Madsen, Aviaja Sigsgaard, Karen Steller Bjerregaard and Christina Fauerby conducted the Danish interviews.

In Ireland, Mr. James Williams, Head of the Survey Unit, Economic and Social Research Institute, Dublin, was responsible for carrying out the analysis of the four-country data; he was assisted by Ann-Marie McCafferty. Mary McCarthy collaborated with the authors in conducting the Irish interviews. Megan Berry organised the Conference, "Fathers and Mothers: Dilemmas of the Work-Life Balance", held at Trinity College in June 2002 at which the preliminary findings of the study were presented; Nicola Connolly contributed to the drafting of tables. Keeley Wynne and Mairead O'Sullivan provided research assistance in the final stages, including responsibility for the painstaking tasks of editing, design, layout and preparation of the manuscript for publication.

The contributions of all of these people were invaluable to the study itself and to the final outcome of this book.

Finally, the authors wish to express their very great thanks to all the individual respondents for their essential contribution to the research, as well as to the many organisations and individuals in all of the countries who participated in the study.

NOTES ON THE AUTHORS

DR. MARGRET FINE-DAVIS

Dr. Margret Fine-Davis is Senior Research Fellow in the Centre for Gender and Women's Studies, Trinity College, Dublin, and was Director of the cross-cultural project, "Fathers and Mothers: Dilemmas of the Work-Life Balance." She was a founder member of the Centre for Women's Studies at Trinity and was its first Acting Director.

Dr. Fine-Davis is a social psychologist with primary research interests in changing gender-role attitudes, social psychological aspects of women's employment, and social indicators. She has conducted numerous studies in these areas, both in Ireland and using cross-national European data, including a time-series analysis published by the Joint Oireachtas (Parliamentary) Committee on Women's Rights, which demonstrated that gender role attitudes in Ireland had shifted significantly during a period of rapid legislative and social change. Her research has also focused on the issue of childcare and its centrality to equal employment opportunities. She was a member of the Irish Government Working Party on Child Care Facilities for Working Parents, which reported to the Government in 1983. She also represented Ireland on Eurostat's Working Party on Subjective Social Indicators, which carried out one of the first series of harmonised surveys in this field. She is currently directing the Work-Life Balance Project, under the EU EQUAL Initiative, which is studying attitudes to work-life balance of the Irish population and experimenting with innovative pilot schemes in the area of flexible working for parents and other groups.

She is a member of the International Editorial Board of the *European Journal of Women's Studies* and was formerly a member of the Editorial Board of the journal, *Social Indicators Research*.

DR. JEANNE FAGNANI

Dr. Jeanne Fagnani is Research Director at the Centre National de la Recherche Scientifique, MATISSE, University of Paris-1, and was the French partner of the cross-cultural project, "Fathers and Mothers: Dilemmas of the Work-Life Balance."
Dr. Fagnani frequently organises or takes part in seminars and workshops on European welfare systems. From 1990 to 1994, she was the person responsible for the research programme funded by the Caisse Nationale d'Allocations Familiales –

CNAF (the National Family Allowance Fund). As an Expert Member of the "European Observatory on National Family Policies" (1994-1997), she had, among other things, to analyse systems of transfers (income tax and family benefits) as far as families were concerned. She has conducted many comparative research projects, funded by the European Commission, in collaboration with European colleagues. In these projects she has investigated, in particular, the interactions between family policy, female employment and labour markets. She has recently made a comparative analysis of family policies in Germany and France and highlighted their impact on their respective fertility level and mothers' employment patterns. She also recently conducted, in collaboration with M. T. Letablier, a study of the impact of the 35-hour work law on the strategies elaborated by young working parents. She is currently the French partner of the European team "Transitions," which is conducting cross-national comparative research funded by the European Commission on the demographic patterns and professional behaviour of people aged 25-39.

PROF. DINO GIOVANNINI

Dino Giovannini is Professor of Social Psychology, Department of Social, Cognitive and Quantitative Sciences, Faculty of Communication Science at the University of Modena & Reggio Emilia (Italy), and was the Italian partner of the cross-cultural project, "Fathers and Mothers: Dilemmas of the Work-Life Balance". Within Social psychology he primarily has focused on the following research areas: social interaction and communication; communicative competence and techniques of communication; emotional involvement; social comparison, social identity, intergroup and interethnic relations; involvement of fathers in children's care and dilemmas of reconciliation between family and work in the parental couple.

During the period 1992-1994 he was the Director of a large research study on "Fathers, mothers and sharing of responsibilities in caring for children" that was funded by the 'Emilia-Romagna' Region. Subsequently, Professor Giovannini continued to conduct research on the various aspects of parental couples' labour, with particular reference to the reciprocal representations of husbands-wives/fathers-mothers regarding childcare, housework, and outside work.

He was the first President of the Executive Committee of the Italian Society of Psychology - Social Psychology Section (1996-99), as well as a member of the Executive Committee in the same Section from January 1999 to December 2001. He was President of the School for Social Workers at the University of Trento (1994-97). He is currently a member of the Committee Course for Primary School Teachers, University of Modena & Reggio Emilia.

PROF. LIS HØJGAARD

Lis Højgaard is an Associate Professor of Sociology at the Institute of Political Science, University of Copenhagen, and was the Danish partner of the cross-cultural project, "Fathers and Mothers: Dilemmas of the Work-Life Balance Prof. Højgaard's major areas of research include research into Gender and Organizational Culture, where she conducts empirical research on workplace culture and gender differentiation, in terms of leadership positions in politics, business and among civil servants and analysis of the gendering of higher education and research. She has also done a study on workplace culture and the gender gap in wages in the private sector and researched the reconciliation of work and family in a number of Danish companies. She is currently the Director of a 5-year research project, "Gender in the Academic Organization," financed by the Danish Research Councils, which is an analysis of gender differences in the scientific community in Denmark. Her own sub-project is an analysis of gender construction in scientific knowledge production.

She has been a member of The Danish National Social Science Research Council since 1998 and on the Board of the Council from 2001. She is Head of the Board of the Danish Academy for Research on Migration (AMID).

HILARY CLARKE

Hilary Clarke was formerly Research Officer in the Research Unit, Centre for Gender and Women's Studies, Trinity College, and part of the Irish research team on the project, "Fathers and Mothers: Dilemmas of the Work-Life Balance." She read Psychology and Philosophy at the University of Leeds, and holds a Masters degree in Women's Studies from Trinity College, Dublin, where her thesis was, "A Comparison of Irish and Swedish Girls' Attitudes towards Men and Women's Work and Family Roles". Ms. Clarke was co-author of the Final Report, "Fathers and Mothers: Dilemmas of the Work-Life Balance" to the European Commission and the Irish Department of Justice, Equality and Law Reform and also co-authored the *Conference Proceedings* relating to the study.

TABLE OF CONTENTS

PREFACE BY GOSTA ESPING-ANDERSEN..V

ACKNOWLEDGEMENTS...IX

NOTES ON AUTHORS..XI

TABLE OF CONTENTS..XV

LIST OF TABLES IN TEXT... XIX

LIST OF FIGURES IN TEXT..XVII

LIST OF TABLES IN APPENDIX.. XXIX

CHAPTER 1: INTRODUCTION.. 1
    OVERVIEW OF BOOK...6

CHAPTER 2: FRANCE.. 9
    SETTING THE CONTEXT: FRENCH FAMILY AND CHILDCARE POLICIES............9
    CHILDCARE ALLOWANCES: REDUCING THE COSTS OF CHILDCARE FOR
    WORKING PARENTS...11
    PARENTAL LEAVE AND CHILD—REARING BENEFIT................................12
    ATTITUDINAL STUDIES.. 14
    WORKPLACE POLICIES IN FRANCE..15
    NEW CHALLENGES: IS THERE A PREDICAMENT FOR FAMILY POLICY?..........18

CHAPTER 3: ITALY...23
    NATIONAL SOCIAL POLICIES...23
    WORKPLACE POLICIES—OBJECTIVE MEASURES...................................28
    ATTITUDINAL STUDIES—SUBJECTIVE MEASURES 32
    STUDIES ON GENDER ROLE ATTITUDES...36

CHAPTER 4: DENMARK..**41**
    DENMARK BY NUMBERS...41
    DANISH RULES OF LEAVE... 45
    LEAVE AND THE LABOUR MARKET.. 47
    GENDER AND WORKING LIFE IN WORKPLACE CULTURES....................... 50
    SCANDINAVIAN EQUALITY MODEL(S)...53

CHAPTER 5: IRELAND..**55**
    NATIONAL SOCIAL POLICIES...55
    CURRENT STATUS OF FAMILY-FRIENDLY ARRANGEMENTS IN IRISH
    WORKPLACES..60
    CHILDCARE IN IRELAND: AN HISTORICAL PERSPECTIVE AND CURRENT
    POLICY ISSUES..62
    ATTITUDINAL STUDIES: CHANGING GENDER ROLES AND SOCIAL POLICIES
    IN IRELAND..68

**CHAPTER 6: A COMPARISON OF THE FOUR COUNTRIES:
AN OVERVIEW**..**75**
    WOMEN'S LABOUR FORCE PARTICIPATION..75
    RELATIONSHIPS BETWEEN FERTILITY AND EMPLOYMENT.......................78
    COMPARATIVE SOCIAL POLICIES...79
    FLEXIBLE WORKING..86
    GENDER ROLES AND ATTITUDES..86
    RESEARCH ON FATHERING.. 87
    CONCLUSION.. 88

CHAPTER 7: METHODOLOGY..**89**
    METHOD..89
    CHARACTERISTICS OF THE SAMPLE..94

CHAPTER 8: CHILDREN AND FAMILY LIFE **97**
    THE EFFECT OF THE BIRTH OF THE YOUNGEST CHILD ON WORK
    AND FAMILY LIFE 97
    DIVISION OF LABOUR WITHIN THE HOUSEHOLD.................................103
    CHILDCARE.. 117
    TIME PREFERENCES...129

CHAPTER 9: THE WORKPLACE...**133**
    WORKPLACE DEMOGRAPHICS...133
    CHANGES IN WORK FOLLOWING THE BIRTH OF THE YOUNGEST CHILD.........138
    POTENTIAL FOR FLEXIBILITY..140
    PERCEPTIONS OF WORKPLACE ATTITUDES......................................146
    WORKPLACE POLICIES..161

CHAPTER 10: COMBINING WORK AND FAMILY LIFE....................**179**
    RECONCILING WORK AND FAMILY..179
    WELL-BEING..192
    CORRELATES OF WELL-BEING..196

CHAPTER 11: SUMMARY AND DISCUSSION....................................**219**
    BACKGROUND..219
    THE STUDY..221
    CHILDREN AND FAMILY LIFE...222
    THE WORKPLACE..228
    COMBINING WORK AND FAMILY LIFE..236
    CONCLUSIONS AND SOCIAL POLICY IMPLICATIONS..............................243

APPENDIX A: TABLES **247**

APPENDIX B: QUESTIONNAIRE...**291**

REFERENCES..**321**

AUTHOR INDEX..**341**

SUBJECT INDEX **345**

LIST OF TABLES IN TEXT

CHAPTER 2: FRANCE..9
   TABLE 2.1. NUMBER OF PLACES IN PUBLIC CHILDCARE FACILITIES FOR
   CHILDREN AGED UNDER THREE YEARS OLD..10
   TABLE 2.2. WHICH IS THE MOST SATISFYING CHILDCARE ARRANGEMENT
   FOR A YOUNG CHILD WHEN BOTH PARENTS ARE ECONOMICALLY ACTIVE?
   (PARENTS WITH AT LEAST ONE CHILD AGED UNDER SIX YEARS OLD)..............15
   TABLE 2.3. PROPORTION OF THE NUMBER OF HOURS PER WEEK
   DEVOTED TO UNPAID AND PAID WORK ASSUMED BY WOMEN (COUPLES,
   AGED BETWEEN 18-64 YRS. OLD)..18

CHAPTER 5: IRELAND..55
   TABLE 5.1. NON-PARENTAL CHILDCARE ARRANGEMENTS FOR
   PRE-SCHOOL CHILDREN OF EMPLOYED COUPLES.....................................58
   TABLE 5.2. MARRIED WOMEN'S LABOUR FORCE PARTICIPATION IN
   IRELAND (%)..64

**CHAPTER 6: A COMPARISON OF THE FOUR COUNTRIES:
AN OVERVIEW**...75
   TABLE 6.1. EMPLOYMENT RATES BY GENDER IN THE
   EUROPEAN UNION (EU15), 2000...76
   TABLE 6.2. PERCENTAGE OF COUPLES LIVING TOGETHER WITH AT LEAST ONE
   CHILD UNDER SIX, WHERE WOMAN WORKS FULL OR PART-TIME AND MAN
   WORK FULL-TIME: CROSS NATIONAL COMPARISONS 1984 & 1999...............77
   TABLE 6.3. CRUDE BIRTH RATES 1980 – 2001 (PER 1000 POPULATION).........78
   TABLE 6.4. TOTAL FERTILITY RATES 1980 – 2001....................................79
   TABLE 6.5. STATUTORY AND OTHER LEAVE PROVISIONS:
   CROSS NATIONAL COMPARISONS..82-85

CHAPTER 7: METHODOLOGY..89
   TABLE 7.1. SAMPLE DESIGN: 4 COUNTRIES..89
   TABLE 7.2. THE INDIVIDUAL COUNTRY SAMPLES....................................90

CHAPTER 8: CHILDREN AND FAMILY LIFE..97
   TABLE 8.1. EFFECT OF THE BIRTH OF THE YOUNGEST CHILD ON WORK AND FAMILY LIFE: MEAN SCORES BY COUNTRY 98
   TABLE 8.2. EFFECT OF THE BIRTH OF THE YOUNGEST CHILD: CHANGES IN THE PROFESSIONAL TASKS OF RESPONDENTS: MEAN SCORES BY COUNTRY AND SEX...100
   TABLE 8.3. EFFECT OF THE BIRTH OF THE YOUNGEST CHILD: CHANGES IN THE RESPONDENTS' RELATIONSHIP WITH THEIR PARTNER: MEAN SCORES BY COUNTRY AND SEX 102
   TABLE 8.4. EFFECT OF THE BIRTH OF THE YOUNGEST CHILD: HOW THE RESPONDENTS' RELATIONSHIP WITH THEIR PARTNER CHANGED: MEAN SCORES BY COUNTRY AND SEX..103
   TABLE 8.5. WHO USUALLY DOES THE SHOPPING FOR FOOD: PERCENTAGE DISTRIBUTIONS BY COUNTRY AND SEX............................105
   TABLE 8.6. WHO USUALLY PREPARES MEALS: PERCENTAGE DISTRIBUTIONS BY COUNTRY AND SEX...106
   TABLE 8.7. WHO USUALLY DOES THE WASHING UP: PERCENTAGE DISTRIBUTIONS BY COUNTRY AND SEX...107
   TABLE 8.8. WHO USUALLY MANAGES HOME LIFE: PERCENTAGE DISTRIBUTIONS BY COUNTRY AND SEX...108
   TABLE 8.9. WHO USUALLY DOES THE WASHING/IRONING CLOTHES: PERCENTAGE DISTRIBUTIONS BY COUNTRY AND SEX............................109
   TABLE 8.10. WHO USUALLY DOES THE CLEANING: PERCENTAGE DISTRIBUTIONS BY COUNTRY AND SEX..110
   TABLE 8.11. WHO USUALLY TAKES THE CHILDREN TO CRÉCHE: PERCENTAGE DISTRIBUTIONS COUNTRY AND SEX.................................111
   TABLE 8.12. WHO USUALLY PLAYS WITH THE CHILDREN: PERCENTAGE DISTRIBUTIONS COUNTRY AND SEX.................................112
   TABLE 8.13. WHO USUALLY FEEDS THE CHILDREN: PERCENTAGE DISTRIBUTIONS BY COUNTRY AND SEX..113
   TABLE 8.14. WHO USUALLY CHANGES NAPPIES/DRESSES THE CHILDREN: PERCENTAGE DISTRIBUTIONS BY COUNTRY AND SEX................113
   TABLE 8.15. WHO USUALLY BATHES THE CHILDREN: PERCENTAGE DISTRIBUTIONS BY COUNTRY AND SEX..114
   TABLE 8.16. WHO USUALLY PICKS UP THE CHILDREN WHEN THEY CRY AT NIGHT: PERCENTAGE DISTRIBUTIONS BY COUNTRY AND SEX.........115
   TABLE 8.17. SUMMARY TABLE SHOWING WHO USUALLY CARRIES OUT DOMESTIC AND CHILDCARE ACTIVITIES: MEAN SCORES BY COUNTRY AND SEX..116
   TABLE 8.18. SUMMARY TABLE SHOWING HOW MUCH HELP RESPONDENTS RECEIVE WITH THE DOMESTIC AND CHILDCARE ACTIVITIES (HELPINDEX): MEAN SCORES BY COUNTRY, SEX AND SES..117

TABLE 8.19. CHILDCARE ARRANGEMENTS FOR THE YOUNGEST CHILD WHEN PARENT IS AT WORK (MOST OFTEN): PERCENTAGE DISTRIBUTIONS BY COUNTRY 118
TABLE 8.20. MEAN COST OF CHILDCARE PER WEEK: MEAN SCORES BY COUNTRY AND SES (IN EUROS)..................................123
TABLE 8.21. SATISFACTION WITH CHILDCARE: MEAN SCORES BY COUNTRY 123
TABLE 8.22. HOW MUCH TIME RESPONDENTS WOULD LIKE TO SPEND WITH THEIR FAMILY: MEAN SCORES BY COUNTRY AND SEX......................130
TABLE 8.23. HOW MUCH TIME RESPONDENTS WOULD LIKE THEIR PARTNER TO SPEND WITH THEIR FAMILY: MEAN SCORES BY COUNTRY AND SEX........131
TABLE 8.24. HOW MUCH PERSONAL TIME RESPONDENTS WOULD LIKE TO HAVE: MEAN SCORES BY COUNTRY..131

CHAPTER 9: THE WORKPLACE..133
TABLE 9.1 COMMUTING TIME: MEAN TIMES BY COUNTRY IN MINUTES 134
TABLE 9.2. MODE OF TRANSPORT USUALLY USED: PERCENTAGE DISTRIBUTIONS BY COUNTRY..135
TABLE 9.3. HOURS RESPONDENT WORKS PER WEEK: MEAN SCORES BY COUNTRY, SEX AND SES...137
TABLE 9.4. SEX OF SUPERVISOR: PERCENTAGE DISTRIBUTIONS BY COUNTRY AND SEX..138
TABLE 9.5. POTENTIAL FLEXIBILITY: PERCENTAGE "YES" BY COUNTRY......141
TABLE 9.6. ACTUAL FLEXIBILITY: PERCENTAGE "YES" BY COUNTRY..........143
TABLE 9.7 HOW MUCH OF THE WORKDAY IS THE RESPONDENT AVAILABLE FOR THEIR CHILD/REN VIA PHONE, MESSAGES, VOICEMAIL, ETC. MEAN SCORES BY COUNTRY, SEX, AND SECTOR..............................145
TABLE 9.8. EASE OF CONTACT WITH YOUNGEST CHILD'S CHILDCARE FACILITY: MEANS SCORES BY COUNTRY AND SES..................................146
TABLE 9.9. POSSIBILITY OF LEAVING WORK TO VISIT YOUNGEST CHILD: MEAN SCORES BY COUNTRY...146
TABLE 9.10. PERCEIVED ACCEPTABILITY BY COLLEAGUES OF RESPONDENT ARRIVING LATE TO/LEAVING EARLY FROM WORK DUE TO CHILDCARE PROBLEMS: MEAN SCORES BY COUNTRY AND SES...................................147
TABLE 9.11. PERCEIVED ACCEPTABILITY BY MANAGERS OF RESPONDENT ARRIVING LATE TO /LEAVING EARLY FROM TO WORK DUE TO CHILDCARE PROBLEMS: MEAN SCORES BY COUNTRY AND SES...................................148
TABLE 9.12. PERCEIVED ACCEPTABILITY OF RESPONDENT BRINGING A CHILD TO WORK BY COLLEAGUES: MEAN SCORES BY COUNTRY, SEX AND SES...148

TABLE 9.13. PERCEIVED ACCEPTABILITY OF RESPONDENT BRINGING A CHILD TO WORK BY MANAGERS: MEAN SCORES BY COUNTRY AND SES..149
TABLE 9.14. HOW WELL COLLEAGUES TAKE INTO ACCOUNT RESPONDENTS' CHILDCARE RESPONSIBILITIES: MEAN SCORES BY COUNTRY AND SEX...149
TABLE 9.15. HOW WELL IMMEDIATE SUPERVISOR TAKES INTO ACCOUNT RESPONDENTS' CHILDCARE RESPONSIBILITIES: MEAN SCORES BY COUNTRY AND SES...150
TABLE 9.16. HOW WELL EMPLOYER TAKES INTO ACCOUNT RESPONDENTS' CHILDCARE RESPONSIBILITIES: MEAN SCORES BY COUNTRY AND SEX.........150
TABLE 9.17. PERCEIVED RESENTMENT OF MEN TAKING EXTENDED LEAVE FOR CHILDCARE: MEAN SCORES BY COUNTRY AND SECTOR............151
TABLE 9.18. PERCEIVED RESENTMENT OF MEN TAKING EXTENDED LEAVE FOR CHILDCARE: MEAN SCORES BY COUNTRY AND SES.................152
TABLE 9.19. PERCEIVED RESENTMENT OF WOMEN TAKING EXTENDED LEAVE FOR CHILDCARE: MEAN SCORES BY COUNTRY AND SES.................153
TABLE 9.20. PERCEIVED RESENTMENT OF WOMEN TAKING EXTENDED LEAVE FOR CHILDCARE: MEAN SCORES BY SES AND SECTOR....................153
TABLE 9.21. PERCEIVED RESENTMENT OF MEN TAKING EXTENDED LEAVE FOR CHILDCARE VS. WOMEN TAKING EXTENDED LEAVE: MEAN SCORES BY COUNTRY AND SEX..154
TABLE 9.22. MEN IN WORK-FAMILY PROGRAMMES PERCEIVED AS 'LESS SERIOUS' ABOUT CAREER: MEAN SCORES BY COUNTRY AND SES................155
TABLE 9.23. MEN IN WORK-FAMILY PROGRAMMES PERCEIVED AS 'LESS SERIOUS' ABOUT CAREER: MEAN SCORES BY SEX AND SECTOR..................156
TABLE 9.24. WOMEN IN WORK-FAMILY PROGRAMMES PERCEIVED AS 'LESS SERIOUS' ABOUT CAREER: MEAN SCORES BY SES AND COUNTRY...156
TABLE 9.25. PERCEIVED ATTITUDES TOWARD MEN VS. WOMEN IN WORK-FAMILY PROGRAMMES: MEAN SCORES BY COUNTRY AND SEX..................158
TABLE 9.26. PERCEPTION THAT TO GET AHEAD EMPLOYEES MUST WORK OVER AND ABOVE THE NORMAL HOURS: MEAN SCORES BY SES AND SECTOR 159
TABLE 9.27. PERCEPTION THAT TO GET AHEAD EMPLOYEES MUST WORK OVER AND ABOVE THE NORMAL HOURS: MEAN SCORES BY COUNTRY, SEX AND SES...159
TABLE 9.28. TO BE VIEWED FAVOURABLY BY TOP MANAGEMENT EMPLOYEES MUST PUT JOB AHEAD OF FAMILY LIFE: MEAN SCORES BY COUNTRY, SEX, SES AND SECTOR...160
TABLE 9.29. PAID MATERNITY LEAVE: AVAILABILITY, USE AND ATTITUDE: PERCENTAGE DISTRIBUTIONS BY COUNTRY AND SEX................162

TABLE 9.30. UNPAID MATERNITY LEAVE: AVAILABILITY, USE AND ATTITUDE: PERCENTAGE DISTRIBUTIONS BY COUNTRY AND SEX 163
TABLE 9.31. PAID PATERNITY LEAVE: AVAILABILITY, USE AND ATTITUDE: PERCENTAGE DISTRIBUTIONS BY COUNTRY AND SEX 164
TABLE 9.32. UNPAID PATERNITY LEAVE: AVAILABILITY, USE AND ATTITUDE: PERCENTAGE DISTRIBUTIONS BY COUNTRY AND SEX 165
TABLE 9.33. AVAILABILITY OF PAID PARENTAL LEAVE: PERCENTAGE DISTRIBUTIONS BY COUNTRY AND SEX 167
TABLE 9.34. AVAILABILITY OF UNPAID PARENTAL LEAVE: PERCENTAGE DISTRIBUTIONS BY COUNTRY AND SEX 167
TABLE 9.35. USE OF PAID AND UNPAID PARENTAL LEAVE BY RESPONDENTS AND THEIR PARTNERS: PERCENTAGE OF 'YES' BY COUNTRY AND SEX 168
TABLE 9.36. ATTITUDES TOWARDS PAID PARENTAL LEAVE: PERCENTAGE DISTRIBUTIONS BY COUNTRY AND SEX 169
TABLE 9.37. ATTITUDES TOWARDS UNPAID PARENTAL LEAVE: PERCENTAGE DISTRIBUTIONS BY COUNTRY AND SEX 169
TABLE 9.38. WHETHER RESPONDENTS WHO DID NOT TAKE PAID PARENTAL LEAVE WOULD HAVE IF IT WERE PAID MORE: PERCENTAGE OF 'YES' BY COUNTRY AND SEX 170
TABLE 9.39. WHETHER RESPONDENTS WHO DID NOT TAKE UNPAID PARENTAL LEAVE WOULD HAVE IF IT WERE PAID: PERCENTAGE OF 'YES' BY COUNTRY AND SEX 170
TABLE 9.40. PART-TIME WORKING: AVAILABILITY, USE AND ATTITUDE: PERCENTAGE DISTRIBUTIONS BY COUNTRY AND SEX 171
TABLE 9.41. JOB-SHARING: AVAILABILITY, USE AND ATTITUDE: PERCENTAGE DISTRIBUTIONS BY COUNTRY AND SEX 172
TABLE 9.42. FLEXIBLE HOURS: AVAILABILITY, USE AND ATTITUDE: PERCENTAGE DISTRIBUTIONS BY COUNTRY AND SEX 172
TABLE 9.43. CAREER BREAKS: AVAILABILITY, USE AND ATTITUDE: PERCENTAGE DISTRIBUTIONS BY COUNTRY AND SEX 173
TABLE 9.44. TERM-TIME WORKING: AVAILABILITY, USE AND ATTITUDE: PERCENTAGE DISTRIBUTIONS BY COUNTRY AND SEX 174
TABLE 9.45. PERSONALISED WORKING HOURS: AVAILABILITY, USE AND ATTITUDE: PERCENTAGE DISTRIBUTIONS BY COUNTRY AND SEX 175
TABLE 9.46. TELE-WORKING: AVAILABILITY, USE AND ATTITUDE: PERCENTAGE DISTRIBUTIONS BY COUNTRY AND SEX 176
TABLE 9.47. FAMILY-FRIENDLINESS OF WORKPLACES: MEAN SCORES BY COUNTRY, SES AND SECTOR 177

CHAPTER 10: COMBINING WORK AND FAMILY LIFE.....................179
    TABLE 10.1. EASE VS. DIFFICULTY IN COMBINING WORK AND FAMILY LIFE: PERCENTAGE DISTRIBUTIONS FOR ALL COUNTRIES BY SEX...............180
    TABLE 10.2. EASE VS. DIFFICULTY IN COMBINING WORK AND FAMILY LIFE: MEAN SCORES BY COUNTRY AND SES...181
    TABLE 10.3. EASE VS. DIFFICULTY IN COMBINING WORK AND FAMILY LIFE: MEAN SCORES BY SECTOR AND SES...181
    TABLE 10.4. THE EXTENT TO WHICH WORKING HOURS CREATE PROBLEMS WITH CHILDCARE ARRANGEMENTS: MEAN SCORES BY COUNTRY..............182
    TABLE 10.5. RESPONDENTS' IDEAL WORKING SCHEDULE: PERCENTAGE DISTRIBUTIONS BY COUNTRY AND SEX...183
    TABLE 10.6. PREDICTORS OF EASE VS. DIFFICULTY IN COMBINING WORK AND FAMILY LIFE: MULTIPLE REGRESSION FOR ALL COUNTRIES...............186
    TABLE 10.6A. ANOVA FOR TOTAL EQUATION TABLE 10.6.........................186
    TABLE 10.7. PREDICTORS OF EASE VS. DIFFICULTY IN COMBINING WORK AND FAMILY LIFE: MULTIPLE REGRESSION FOR ALL COUNTRIES...............188
    TABLE 10.7A. ANOVA FOR TOTAL EQUATION TABLE 10.7.........................188
    TABLE 10.8. PREDICTORS OF EASE VS. DIFFICULTY IN COMBINING JOB AND FAMILY LIFE: MULTIPLE REGRESSION FOR IRELAND ONLY................190
    TABLE 10.8A. ANOVA FOR TOTAL EQUATION TABLE........................190
    TABLE 10.9. PREDICTORS OF EASE VS. DIFFICULTY IN COMBINING JOB AND FAMILY LIFE: MULTIPLE REGRESSION FOR ITALY ONLY....................191
    TABLE 10.9A. ANOVA FOR TOTAL EQUATION TABLE 10.9.........................191
    TABLE 10.10. SATISFACTION WITH PRESENT STATE OF HEALTH: MEAN SCORES BY COUNTRY AND SEX..192
    TABLE 10.11. SATISFACTION WITH PRESENT WORK: MEAN SCORES BY COUNTRY AND SEX...193
    TABLE 10.12. SATISFACTION WITH PRESENT WORK: MEAN SCORES BY SEX AND SES...193
    TABLE 10.13. SATISFACTION WITH FAMILY LIFE: MEAN SCORES BY COUNTRY AND SEX...194
    TABLE 10.14. SATISFACTION WITH PARTNER: MEAN SCORES BY COUNTRY AND SEX...194
    TABLE 10.15. SATISFACTION WITH LIFE IN GENERAL: MEAN SCORES BY COUNTRY AND SEX...195
    TABLE 10.16. SUMMARY TABLE OF SATISFACTION LEVELS: MEAN SCORES BY COUNTRY..195
    TABLE 10.17. RELATIONSHIPS BETWEEN TIME-RELATED VARIABLES AND MEASURES OF WELL-BEING: CORRELATIONS FOR ALL COUNTRIES, MALES AND FEMALES...198

TABLE 10.18. Relationships between Time-related Variables and Measures of Well-being: Correlations for All Countries, Males only..200
TABLE 10.19. Relationships between Time-related Variables and Measures of Well-being: All Countries, Females only...............201
TABLE 10.20. Relationships between Variables related to Domestic Help/Childcare and Measures of Well-being: Correlations for All Countries, Males and Females....................202
TABLE 10.21. Relationships between Variables related to Domestic Help/Childcare and Measures of Well-being: Correlations for All Countries, Females Only............................203
TABLE 10.22. Relationships between Variables related to Domestic Help/Childcare and Measures of Well-being: Correlations for All Countries, Males Only..............................204
TABLE 10.23. Relationships between Perceived Attitudes in the Workplace and Measures of Well-being: Correlations for All Countries...206
TABLE 10.24. Relationships between Perceived Attitudes in the Workplace and Measures of Well-being: Correlations for All Countries, Males Only..207
TABLE 10.25. Relationships between Perceived Attitudes in the Workplace and Measures of Well-being: Correlations for All Countries, Females Only 208
TABLE 10.26. Relationships between Measures of Family Friendliness of the Workplace: Combining Work and Family and Measures of Well-being: Correlations for All Countries 212
TABLE 10.27. Relationships between Measures of Family Friendliness of the Workplace, Combining Work and Family and Measures of Well-being: Correlations for All Countries, Males Only 213
TABLE 10.28. Relationships between Measures of Family Friendliness of the Workplace, Combining Work and Family and Measures of Well-being: Correlations for All Countries, Females Only 214
TABLE 10.29. Relationships between Measures of Well-being: Correlations for All Countries...216
TABLE 10.30. Relationships between Measures of Well-being: Correlations for All Countries, Males Only..............................217
TABLE 10.31. Relationships between Measures of Well-being: Correlations for All Countries, Females Only...........................218

LIST OF FIGURES IN TEXT

CHAPTER 8: CHILDREN AND FAMILY LIFE 97
    FIGURE 8.1. SUMMARY FIGURE SHOWING PERCENTAGE OF RESPONDENTS USING DIFFERENT GROUPED TYPES OF CHILDCARE: PERCENTAGE DISTRIBUTIONS BY COUNTRY 119
    FIGURE 8.2. MEAN NUMBER OF HOURS YOUNGEST CHILD IS IN CARE PER DAY AND PER WEEK: MEAN SCORES BY COUNTRY 120
    FIGURE 8.3. MEAN COST OF CHILDCARE PER WEEK BY COUNTRY (IN EUROS) 122
    FIGURE 8.4. PERCENTAGE OF PEOPLE THAT USE ALTERNATIVE CHILDCARE ARRANGEMENTS 129

CHAPTER 9: THE WORKPLACE 133
    FIGURE 9.1. HOURS RESPONDENT WORKS PER WEEK: MEAN SCORES BY COUNTRY AND SEX 136
    FIGURE 9.2. WHETHER RESPONDENTS MODIFIED THEIR WORKING TIME: PERCENTAGE DISTRIBUTIONS BY COUNTRY AND SEX 139
    FIGURE 9.3. PERCENTAGE OF PARENTS WHO EVER BRING A CHILD TO WORK DUE TO CHILDCARE PROBLEMS: PERCENTAGE DISTRIBUTIONS BY COUNTRY AND SEX 144
    FIGURE 9.4. USE OF MATERNITY AND PATERNITY LEAVE BY COUNTRY: PERCENTAGE DISTRIBUTIONS BY COUNTRY 166
    FIGURE 9.5. RELATIVE FAMILY-FRIENDLINESS OF WORKPLACE: MEAN SCORES BY SECTOR, SES, AND COUNTRY 177

CHAPTER 10: COMBINING WORK AND FAMILY LIFE 179
    FIGURE 10.1. ACTUAL AND PREFERRED WORKING PATTERNS OF EUROPEAN COUPLES (ADAPTED FROM BIELENSKI & KAUPPINEN, 1999, P. 6) 184

LIST OF TABLES IN APPENDIX

APPENDIX A: TABLES

TABLE A1. AGE BY COUNTRY: MEAN SCORES..................................247
TABLE A2. MARITAL/COHABITATION STATUS: PERCENTAGE DISTRIBUTIONS BY COUNTRY...247
TABLE A3. SOCIO-ECONOMIC STATUS: PERCENTAGE DISTRIBUTIONS BY COUNTRY..248
TABLE A4. LEVEL OF EDUCATION: PERCENTAGE DISTRIBUTIONS BY COUNTRY...249
TABLE A5. SECTOR RESPONDENT WORKS IN: PERCENTAGE DISTRIBUTIONS BY COUNTRY...249
TABLE A6. NUMBER OF CHILDREN IN RESPONDENTS' FAMILY: PERCENTAGE DISTRIBUTIONS AND MEAN SCORES BY COUNTRY..............250
TABLE A7. AGE OF YOUNGEST AND NEXT YOUNGEST CHILD: MEAN AGES BY COUNTRY...250
TABLE A8. CHANGES IN THE WAY RESPONDENTS ORGANISED THEIR DAY: PERCENTAGE DISTRIBUTIONS BY COUNTRY..................................251
TABLE A9. CHANGES IN THE LIFE HABITS OF RESPONDENTS: PERCENTAGE DISTRIBUTIONS BY COUNTRY..251
TABLE A10. CHANGES IN THE PROFESSIONAL TASKS OF RESPONDENTS: PERCENTAGE DISTRIBUTIONS BY COUNTRY..252
TABLE A11. CHANGES IN THE AMOUNT OF DOMESTIC CHORES OF RESPONDENTS: PERCENTAGE DISTRIBUTIONS BY COUNTRY......................252
TABLE A12. CHANGES IN THE FRIENDSHIPS OF RESPONDENTS: PERCENTAGE DISTRIBUTIONS BY COUNTRY..253
TABLE A13. CHANGES IN THE FREE TIME OF RESPONDENTS: PERCENTAGE DISTRIBUTIONS BY COUNTRY..253
TABLE A14. CHANGES IN THE RESPONDENTS RELATIONSHIP WITH THEIR PARTNER: PERCENTAGE DISTRIBUTIONS BY COUNTRY....................253
TABLE A15. HOW THE RESPONDENTS RELATIONSHIP WITH THEIR PARTNER CHANGED: PERCENTAGE DISTRIBUTIONS BY COUNTRY...............254
TABLE A16. CHILDCARE ARRANGEMENT FOR YOUNGEST CHILD WHEN PARENT IS AT WORK (NEXT MOST OFTEN): PERCENTAGE DISTRIBUTIONS BY COUNTRY...255
TABLE A17. CHILDCARE ARRANGEMENT FOR YOUNGEST CHILD WHEN PARENT IS AT WORK (THIRD MOST OFTEN): PERCENTAGE DISTRIBUTIONS BY COUNTRY...256

TABLE A18. MEAN NUMBER OF HOURS YOUNGEST CHILD IS IN CARE PER DAY AND PER WEEK: MEAN SCORES BY COUNTRY..........................257
TABLE A19. THE SECOND YOUNGEST CHILD'S CHILDCARE ARRANGEMENTS WHEN PARENT IS AT WORK (MOST OFTEN): PERCENTAGE DISTRIBUTIONS BY COUNTRY..258
TABLE A20. THE SECOND YOUNGEST CHILD'S CHILDCARE ARRANGEMENTS WHEN PARENT IS AT WORK (NEXT MOST OFTEN): PERCENTAGE DISTRIBUTIONS BY COUNTRY...259
TABLE A21. THE SECOND YOUNGEST CHILD'S CHILDCARE ARRANGEMENTS WHEN PARENT IS AT WORK (THIRD MOST OFTEN): PERCENTAGE DISTRIBUTIONS BY COUNTRY...260
TABLE A22. REASONS FOR HAVING CHOSEN A CHILDCARE CENTRE/ CRÉCHE: PERCENTAGE DISTRIBUTIONS BY COUNTRY............................261
TABLE A23. REASONS FOR NOT HAVING CHOSEN A CHILDCARE CENTRE/ CRÉCHE: PERCENTAGE DISTRIBUTIONS BY COUNTRY............................262
TABLE A24. REASONS FOR DISSATISFACTIONS WITH CHILDCARE ARRANGEMENTS: PERCENTAGE DISTRIBUTIONS BY COUNTRY AND SEX........263
TABLE A25. USE OF RESPONDENT'S OWN SICK LEAVE AS AN ALTERNATIVE CHILDCARE ARRANGEMENT: PERCENTAGE DISTRIBUTIONS BY COUNTRY.....264
TABLE A26. USE OF RESPONDENT'S OWN SICK LEAVE AS AN ALTERNATIVE CHILDCARE ARRANGEMENT: MEAN SCORES BY SEX AND SES..................264
TABLE A27. USE OF PARTNERS' SICK LEAVE AS AN ALTERNATIVE CHILDCARE ARRANGEMENT: PERCENTAGE DISTRIBUTIONS BY COUNTRY......265
TABLE A28. USE OF PARTNERS' SICK LEAVE AS AN ALTERNATIVE CHILDCARE ARRANGEMENT: MEAN SCORES BY COUNTRY AND SEX...........265
TABLE A29. USE OF RESPONDENT'S OWN ANNUAL LEAVE AS AN ALTERNATIVE CHILDCARE ARRANGEMENT: PERCENTAGE DISTRIBUTIONS BY COUNTRY 265
TABLE A30. USE OF RESPONDENT'S OWN ANNUAL LEAVE AS AN ALTERNATIVE CHILDCARE ARRANGEMENT: MEAN SCORES BY COUNTRY AND SEX..266
TABLE A31. USE OF PARTNERS' ANNUAL LEAVE AS AN ALTERNATIVE CHILDCARE ARRANGEMENT: PERCENTAGE DISTRIBUTIONS BY COUNTRY......266
TABLE A32. USE OF PARTNERS' ANNUAL LEAVE AS AN ALTERNATIVE CHILDCARE ARRANGEMENT: MEAN SCORES BY COUNTRY, SEX AND SECTOR...267
TABLE A33. USE OF RESPONDENTS' FLEXI-TIME AS AN ALTERNATIVE CHILDCARE ARRANGEMENT: PERCENTAGE DISTRIBUTIONS BY COUNTRY......267
TABLE A34. USE OF RESPONDENTS' FLEXI-TIME AS AN ALTERNATIVE CHILDCARE ARRANGEMENT: MEAN SCORES BY COUNTRY AND SES...........268
TABLE A35. USE OF RESPONDENTS' FLEXI-TIME AS AN ALTERNATIVE CHILDCARE ARRANGEMENT: MEAN SCORES BY SEX, SECTOR AND SES.......268

TABLE A36. USE OF RESPONDENTS' FLEXI-TIME AS AN ALTERNATIVE CHILDCARE ARRANGEMENT: MEAN SCORES BY COUNTRY, SES, SEX AND SECTOR..269
TABLE A37. USE OF PARTNERS' FLEXI-TIME AS AN ALTERNATIVE CHILDCARE ARRANGEMENT: PERCENTAGE DISTRIBUTIONS BY COUNTRY.....269
TABLE A38. USE OF PARTNERS' FLEXI-TIME AS AN ALTERNATIVE CHILDCARE ARRANGEMENT: MEAN SCORES BY COUNTRY AND SES..........270
TABLE A39. USE OF RESPONDENTS' PARENTAL LEAVE AS AN ALTERNATIVE CHILDCARE ARRANGEMENT: PERCENTAGE DISTRIBUTIONS BY COUNTRY.....270
TABLE A40. USE OF RESPONDENTS' PARENTAL LEAVE AS AN ALTERNATIVE CHILDCARE ARRANGEMENT: MEAN SCORES BY COUNTRY AND SECTOR.......271
TABLE A41. USE OF PARTNERS' PARENTAL LEAVE AS AN ALTERNATIVE CHILDCARE ARRANGEMENT: PERCENTAGE DISTRIBUTIONS BY COUNTRY......271
TABLE A42. USE OF PARTNERS' PARENTAL LEAVE AS AN ALTERNATIVE CHILDCARE ARRANGEMENT: MEAN SCORES BY SEX AND SES...................271
TABLE A43. USE OF PARTNERS' PARENTAL LEAVE AS AN ALTERNATIVE CHILDCARE ARRANGEMENT: MEAN SCORES BY SECTOR AND COUNTRY.......272
TABLE A44. USE OF RESPONDENTS' INFORMAL ARRANGEMENTS WITH EMPLOYER AS AN ALTERNATIVE CHILDCARE ARRANGEMENT: PERCENTAGE DISTRIBUTIONS BY COUNTRY...272
TABLE A45. USE OF RESPONDENTS' INFORMAL ARRANGEMENTS WITH EMPLOYER AS AN ALTERNATIVE CHILDCARE ARRANGEMENT: MEAN SCORES BY COUNTRY AND SES..273
TABLE A46. USE OF RESPONDENTS' INFORMAL ARRANGEMENTS WITH EMPLOYER AS AN ALTERNATIVE CHILDCARE ARRANGEMENT: MEAN SCORES BY COUNTRY, SES, SECTOR AND SEX.....................................273
TABLE A47. USE OF PARTNERS' INFORMAL ARRANGEMENTS WITH EMPLOYER AS AN ALTERNATIVE CHILDCARE ARRANGEMENT: PERCENTAGE DISTRIBUTIONS BY COUNTRY..274
TABLE A48. ALTERNATIVE CHILDCARE ARRANGEMENTS— OTHER RELATIVE: PERCENTAGE DISTRIBUTIONS BY COUNTRY...................274
TABLE A49. ALTERNATIVE CHILDCARE ARRANGEMENTS— NEIGHBOUR/BABYSITTER: PERCENTAGE DISTRIBUTIONS BY COUNTRY.........275
TABLE A50. HOW MUCH TIME RESPONDENTS WOULD LIKE TO SPEND WITH THEIR FAMILY: PERCENTAGE DISTRIBUTIONS BY COUNTRY...............275
TABLE A51. HOW MUCH TIME RESPONDENTS WOULD LIKE THEIR PARTNER TO SPEND WITH THEIR FAMILY: PERCENTAGE DISTRIBUTIONS BY COUNTRY...276
TABLE A52. HOW MUCH PERSONAL TIME RESPONDENTS WOULD LIKE TO HAVE: PERCENTAGE DISTRIBUTIONS BY COUNTRY 276
TABLE A53. MEAN NUMBER OF HOURS PARTNER WORKS PER WEEK: MEAN SCORES BY COUNTRY AND SEX..277

TABLE A54. WHETHER OR NOT RESPONDENT NORMALLY WORKS TYPICAL HOURS: PERCENTAGE DISTRIBUTIONS BY COUNTRY....................277
TABLE A55. WHETHER PARTNERS OF RESPONDENTS MODIFIED THEIR WORKING TIME: PERCENTAGE DISTRIBUTION BY COUNTRY AND SEX.........277
TABLE A56. WHEN PARTICIPANTS ALTERED THEIR WORKING TIME, DID THEY INCREASE OR DECREASE IT? PERCENTAGE DISTRIBUTIONS BY COUNTRY AND SEX...278
TABLE A57. PERCENTAGE OF RESPONDENTS AND PARTNERS WHO TEMPORARILY INTERRUPTED THEIR WORKING ACTIVITY: PERCENTAGE DISTRIBUTIONS BY COUNTRY AND SEX...278
TABLE A58. HOW MUCH OF THE WORKDAY IS THE RESPONDENT AVAILABLE FOR THEIR CHILDREN, VIA PHONE, MESSAGES, VOICEMAIL, ETC.: PERCENTAGE DISTRIBUTIONS BY COUNTRY AND SEX......................279
TABLE A59. RESPONDENT'S ABILITY TO KEEP IN CONTACT WITH CHILDMINDER/CRÉCHE/NURSERY/ETC. DURING THE DAY FOR CHILD 1: PERCENTAGE DISTRIBUTIONS BY COUNTRY AND SEX.............................279
TABLE A60. RESPONDENT'S ABILITY TO KEEP IN CONTACT WITH CHILDMINDER/CRÉCHE/NURSERY/ETC. DURING THE DAY FOR CHILD 2: PERCENTAGE DISTRIBUTIONS BY COUNTRY AND SEX.............................280
TABLE A61. REASONS FOR DIFFICULTY IN CONTACTING THE YOUNGEST CHILD: PERCENTAGE DISTRIBUTIONS BY COUNTRY 280
TABLE A62. RESPONDENT'S ABILITY TO GET AWAY FROM WORK TO VISIT CHILD'S CHILDMINDING FACILITY/CRÉCHE/NURSERY/ ETC. FOR CHILD 1: PERCENTAGE DISTRIBUTIONS BY COUNTRY AND SEX 281
TABLE A63. RESPONDENT'S ABILITY TO GET AWAY FROM WORK TO VISIT CHILD'S CHILDMINDING FACILITY/CRÉCHE/NURSERY/ ETC. FOR CHILD 2: PERCENTAGE DISTRIBUTIONS BY COUNTRY AND SEX 281
TABLE A64. REASONS FOR DIFFICULTIES IN LEAVING WORK TO VISIT CHILD: PERCENTAGE DISTRIBUTIONS BY COUNTRY 282
TABLE A65. EASE VS. DIFFICULTY IN COMBINING WORK AND FAMILY LIFE: PERCENTAGE DISTRIBUTIONS BY COUNTRY AND SEX 283
TABLE A66. DO THE HOURS THAT YOU WORK CREATE PROBLEMS IN YOUR CHILDCARE ARRANGEMENTS? PERCENTAGE DISTRIBUTIONS BY COUNTRY AND SEX 284
TABLE A67. SATISFACTION WITH PRESENT STATE OF HEALTH: PERCENTAGE DISTRIBUTION BY COUNTRY AND SEX 285
TABLE A68. SATISFACTION WITH PRESENT WORK: PERCENTAGE DISTRIBUTION BY COUNTRY AND SEX 286
TABLE A69. SATISFACTION WITH FAMILY LIFE: PERCENTAGE DISTRIBUTION BY COUNTRY AND SEX 287

TABLE A70. SATISFACTION WITH RELATIONSHIP WITH PARTNER: PERCENTAGE DISTRIBUTIONS BY COUNTRY AND SEX 288
TABLE A71. SATISFACTION WITH LIFE IN GENERAL: PERCENTAGE DISTRIBUTIONS BY COUNTRY AND SEX………………………...…………..289

CHAPTER 1

INTRODUCTION

Demographic changes throughout Europe have led to a changing social situation requiring new social policies. The increasing labour force participation of women, particularly of women in the childbearing years, has been accompanied by increasing needs for childcare, flexible working arrangements and greater demands for equality in the workplace. EU policy in the equality area has played a significant role in starting the process of harmonising social legislation in the member countries so that countries that were lagging behind have been forced to catch up with countries more advanced in this area. However, this process has only just begun and there is still a long way to go.

The challenge which still faces even the most advanced of the EU member states is how to facilitate more egalitarian sharing of roles, that is, how to relieve women of the double burden of employment and domestic tasks, while encouraging men to take an active part in family and domestic life.

Alongside the ever increasing labour force participation of mothers with young children, the question of how to help working parents combine their job with their family life is high on the social policy agenda (European Commission, 1995).). Flexibility in the provision of childcare and the development of family friendly initiatives at work are seen as crucial to the development of policies which facilitate the reconciliation of work and family life (European Commission, 1997). Given that more than two-thirds of the working population in the EU are either married or living with a partner (Bielenski & Kauppinen, 1999), this issue is clearly of concern to a very great number of people.

It is currently widely recognised that balancing work and family responsibilities is a matter of urgent concern and that "family policies" are required to address such issues. Moreover, promoting equal opportunities for women and men in the labour market – one of the main objectives of the Commission's Equal Opportunities Unit – has gone hand in hand with a growing emphasis on fathers' involvement in family life.

At the same time, the 1990s stand out as a time of technological, economic and social change, broad trends that made their mark on the work-family interface. Against such a background, we wanted to contribute to the debate and to explore how dual-earner couples living with young children elaborate strategies to combine their job with their family responsibilities and how the difficulties they may have to cope with impact on their well-being.

Several reasons justify the choice of Ireland, France, Denmark and Italy. First, in each of these countries, the policy objective of reconciliation of employment and family life has gradually moved onto the political agenda. Despite considerable variations in the political impact of the issue, and also in the public provision of services provided to families, a range of measures has been progressively implemented to reduce the conflicts between paid work and family life. Second, each has different welfare regimes (Esping-Andersen, 1990; Pierson, 2001) and this has strong implications for how far these different countries place the onus for reconciling employment and family life on public policy and how much on individuals, families and employers. France and Italy are part of the cluster of countries whose welfare regimes are qualified 'conservative', (sometimes termed 'Christian democratic' or 'Bismarckian'). Among others, they include the following features: high levels of spending, high levels of payroll tax financing and explicit or implicit family policies. However, France differs from the other conservative welfare states when social care is taken into account. Ireland, like the UK, is classified in the liberal cluster and Denmark in the social democratic one (*Ibid.*). They devote different proportions of their social protection system to family policy[1]. On the one hand, Denmark and France have a well established and long-standing early childhood system, while on the other, in Italy public provision for childcare varies according to the region, but is generally scarce, and in Ireland it lags behind.

Third, labour force participation rates and employment patterns of mothers still vary according to the country, Denmark showing the closest gender gap in terms of working hours and professional trajectories between men and women. Italy has traditionally had lower rates of female participation, yet this has been changing, particularly in Northern Italy and has, at the same time, the lowest fertility rates in the world (like Spain). Ireland has traditionally had lower rates of female employment, however, in the last three decades the labour force participation of married women has increased geometrically. The economy has recently experienced a boom and there has been an even greater demand for female labour. France is well known for having promoted the model of the "working mother" and a high proportion of mothers are in paid work, however, this is still less than the remarkably high rates which are evident Denmark.

Moreover, there are a lot of commonalities between these countries. All are currently grappling with similar issues, due to the convergence of economic and social conditions in the Community and their Welfare states are undergoing quite

---

[1] Respectively Denmark, France, Ireland and Italy devote 13 per cent, 9 per cent, 13 per cent and 3.6 per cent to family and children (Eurostat, 2002).

significant changes (Pierson, 2001). Decision-makers have to tackle a number of issues (reform of pension systems, rise in unemployment, fighting poverty and social exclusion, public deficits, etc.), and are confronted by a number of dilemmas: against the background of cost containment and "recalibration of welfare states" (*Ibid.*), they have to make trade-offs and find compromises. In this context, room for manoeuvre may be felt to be narrow and priorities need to be made. However, it is notable that in some countries a higher priority is given to public provision of childcare facilities and related schemes aimed at helping working parents.

In this context, it is relevant to investigate strategies dual-earner couples with young children adopt to maximize the resources they draw upon and to mitigate constraints. However it has been largely documented that they affect parents quite differently depending on their place in the social structure: high-income dual-career couples and low skilled workers often face different pressures and difficulties. Occupational status is hence at the core of our analysis. Emphasis throughout the book is also put on changes that have been thrust upon parents just after the birth of the youngest child. In this field, working parents are dependent on the kind and level of support provided by society, which raises the question of whether or not children are considered as "public" and/or "private" goods. In our analysis, we will assess if families can rely – and to what extent – on public support or if they are obliged to juggle with different alternatives that may sometimes aggravate the management of their daily life.

While the increasing labour force participation of women in the childbearing years has been accompanied by increasing needs for childcare, flexible working arrangements and greater demands for equality in the workplace, concomitantly, the caring issue (Lewis, 1995) has come to the forefront of the socio-policy agenda. Lack of professional care (linked to training-programmes of the carers) or of adequate care which fits in with working hours might explain the trade-offs made by parents in their professional life, in particular the time they accept to devote to their job. Along this line, we decided to also focus on attitudes towards childcare arrangements, family-friendly measures at the workplace and on their impact on reported well-being. We hypothesized for example that satisfaction with childcare arrangements would be positively correlated with parents' well-being, and that this would impinge more on mothers than on fathers.

Flexibility is often said to enhance equal opportunities between women and men. However, it might be largely employer driven and can result in negative outcomes for the parent (Burchell and Fagan, 2002). Recent research and data have demonstrated that there is a significant proportion of wage-earners with work schedules that include working nights, weekends or variable start and finish times (Merllié and Paoli, 2000). Studies of changing labour markets suggest that, by introducing and extending flexible working practices, employers are seeking to increase the productivity of labour, efficiency and performance, and are not paying sufficient attention to the impact of imposed flexibility on families. The hidden costs of these practices are high. For instance, research conducted by Burchell and Fagan (*op. cit.*), using a multiple regression analysis, shows that as far as satisfaction with work-life balance is concerned, the three most important variables point to the negative aggregate effects of unsociable hours and long hours.

On the other hand, flexible work schedules that have been negotiated between employers and employees might offer some scope for a better work/family life balance. Spatial constraints are also taken into account as they may limit the room for manoeuvre of working parents, in particular in big metropolitan areas like Paris, Copenhagen and Dublin where commuting can be very time-consuming. Therefore we also explored how working parents deal with these organisational and spatial patterns.

A spate of literature also provides evidence that the boundaries between family life and work are blurring. Thanks to the new technologies, a growing number of highly qualified workers are working from home. How do these working patterns impact on the family relationships? Do fathers take advantage of this to spend more time with their children and care for them? It is often argued that there is a gap between the public and the private sectors as far as family-friendly measures are concerned. Holding a stable job in the public sector where trade unions are generally stronger would provide employees with more flexible opportunities. It would be easier to claim their rights to parental leave, sick leave or time off to look after children. However, being a public servant has different implications from one country to another. In Denmark, for instance, the public sector is now required to increase productivity, which may impact on the interplay between work and family. Thus a key aspect of our analysis was to examine issues of work-life balance in different institutional settings and socio-economic contexts.

The present study has brought together an international team of researchers, each of whom has tackled these issues from a somewhat different vantage point: Højgaard (Denmark), from the viewpoint of working practices (e.g., Højgaard, 1998); Giovannini (Italy), from the perspective of parental, particularly fathers', attitudes towards sharing roles (e.g. Giovannini, 1998); Fagnani (France) with emphasis on the role of childcare policy and the effects of specific policies (e.g., Fagnani, 1998a); and Fine-Davis (Ireland) from the perspectives of social attitudes, values and policy preferences (e.g., Fine-Davis, 1988a).

This team of researchers represents countries that have traditionally been at different points on the continuum, and yet are all currently grappling with similar issues, due to the convergence of social conditions in the Community. As two of the participating countries are more advanced than the other two in terms of social policy and specifically childcare provision, it was felt that the instruments used in previous research in Denmark and France would be able to anticipate attitudes and policies emerging in Ireland and Italy. While Italy may in many ways be analogous to Ireland, the kind of research, particularly on fatherhood and fathers' contribution to childrearing and domestic tasks carried out by Giovannini and his colleagues in the 1990s (e.g. Giovannini, 1998; Giovannini and Molinari, 1994) was groundbreaking and had a unique contribution to make to international research.

It was the aim of the project to use the varied expertise of this group to identify the key issues concerning the reconciliation of work and family roles, with particular emphasis on how to involve men more in domestic and family activities. The purpose of the study was to explore people's attitudes and experiences in coping with balancing work and family, with particular reference to the different perspectives of men and women. Attitudes towards and experience of different workplace social policies was also explored. Another major purpose of the study was to develop new social indicators to measure issues of work life balance, which could be utilised in studies with larger more representative samples.

The immediate goals of the project were several: The first was to systematically examine the latest research findings and instruments in the four countries, each of which represents a different "experience" of the evolving gender role process. The second was to compare and synthesise the findings, leading to the development of a composite instrument which would provide a mechanism for data collection, in the first instance, in the present study, but which could then subsequently be used in individual member states or at EU level. Such an instrument would constitute a measuring tool to assess attitudes and policies at individual country or EU level concerning redistribution and sharing of gender roles.

In the book we present material in two stages. In the first, we provide an overview of the latest research findings relevant to the area in the four countries, as well as some comparison and synthesis of the situations in these countries. In the second stage of the book we present the comparative results of an empirical survey carried out simultaneously in France, Italy, Denmark and Ireland, which provides an analysis of people's dilemmas and coping strategies in four different countries of the EU. It is our hope through this collective research to contribute to a better understanding of the realities of life, including the tradeoffs and compromises, made by young working parents in their attempt to exercise the roles of parent and worker. We also hope to demonstrate the dramatic role played by public, social and family policies in facilitating access to equal opportunities and quality of life. Finally and most importantly, we hope to shed light on those factors which are associated with work-life balance and well-being, so that workplace policies as well as social policies at the more macro level may be further developed in order to enhance opportunities for women and men to optimally combine their multiple roles of worker, parent and individual.

CHAPTER 1

OVERVIEW OF THE BOOK

The book is organised in several sections. In the first major section, "Work-Life Balance: Review of Current Issues, Policies and Research," we present four separate literature reviews for France, Italy, Denmark and Ireland. These were carried out individually by the authors and their assistants. The purpose of the literature reviews was to provide an overview of recent research, primarily 1990 to the present, with some earlier studies included if of particular significance. These reviews broadly covered the following areas:

(a) National social policies concerning leave arrangements and flexible working;
(b) Workplace policies concerning flexible working and studies concerning their prevalence and effects;
(c) Attitudinal studies concerning work-life balance, childcare and gender role attitudes.

While each review covers broadly similar areas, each is also unique in painting a picture of an individual country – highlighting the key issues in that country. For example, the French literature review refers more extensively to childcare policy, because France has a highly developed social policy in this area.

The literature reviews thus present an overview of current policy and research relevant to work life balance, which forms a backdrop to the present study and places it in its European context. A second major purpose of the literature review was to identify instruments and items from previous research, which had been used to measure the topics of the current research. These were examined and a selection made. A new instrument was then constructed which reflected the best of the items located in previous research from Denmark, Italy, France and Ireland.

Following the four country literature reviews, we present a chapter synthesising the key points to emerge from these reviews in light of key demographic trends in the four countries. In this section we highlight the major issues that have been found cross-culturally to be relevant to reconciliation of work and family life of working parents with young children and the attainment of work life balance. It is these issues that formed the basis of the study that we subsequently carried out.

In the second major section, "The Study," we present the Method and Results of the comparative study that we carried out in 2001-2002 in the four countries. The results are presented under several headings: "Children and Family Life," "The Workplace," and "Combining Work and Family Life."

In the first of these sections (Chapter 8), "Children and Family Life," we initially present results on the effect of the birth of the youngest child on the work and family life of the parents and the division of labour within the household. While much

INTRODUCTION

previous research has been carried out on the latter topic, we present here some new measures including an index of help in the household (HELPINDEX). We then examine the childcare arrangements for the youngest and next youngest child and related issues, such as cost and satisfaction with childcare.

Chapter 9 concerns the workplace environment of the working parents in the sample. We begin with descriptive information, covering issues of time and commuting. We then examine the nature of the workplace in terms of its potential and actual flexibility for working parents.

Next, attitudes in the workplace are examined. These include perceived attitudes of colleagues, immediate supervisor and employer concerning one's childcare responsibilities – is the attitude sympathetic and understanding or harsh and unaccepting? A key set of questions in this section concerned attitudes in the workplace toward people who avail of "family friendly" policies, such as extended leave for care for newborn children, part-time working, job sharing, etc., in an attempt to see if such individuals are perceived in a less favourable light, for example, as "less serious" about their career. Similarly, attitudes towards the long-hours culture and "presenteeism" were explored as potential barriers to work-life balance.

In this chapter we also present results concerning workplace policies. This includes respondents' reports concerning the existence of a range of family friendly workplace policies, the extent to which respondents availed of these, as well as their attitudes towards the policies.

Most of the results were analysed in a comparative way to examine country differences, as well as similarities. Sex was a stratification characteristic, thus allowing sex differences to be explored throughout. The sample was further stratified by socio-economic status (SES) and sector of employment (public vs. private). Using these four stratification characteristics: 1) Country (France, Italy, Denmark and Ireland); 2) Sex (male/female); 3) Socio-economic status (Low/High); and 4) Sector (public/private), we built overlapping factorial designs, enabling us to use 3- and 4-way analysis of variance (ANOVA) to tease out the significant main effects and interaction effects of each of these key independent variables on a large array of dependent measures.

Chapter 10 presents the results concerning "Combining Work and Family." Building upon many of the measures presented in the preceding sections, this chapter examines the predictors of successfully combining work and family life. The most significant predictors of ease *vs.* difficulty are presented for the combined four-country sample and then for males and females separately. Individual country differences are also discussed.

Results concerning several classic measures of perceived well-being are also included in this chapter: i.e., satisfaction with work, health, partner/spouse, family life and life in general. Country differences are examined for each of these measures and their correlates are also explored in detail, drawing upon the key sets of variables presented earlier, including time variables, attitudes in the workplace, extent of domestic help received, etc. Policies in the workplace, such as potential and actual flexibility and overall "family friendliness" of the workplace are also examined in relation to the various measures of perceived well-being. The overall purpose of this chapter is to identify which variables are significantly related to 1) successfully combining work and family life, and 2) to well-being in various life domains.

The final chapter, Chapter 11, presents a summary and discussion of the main findings, relating these to previous research in the area, both in Europe and elsewhere.

CHAPTER 2

FRANCE

In comparative and cross-national research, France is always one of the clusters of countries with policies that provide extensive support for maternal employment. Shaver and Bradshaw (1995) have demonstrated that support for the dual breadwinner family is much more generous in France than in most European countries. When childcare costs are taken into account, France ranks top of fifteen countries in support for this model. As a matter of fact, in France, there is a strong tradition of policies to help to combine paid work and family responsibilities.

However it is worth noting that relatively little research has been devoted to the work/life balance issue *per se*. It contrasts with the fact that social scientists in the 1980s and 1990s generated a flurry of important and interdisciplinary research into the causes of growing labour force participation of married women and young mothers (Glaude, 1999; Marry, 1998; Maruani, 2000). Much less attention has been paid to how working mothers and fathers combine a job and a family life and rely or not on the different schemes provided by the family and social policies. Research devoted to the strategies elaborated by dual-earner couples in order to achieve their employment aspirations while rearing young children are much less common than research investigating the complex bundle of factors explaining the gender discrimination in the labour market (Meurs and Ponthieux, 2000).

However, the issue of the reconciliation of professional and family life - largely echoed in the media - is high on the political and social agenda and decision-makers are becoming aware of the paramount importance of improving the schemes which have been progressively put in place by the family policy since the seventies.

1. SETTING THE CONTEXT: FRENCH FAMILY AND CHILDCARE POLICIES

1.1. A Generous and Sophisticated Childcare Policy

France has a well established and long-standing early childhood system and public provision for infant care has always been regarded as an ongoing and normal service (Fagnani, 2000; Martin, 1998; Norvez, 1990). To ease the serious shortage of childcare facilities, a policy of investment in and equipment of childcare services has been developed over the last three decades, initially through the so-called '*contrats-crèches*' and later, the '*contrats-enfance*': departmental family allowance funds (*Caisse d'Allocations Familiales*, CAF) and their national organization (CNAF) – the branch of the Social Security system responsible for family policy - subsidize services in general and stimulate development through the "*contrat enfance*" programme in which CAFs sign and co-finance agreements with local authorities to support the expansion of services for children under six years.

Compulsory school age is six years old. Services below that age are split: - '*Crèches collectives*' are publicly subsidised day care centres where children under three years old are cared for by trained staff. They are supervised by 'Protection Maternelle et Infantile' (PMI), a statutory service responsible for health care of children under six years old with supervisory responsibility for all public and private childcare provisions. 'Crèches familiales' are services that organise and monitor childcare by licensed (or registered) childminders, paid by local authorities and monitored by qualified state infant care personnel. These childminders care for children (no more than three children) in their own home but they regularly convene for staff meetings in public facilities. In crèches, fees are income-related.

Since the early 1980s, the number of childcare places in crèches has increased regularly, to reach a total of 200,000 in 2000 (Table 2.1). Around 9% of children aged under three are cared for in crèches. To justify the limits in funding allocated for the building and running of crèches, policy-makers often emphasise the high costs of crèches for both municipalities and the Social Security Department.

Table 2.1. Number of Places in Public Childcare Facilities For Children Aged Under Three Years Old

TYPE OF FACILITIES	NUMBER OF PLACES
Nursery school ('école maternelle')	255,000 (56%)
Collective Crèches	138,400 (30.5%)
Other types of 'Crèches'	61,000 (13.5%)
Total number of places in public childcare provision (full-time)	**454,500 (100%)**
'Haltes-garderies' (Only on part-time basis)	68,100

Source: DREES, Ministère de l'Emploi et de la Solidarité, 2000

1.2. A Specific French Institution: 'École Maternelle'

The education system is responsible for an extensive network of nursery schooling ('*écoles maternelles*') for children aged two to six years. This service is the responsibility of the National Ministry of Education, although local authorities are responsible for providing various inputs, including non-teaching staff and supervision during the midday break; they also provide some out-of-school childcare. Nursery education is free to parents. Open 35 hours per week, schools are routinely closed on Wednesdays, but are supplemented by a half-day Saturday session. All of these schools have canteen facilities and canteen-fees are income-related. Around 260,000 children aged two (36% of those aged two) and 98% of children aged three already attend "écoles maternelles".

2. CHILDCARE ALLOWANCES: REDUCING THE COSTS OF CHILDCARE FOR WORKING PARENTS

2.1. The Allowance for Childcare in the Home (AGED)

This allowance – *Allocation de garde d'enfant à domicile (AGED)* was established in 1986. It covers part of the social security contributions, which must be paid by a family who employs someone at home to care for their child/ren aged under six. Families are eligible if both parents (or the lone parent) are economically active. Recipients of AGED are able to deduct 50% of the actual costs of care from their income tax. By the end of June 2002, there were 60,000 recipients.

2.2. The Allowance to Employ an Approved Childminder (AFEAMA)

'*Aide à la Famille pour l'Emploi d'une Assistante Maternelle Agréée*' (AFEAMA) was created in 1990. It is an allowance provided to working parents who have at least one child aged under six cared for by a registered childminder. Its amount covers the social security contributions to be paid by the employer of the registered childminder. An additional financial contribution is also given to the family. The number of recipients reached 580,000 by the end of June 2002. This childcare arrangement has become the most frequently used by dual-earner (and lone parent) families, with at least one child under three, who opt for "formal childcare".

2.3. Maternity Leave

Working mothers receive 16 weeks statutory maternity leave on full pay. This leave is paid by her health insurance, which is funded by statutory contributions from both employer and employee. If the working mother is giving birth to her third child (or more), then maternity leave is extended at full pay from 16 weeks to six months.

The socialist government, headed by Premier Jospin, introduced some changes in family policy. As a matter of fact, surveys and public opinion polls have provided evidence that many working mothers had to deal with many difficulties in organising childcare, and that a growing proportion of parents were complaining about the shortcomings and shortage of services and public facilities.

Therefore, the government wanted to give priority to issues of work/life balance that were high on the social and political agenda. Moreover, a spate of literature had argued that fathers play an important part in the emotional and cognitive development of children. Many experts also put emphasis on the necessity of a father's presence at home after a birth. Along this line, Ministry Ségolène Royal, in charge of family affairs in 2000-2001, firmly stated that it was important to promote equality at home and to provide men with the opportunity to look after their toddler if they wanted to.

2.4. The creation of a statutory paternity leave

In this context, the right of fathers to make a commitment to family life has made its mark on the social and political debate: fathers have now been granted (since January 2002) two weeks' statutory paternity leave (before it was only three days), on full pay (up to a ceiling of 2,352 Euros per month by 2002, paid by the social security)[1]. From a symbolic point of view, it is a turning point in the history of French family policy: for the first time the issue of fathering has come to the forefront of the family policy arena. This is a social recognition of the important role fathers are assumed to play in the family, and it will contribute to supporting the idea at the workplace that a man is not only a worker but also a father. It also illustrates growing public awareness that in order to achieve equality at work, it is necessary to encourage the equal sharing of family obligations and domestic work.

3. PARENTAL LEAVE AND CHILD-REARING BENEFIT

The parental leave scheme was established in 1977. The French parental leave scheme (Congé Parental d'Education - CPE) was set up as part of employment legislation in 1977. The objective was to "diversify childcare", and to improve the situation of the "woman who wishes to raise her child herself". Since then, parental

---

[1] 21 days if they are multiple births. This leave cannot be divided, 11 days must be taken in a row and within a four month period following the birth (art. L. 122-25-4 du Code du travail). All economically active fathers are eligible.

leave has been progressively extended, alongside the expansion of public childcare provision. All the changes have reflected progressive adaptation both to the changing economic context and to the need to adopt a more gender-neutral approach at a time when public opinion was becoming more sensitive to gender discrimination. CPE currently allows all salaried employees, male or female, who have worked for at least one year in the company before the birth of a child, to cease employment totally or to work on a part-time basis (between 16 and 32 hours per week and the employee is not allowed to work somewhere else), in order to care for a new-born child, irrespective of its birth order. According to employment legislation, the employee who is on leave can only be dismissed or made redundant if it is for reasons not connected to her (or his) leave. After completing their leave (when the child reaches three years of age), an employee must be reinstated without a reduction in pay in the same position or in a similar one, and is eligible for retraining with pay. Parental leave is not paid. However, it is possible to be on parental leave and also receive the Child Rearing Benefit (Allocation Parentale d'Education - APE) if the parent is eligible.

APE is provided to parents (the mother or the father) with at least two children, the youngest aged less than three. It is not income-related and not taxable. In 2001, its amount was FF 3,131 a month. This benefit is provided until the youngest child reaches the age of three, but only if one of the parents (the mother or the father) stops work completely or works on a part-time basis. If a parent works part-time, the amount of the benefit is reduced.

Of the working parents who take unpaid Parental Leave, an overwhelming 98% of them are mothers. Most mothers take some Parental Leave, though take-up is much higher among mothers at the lower end of the economic spectrum (Gallou & Simon, 1999).

3.1. Some Characteristics of the Recipients

Mothers who were in employment just before taking maternity leave are more likely to claim APE if they are entitled to CPE because they have a job guarantee. Against the background of high unemployment among women, most of the working mothers who are not entitled to CPE cannot take the risk of losing their job except if their partner has secure employment. This hypothesis receives support from research conducted among mothers with three children who were receiving APE (Fagnani, 1995) and from a survey recently conducted by CREDOC (Gallou and Simon, 1999) based on a representative national sample of former recipients of APE having two children. Among those who had a job just before receiving APE and who resume their job immediately afterwards, 60% were on parental leave (CPE).

Why are take-up levels of APE so high? The changes in APE eligibility since July 1994, which extended eligibility to parents with two children and introduced the option of part-time work from the beginning of the payment period, have contributed to a dramatic increase in the number of recipients, reaching 530,000 in December 2000 compared to 275,000 in December 1995. Not surprisingly, the economic activity rate of mothers with two children, the youngest aged less than three years, has decreased from 69% in 1994 to 53% in 1998. It has been estimated that between 1994 and 1997, about 110,000 working mothers with two children have retired from the labour market to take advantage of APE (Allain & Sédillot, 1999).

Most mothers who are highly qualified and career-oriented either do not claim parental leave at all or do so only on a part-time basis (e.g. working four days a week, and taking Wednesday off because school is closed on this day). Thus, female managers and professionals represent only 3% of the former recipients of APE, compared to 13 % of the total female workforce.

4. ATTITUDINAL STUDIES

4.1. Attitudes to Caring Responsibilities: Who Should Take Care of the Young Child?

Traditional norms are still very influential in the family sphere. A recent public opinion survey (CREDOC, 2001) showed that among men and women, half of them think that when children are young, one of their parents should give up work temporarily. Thirty-two per cent think that this parent should be the mother; only 15% think it should be the parent who earns the lowest income, leaving just a very few who think it should be the father. Thirty-eight per cent think that they should reduce the number of working hours and only 11% think that both parents should reduce their working time.

Therefore, most of the parents think that when the child is very young, the best solution is to provide one of the parents with opportunities to stop working temporarily or to reduce working time. Fully 69% of proponents of both solutions think that it should be the mother and 34% think it should be the parent who earns the lowest income. Traditional attitudes have been declining over the nineties, however they remain predominant.

4.2. Attitudes towards Childcare Arrangements

However, when both parents remain in employment after the birth of the child or maternity leave, either because they are obliged or by choice, which is the most satisfying childcare arrangement for them? A CREDOC survey (2001) shows that the registered childminder is at the top of the ladder. As a matter of fact, this childcare arrangement is the most convenient for them because it is more flexible than the crèche and a childminder more easily accepts looking after the child when he (she) is ill. It is also a 'mother like' arrangement'. Accordingly it is the most common formal childcare arrangement for children under three.

As illustrated in Table 2.2, relying on grandparents is a satisfying solution for one out of five persons having at least one child aged under six years of age. Relying on a nanny at home is not often mentioned, because it is a very expensive solution for parents who cannot fully take advantage of the tax deduction (see above, the issue related to AGED).

Table 2.2. *Which is the most satisfying childcare arrangement for a young child when both parents are economically active? (Parents with at least one child aged under six years old)*

Childcare Arrangement	Percentage
Registered childminder	**38.5**
Collective crèche	20.0
Grand-parents	19.0
Nanny at home	7.2
Family crèche	5.1
Non-Registered childminder	**3.3**
Halte-garderie	3.3
Other	2.3
Don't know	1.3
TOTAL	**100.0**

Source: CREDOC, 2001

5. WORKPLACE POLICIES IN FRANCE

It should be emphasised that French employers partly finance family policies through their social contributions and they mostly think that it is not up to them to provide their employees with childcare. They argue that the State, through its institutions, has the obligation to provide families and working parents with services aimed at helping them to combine a job with their childrearing responsibilities. Against this background, French employers are only expected in this field to submit to the legislation related to parental and maternity leave. And most of them don't feel the need to implement extra-statutory schemes at the workplace to help working parents.

Large firms are only required to consider the gender equality issue: some of them have a written Equal Employment Opportunities statement and all are required to produce an annual report on the situation of women's employment in the company (Lanquetin et al., 2000).

However, as demonstrated by researchers (Hantrais and Letablier, 1996; Evans, 2001), gender equity policies might not fit well with family-friendly policies, because of the enduring asymmetry between the sexes in family involvement.

Some hospitals and a few big companies have their own childcare centre either because they need to provide their employees with flexible childcare arrangements if they want them to accept atypical working schedules (nurses, for example) or because they want to retain highly qualified staff and to reduce turn-over rates by offering them 'family-friendly' measures or 'perks' which are targeted at employees having children (IBM, Hewlett- Packard, EDF, the National electricity supplier company, for example) (extra-statutory maternity leave, outdoor activities for children, 12 days off when a child is ill instead of the compulsory three days). A lot of large companies also provide their employees with summer camps or outdoor activities for children on Wednesdays (when school are closed).

5.1. Companies and the Parental Leave Scheme (CPE)

Little research has been devoted to this issue (Van de Walle, 1997). However, it seems that the attitudes of employers vary according to the economic sector, the qualification of staff, the proportion of female workers, the size of a company and its economic performance. The divergence between the public and private sector is also strong. The workplace culture in the private sector makes it difficult for a man, in particular at management level, to take parental leave or even to reduce his hours of work.

A recent qualitative research project on parental leave - based on in-depth interviews with employers and employees - has investigated the ways in which companies implement parental leave and what goals they pursue (*Ibid.*). Fifteen private and public employers were included, and around 30 in-depth interviews were conducted with employees who had taken parental leave. The following typology of employers was developed:

- Supportive employers, prosperous companies or public employers which want to retain highly-trained and experienced women who tend to leave after having a baby, and where recruitment and retention of female staff remain important motivating forces (e.g. hospitals confronted with a shortage of nurses). Employers in this case consider CPE as a means of improving human resources management. These companies can also afford to implement such a family-friendly policy.
- Companies where human resources management is reluctant to provide CPE but feels obliged to follow the law. Sometimes they try to discourage the employee from claiming it. Information about CPE is either poorly disseminated or not at all. These companies do not

refuse to provide CPE but warn the employee of the risks involved. In these companies, employees are supposed to devote all their time to their job. Consequently, CPE is perceived as a legal requirement, which complicates the management of human resources.

- Companies which need to reduce staff numbers or reduce their hours of work, with pro-rata salary. In this case, employees not only can take CPE but they can be encouraged or even required to do so to avoid being made redundant. In this context, CPE is a component or an instrument of employment policy and a means of cutting costs. For example, to stave off redundancy, an extended leave arrangement of three to six years for the third child is available at a large food manufacturer and is paid at half the minimum wage (about 2,600 F). Half of the leave period counts towards years of service and the employee can return to the same or a similar position.

5.2. Fathers at the Workplace

So far, in France, the drive to raise the presence of mothers in the workplace has not been accompanied by a drive to raise the presence of fathers in the home. The result is that although female (mothers') participation rate in the labour market is amongst the highest in Europe, with the notion of 'the working mother' fully integrated into family policy (Fagnani, 2000), fathers' participation rate in the home ranks amongst the lowest, as demonstrated by the Eurostat surveys on time-use diaries.

Research is overdue into the impact of fathers' presence or absence on family relationships and on the children's welfare, owing to the long working hours that prevail today, in particular as far as high and middle management and professionals are concerned (Fermanian, 1999). However, qualitative research has put emphasis on the fact (Castelain-Meunier, 1998; Neyrand, 1999) that many young fathers would like to play a bigger part in their children's lives. This mirrors the cultural changing attitudes between generations that have occurred over the last decades. However most of the large companies tend to view seniority at work as irreconcilable with a high degree of family commitment.

6. NEW CHALLENGES: IS THERE A PREDICAMENT FOR FAMILY POLICY?

6.1. The Gendered Division of Work: An Enduring Asymmetry Between the Sexes in Family Involvement

Traditional value systems underlying the behaviour of both men and women in the family sphere and in the professional sphere still play an important role in France. Recent research has confirmed that the unequal gender distribution of domestic and child-raising tasks within the family still persists, as Table 2.3 illustrates (Anxo *et al.*, 2000; Barrère-Maurisson *et al.*, 2000 and 2001; Brousse, 1999).

Table 2.3. Proportion of the number of hours per week devoted to unpaid and paid work assumed by women (Couples, aged between 18-64 years old)

Year	PERCENTAGE OF HOURS DEVOTED TO WORK			TOTAL
	Paid work	Domestic chores	Caring for children or old people	
1986	33%	74%	74%	**53.4%**
1999	36%	68%	69%	**51.6%**

Source: Budget-time surveys 1986 and 1999, INSEE, Brousse, 1999

Time-budget surveys made by INSEE in 1999 show that mothers still work twice as many hours in the home as fathers. Changes over the period 1986 – 1999 have been modest. However, one noted cultural change is that fathers have become more involved in decisions regarding the education of their children, as opposed to merely being involved later in decisions regarding career.

The unequal sharing of domestic tasks partly explains (but also mirrors) the fact that in the majority of dual-earner couples with children the woman devotes less time to her job than her partner (Fermanian and Lagarde, 1998), as soon as they have a young child. Among highly educated couples (Fermanian, 1999) both of them working full-time at the management level, it has been shown that the mother most always comes back home earlier than the father. As a matter of fact, even career-oriented women who can afford to hire someone at home for cleaning and caring, still assume the mental burden of the organisation of family life (Laufer, 1998; Marry, 1998). Family policy does contribute to reinforce this gender division of work, in particular through the APE scheme, which is not designed to encourage fathers to stop work temporarily. Moreover, in public childcare facilities, the staff is only female. Childminders are also only women's jobs. All these characteristics reinforce the idea that caring for children is a woman's issue.

6.2. New Services in Childcare Provision: What is at Stake?

As a result of the changes in the working patterns of women and men, there is a growing effort to meet the demands of parents confronted by atypical and flexible working hours. Along this line, some new services have been created by non-profit associations or agencies, which can be partly funded by the local Family Allowance Fund (CAF). However, improving the regulation and training of staff employed in this market-based sector of childcare is at stake. The National Ministry of Family is also currently encouraging local authorities to develop more flexible childcare services. Some *crèches* are already operating until late in the evening. However the staff working in these facilities (mostly women) are very reluctant about these changes which impact on their own daily life.

6.3. The New Law that Mandates a 35-Hour Week: Does it Improve the Possibilities of Combining a Job with Family Life?

Theoretically, the French adoption of a 35-hour working week (calculated on an average over the year, which means that employees can work 40 hours a week or more for a few months and much less during other periods of time) was part of the search for a better work-life balance. It was also intended to create employment. It is too early to really assess the impact of the 35-hour law on the daily life of working parents. So far, only big companies have been required to implement the law. Small and medium sized companies are currently negotiating, among other things, the new working schedules with the representatives of their employees or directly with the employees. The jigsaw of smaller-scale studies does however already suggest a number of broad conclusions.

First, it is important to keep in mind that most of the employers were very reluctant toward this law and strongly opposed the view of the government when the law was passed by 1999. However, employers have been obliged to come to terms with the implementation of the law. Therefore, in exchange and to offset the drawbacks of this law, they have tried to increase flexibility at the workplace. In the banking sector or in the retail sector, for example, they have made an agreement, which entails an extension of the opening hours. As a result, many employees are now obliged to work later in the evening or to work on Saturdays which can force or encourage some mothers of young children to stop working until the children are old enough to become autonomous.

Recent research (Fagnani & Letablier, 2003a) examined the perception by parents of young children of the impact of the law on their work and family life balance. It relied upon responses to questions on the 35 hours drawn from an original survey—carried out two years after the implementation of the first law—on the reconciliation between work and family life, using a representative sample of recipients of family allowances. The survey provided information about the judgement of parents, fathers or mothers, concerning changes induced in the management of their daily life.

Six out of ten respondents reported a positive impact on their work/life balance. The degree of satisfaction was higher where the organisation of work was regular and based on standard working hours. Satisfaction was also highly correlated with the negotiation process in the workplace. However, the reduction of working time revealed inequalities between workers: between those employed in sheltered economic sectors and "family-friendly" companies with a tradition of social dialogue, and those facing severe constraints in the workplace, or who had had to accept unsocial or flexible hours of work in exchange for a reduction of working time, without any consideration for their family obligations. This widened the gap between these two groups of workers irrespective of gender and professional status.

Another survey was conducted at the end of 2000- beginning of 2001, among 1,618 salaried people (with or without children) working in companies having implemented this law for at least one year (Estrade *et al.*, 2001). The following results are quite instructive:

- Three out of four female managers (with or without children) deem that their daily life (at work and out of work) has been improving. This is the case for only 40% of women with low qualified jobs.
- 40% of employees complain that work has become more intense and that they have to do the same amount of work in a shorter time span than before.
- As far as the reconciliation of family and professional life is concerned, diversity is also the rule: nearly half of the parents having children under 12 years report that they have been spending more time with their children since the reduction of their working hours.
- Around a third of employees declare that combining work and family life is easier than before the reduction of working time (32 % of men, 38 % of women). Fifty-seven per cent declare that nothing has changed.
- It is illustrative that the gender division of work has not been affected by the reduction of the working time. Women still assume the main burden of household chores and devote more time than before to

cleaning, doing some tidying up, cooking and gardening. Men spend more time doing odd jobs, gardening and some shopping.

The consequences for employees vary according to the economic sector, the modalities of the agreement signed between social partners, whether the company is in dire straits or not, etc. Nevertheless, it should be emphasised that small firms currently had to deal with a lot of difficulties in putting the law into practice.

Dominique Méda (2001), an essayist, has recently published a book, which devotes a large amount of space to endorsing the view that employers should take into further consideration the private life of their employees. In particular, she argues that trade unions and employers are turning a blind eye to the rights and obligations of working parents and that it is detrimental to the gender equality objective. She also challenges the common view that part-time managers are ineffective. However, against the background of an increase in redundancies in the private sector, it seems unlikely that French policy-makers will further develop the legislation regarding these issues. The announcement of the two-weeks paternity leave was strongly criticised by the employers whose attitudes mirror the fact that the issue of reconciling paid work and unpaid work is still not high on the economic and political agenda.

CHAPTER 3

ITALY

1. NATIONAL SOCIAL POLICIES

In Italy, family policies are not an explicit and unitary formulation and it is difficult to establish the extent of their institutionalisation at the national level. In other words, social-policy interventions affecting households show a high degree of fragmentation at different institutional levels. The subject of "Parental leave" has been recently systematised by the so-called "*Testo Unico*" act of law, n. 151/2001: it is an effective juridical tool, that further renovates the new parameters introduced by Act No. 53/2000 (see paragraph 1.2).

1.1. Childcare

The majority of recent studies on the Italian care-system agree that care-activities are almost entirely delegated to the family, and within the family the gendered division of labour continues to be very traditional, such that women in general – working and non-working women – are the main care-providers (Trifiletti, 1996; De Simone and Villa, 1998; Saraceno, 1998). According to these studies, the family - with its gendered and generational division of responsibilities and labour, as well as its asymmetrical structure of interdependencies – can be seen as the "implicit partner" of Italian social policies.

From a legislative point of view childcare represents an issue in which different normative interventions intersect. If we consider care-work carried out inside families, the main legislative intervention concerns the issue of insurance against domestic accidents for housewives. Act No. 493/1999 regarding exclusively the relationship between the state and citizens, regulates the protection of health inside the home and introduces the obligation of insurance against domestic accidents in order to protect those who freely carry out care-work (and hence childcare) without a contract, in recognition of the social and economic value of this work. The main effect of the Act is that it equates domestic accidents with accidents at work. Furthermore, it recognises that the domestic/care-work to be protected can be carried out both by women and men and both in "*de-jure*" and in "*de-facto*" families.

If we consider the institutional provision of childcare, in Italy there are two kinds of public pre-school services: crèches or day care (*asilo nido*) for children from three months to three years old and kindergartens (*scuola materna*) for children three to five years old. Crèches differ greatly from kindergartens in terms of their conceptualisation as services to families (the former) or as universal educational rights for the children (the latter), funding status, take-up rate, and extent of provision within the country.

The existing Italian legislative literature on childcare focuses mainly on crèches, as they represent a crucial service-tool for the life of many Italian families and an area where important changes have recently been made (Trifiletti, 1996; Ferrucci, 1998; Rauti, 1998; Saraceno, 1998). In this area, there are two acts, which can be referred to as key factors of public intervention. Act No. 1044/1971, subsequently integrated and modified by Act No. 891/1977, introduces crèches for children up to three years old, as public services run by Municipalities at a local level. In Act No. 1044/1971 crèches are defined as "individual-demand services" and not as universal services, as opposed to schools (compulsory) and public kindergartens. Service - providers establish fees to be paid on a sliding scale according to the income of parents, in order to cover part of the service cost. On this subject, Ferrucci (1998) points out that the persistence in Italy of access-criteria to this service, by favouring some occupational groups, risks penalising households strongly, where parents, and especially mothers, carry out atypical and unstable activities.

No organic provisions at a national level and no further developments have taken place on the matter of crèches since the 1970s. On this subject, Saraceno (1998) highlights the fact that a particular idea of family and household responsibilities - when children are very young – persists at a national level. According to the author, this idea is orientated to a rigid gendered division of labour and is linked to a residual definition of this service-area.

Specific infancy-protection is the objective of Act No. 285/1997, which promotes rights and opportunities for children and adolescents. The Act puts into place a national fund for children and adolescents to be used in order to finance several projects, especially in urban areas, to be realized at different (i.e. local, regional and national) levels. Such projects are aimed to promote rights, quality of life, development, individual achievement and the socialisation of children and adolescents.

1.2.Maternity, Paternity, and Parental Leave

Given that in Italy a satisfactory system of childcare services is lacking, especially for infancy, as argued in the previous section, the provisions regarding maternity leave are, in practice, the only ones in force that give actual support to parents (in particular to working women) in their task of bringing up children. In the present section, the description of current Italian provisions on maternity, paternity, and parental leave are collated, as the reference-legislation is the same for each measure.

The provisions regarding maternity leave represent one of the most important and innovative measures – also considered as more generous than the minimum criteria established by the European Union - aimed at helping mothers to cope with their dual responsibility. There is a general consensus in the literature that in Italy the degree of protection for working mothers is high. The tendency in most recent years has also been to extend progressively the provision on maternity leave to non-waged employment (self-employed women, as well as professional women) (De Simone and Villa, 1998; Saraceno, 2001).

Maternity leave is regulated by Act No. 1204/1971 and Act No. 903/1977, whose normative bodies have been significantly integrated and changed by the recent Act No. 53 of 8 March 2000. In particular, the law on maternity leave, enacted in 1971, establishes maternity protection measures for all employees, both in the private and public sector. Furthermore, a five-month period of compulsory leave (paid at 80%) and an optional-leave period lasting a further six months (paid at 30%) were introduced. The subsequent Act, No. 903/1977 extends optional-leave to the father who can benefit from it instead of the mother, on the condition that the parents are legally married and both are employees. De Simone and Villa (1998) point out in their study that optional-leave has a relatively low take-up rate since women prefer to go back to work and make use of the provision for working mothers with very young children, which allows for a reduction in their daily working hours, but with no reduction in earnings.

The enactment of Law No. 53 of 8 March 2000 has substantially modified the protection recognising working parents during the period of compulsory and optional-leave (for further elaboration of this area, see Del Punta (2000), Gheido and Casotti (2000), Bozzao (2001), Saraceno (2001), Calafà (2001) and Gottardi (1999)). Regarding compulsory leave, changes refer to both the working mother and the working father. The mother is allowed to make use of some flexibility in her choice of the time-period, provided that its length remains five months, while the father has an autonomous right to the interruption of labour during the first three months of the life of his child, under specific conditions of absence or non-ability of the mother. There are no changes as far as economic treatment recognised for compulsory leave is concerned. It remains the same at 80% of the salary. Moreover, some specific contracts provide the full payment of salaries: historically those in the public sector, but also in big industries, insurance companies, banks, and so on.

As already mentioned, all the matters regarding "Maternity and Paternity in the working places" strongly reformed with the Act No. 53/2000, are nowadays concentrated within the "*Testo Unico*" Act of Law, n. 151 of 26 March 2001, as amended by Act n. 115 of 23 April 2003. Therefore, all the legal provisions concerning maternity and paternity protections, parental rights and absences from the workplace, can be found in one piece of law. The "*Testo Unico*" is the end point of a long list of legislative productions, begun in Italy in 1902, with the Act n. 242 containing the compulsory maternity leave for 30 days after the birth.

If the overall picture of compulsory leave drawn in Act. No. 53 remains unchanged in comparison to previous legislation; significant innovations have been introduced for parental leave, by contributing to modifying the position of the working father strongly, relative to abstention from work. Under "parental leave" three forms of labour interruption can be distinguished:

- Optional-leave;
- Daily leave;
- Leave for caring of a sick child.

Previous legislation allocated a six-month period to the working mother for optional-leave, as an extension of her compulsory leave. This was to be taken during the first year of the life of her child and the compensation was at 30% of salary. From the enactment of Law No. 53 (8 March 2000) both parents can now benefit from optional-leave for a continuous or segmented period, without needing to justify it and by paying attention exclusively to single and joint duration. In particular, the father is entitled to optional-leave even though the mother is not, if she is a domestic worker, home help, housewife, or professional worker, for example. In relation to the length of optional-leave, there is no change for working mothers, while an incentive of an extra month (for a total period of seven months) is given to fathers who have taken advantage of their three-month compulsory leave. Both parents can benefit from the optional-leave during the first eight years of the life of their child. The payment coverage rate remains unchanged at 30% for the first three years of life of the child.

With regard to daily leave, previous legislation established so-called "leave for breast-feeding", consisting of one or two hours according to whether daily working hours are equal to or fewer than six hours. With the changes introduced by Act No. 53/2000, working fathers are also entitled to daily leave and to the relative economic and normative treatment, in the following cases:

- The employed working mother chooses not to benefit from them;
- The mother is not an employee;
- The father has exclusive custodial responsibility for his child.

In the case of twin-delivery, leave periods can be doubled and additional hours can be used also by the father.

In relation to leave for the care of a sick child, according to the previous legislation, the mother was entitled to leave during periods of illness of her child up to the first three years of her/his life. As from Act No. 53/2000 both parents can alternatively make use of leave in order to care for their child. In the first three years of the life of the child, there are no time limits to parental leave; this leave is not paid, but working parents are entitled to figurative contributions (*contributi figurativi*). If the child is between three and eight years old, parental leave is limited to five working days a year for each parent; this leave is not paid and the working parent is entitled to a reduced coverage of contributions (*copertura contributiva ridotta*), the same as it is provided for optional-leave.

Bozzao (2001) summarises the important general changes introduced by the new legislation about maternity, paternity and parental leave in the concluding section of her work. First of all, Act No. 53/2000 sets up, on a permanent basis, full equality between the position of the working mother and that of the working father. Besides compulsory leave, optional-leave is also given to the father, without the need for the mother (who is an employee) to renounce her entitlement. Furthermore, entitlements to compulsory and optional-leave are extended to a wider variety of working parents, i.e. professional workers. Moreover, as shown by Act No. 53/2000, a legislative trend towards a "progressive socialisation" of costs linked to the provisions granted by the protection system of families has taken place. This is confirmed by the gradual transition of provisions' funding from a system based on employers' contributions to a system based on public taxation. Both the extension of the subjective sphere of beneficiaries and the changes in the funding system point to a new legislative tendency which moves from family protection to citizenship rights, the entitlements being linked to each individual as a member of a civil community.

1.3.Flexible Working Patterns

During the 1990s profound changes were introduced within labour legislation, with the primary aim of sustaining employment levels. The enacted interventions have also contributed to diversifying working hours even though they were designed to shorten time-schedules and encourage forms of work-sharing. However, the current legislative framework remains characterised by a high level of fragmentation as a consequence of the superimposition of provisions deriving from different sources. What follows is an attempt to identify key legislative measures that have marked the process of 'flexibilisation' - the de-standardisation of labour-relations and working time-schedules.

One of the most important forms of atypical labour-relations is represented by part-time work. It is defined as an arrangement of employment characterised by a reduced time-schedule in comparison to that established by law or collective bargaining. Moreover, a proportionally lower wage corresponds to it.

Act No. 863/1984, besides part-time work, also regulates the "*Contratti di solidarietà*", the Italian version of job sharing. Under this scheme, firms and workers may agree to cut down hours, days or months of work - partially compensated by labour redistribution to newly recruited or other employees - in order to avoid lay-offs in periods of economic crisis. Firms who signed *contratti di solidarietà* since 1993 now receive (i) a subsidy amounting to 25% of wage-savings on account of reduced activity (ii) a discount on social security contributions. Workers on *contratti di solidarietà*, on the other hand, are entitled to 75% of wages lost on account of the reduction of working time.

Another version of flexible working patterns is tele-work. It includes all forms of work that are carried out in a place that is different from the workplace. It can be carried out at home or in satellite-equipped places or in a non-determined place, such as in the case of mobile work (*lavoro mobile*). It implies the availability of an electronic connection with the firm. Tele-work is regulated by the Decree with the force of Law No. 626/1994. Tele-work is regulated by collective agreements that have controlled its introduction, often on an experimental basis. In addition to required production levels, wage conditions, cost coverage, privacy protection, etc., collective agreements usually establish typical conditions linked to working schedules. Therefore, the regulation of tele-work shows interesting implications for working-time issues (see Piazza *et al.,* 1999).

2. WORKPLACE POLICIES—OBJECTIVE MEASURES

In Italy, the majority of measures for supporting the reconciliation of work and family-life are an outcome of public intervention in diversified forms. Numerous local governments and primarily the state, have offered several means of reconciliation especially tailored for female employees. Private employers, companies and organisations, on the other hand, have delayed their active involvement in promoting reconciliation policies. Moreover, even trade unions have had difficulty in assuming a gender-based perspective aimed at the reconciliation between family and professional work life. A consequence of this situation is that in Italy, the literature on the experience of reconciliation policies at the company level is rather sketchy and poorly developed.

2.1. Current Status of:

2.1.1. Childcare
In Italy childcare as an integrative service provided by companies or organisations is not a widespread phenomenon. The poor status of concrete workplace measures for relieving parents of care burdens is due to the fact that these facilities are viewed with suspicion by firms and local governments. Therefore, the author has been

unable to identify a single Italian study that deals systematically with the rare companies' experiences of providing childcare.

2.1.2. Flexible Working Patterns
On the basis of studies considered in the present section, working time schedules experimented with at the workplace during recent years as an alternative to standard working time (eight hours a day for five working days a week, for around forty-seven weeks a year) can be classified as follows:
- Part-Time Work
- Elasticity of Daily Working Schedules
- Work Permits, Parental Leave, Leave of Absence
- New Forms of Shift Work
- Flexitime and Year-Based Working Schedules (Annualizzazione degli Orari)
- Job-sharing

2.2. Studies of Experiences with Flexible Working Patterns in Companies/ Organisations

Italian studies concerning experiences with flexible working patterns in companies and organisation can be categorised into three groups:
- General descriptive studies;
- Descriptive company case studies;
- Empirical research works on specific company case studies.

2.3. General Descriptive Studies

Grecchi (1999) carried out a study, which gathered the opinions of the key actors such as the Minister of Labour and Social Security, the Associations of employers and trade unions, and the experiences of companies and organisations through managers' reports, together with cases of experimentation of equal opportunities for men and women. In particular, through semi-structured questionnaires and interviews with managers, data has been gathered on actual cases of companies which have put into place working time arrangements that allow women and men to reconcile their professional and family life. The aim of the study was to demonstrate that equal opportunities for men and women in the labour market, is a positive factor for the company's competitiveness and not an obstacle to it. In other words, the leading hypothesis of the study was that optimising female resources at the workplace can assist companies in facing the globalisation challenge.

2.4. Descriptive Company Case Studies

Bergamaschi, Omodei Zorini and Schweizer (1995) explored the relationship between women and work through female "health status", and described workplace policies operated by three companies employing both clerical and factory-worker female workers. The analysis of these company cases was through information (relating to the composition and the re-distribution of labour force, the policies of trade unions and industrial relations) derived from newspapers, publications of the trade unions and the company, and interviews with managers and member of trade union organisations at the workplace.

Bianchi (2000) carried out a specific investigation on the reconciliation between family, care-work and paid work for women within the context of the Autonomous Province of Bolzano and the region Alto-Adige. The interventions relating to family-work reconciliation were analysed in terms of the personnel policies utilised by Bolzano, and by identifying some proposals for improving the conditions for female workers.

A third group of descriptive study cases is offered by those presented at the national conference on "Le famiglie interrogano le politiche sociali" that took place in Bologna during 1999. Mantovani (1999) reports on the experience within private production sectors, specifically relating to the measures implemented for the support of role reconciliation at TIM, a telecommunication company that introduced a specific programme ("Tim Mamma") in 1998, aiming to nurture the professional and cultural relationship between the company and female workers during pregnancy and the first years of the child.

The experience of the Elettrolux-Zanussi group relating to positive actions favouring family-work reconciliation is presented by Cazzaniga (1999). The company realized specific measures concerning the flexibilisation of working time of female workers and a childcare programme. Within the report presented by Riva (1999) on the case of Du Pont one can find a description of the specific measures relating to the flexibility of the working time and space and programmes of personal and family care adopted on the workplace, together with a reflection on how to increase the effectiveness of these instruments.

2.5. Empirical Research Works on Specific Company Case Studies

Within the public sector, we find a report by Vilde (1999) who accounts for the experience of the Province of Milan, by giving information about family-friendly measures, the company and the female working conditions. Bertozzi (1999) describes the experience of the Municipality of Forlì, by providing detailed data on the project for the reduction of working time and the income integration of mothers and fathers and a specific research report on the experience of the Municipality regarding an ADAPT Project on the flexibility of working time.

The study by Bergamaschi, Chiesi, De Filippi and Sogni (1993) has been carried out at Italtel (Milan), a company that was subject to a profound re-structuring process during the 1980's. Particular attention was paid to the role played by the measures concerning the flexibilisation of working time within the company's restructuring strategies. The analysis of working-time regimes introduced in the company was carried out by focusing particularly on family-life conditions that have been considered by the authors as an important explicative factor.

Research by Filippi (1997) and Bassi, Casotti and Sbordone (2000) illustrate two cases of co-operatives. The first relates to the co-operative of "Insieme Si Può" in the North-East of Italy. It is a co-operative of labour and social and training services where a majority of women work. Filippi identifies the following three areas: labour, family (through an analysis of the conditions of different typologies of women) and family-work life reconciliation. The second piece of research focused on the experience of the "Consorzio Solidarietà Sociale" of Forlì-Cesena that gathers different social co-operatives together at a local level. The study offers evaluative monitoring results – collected by both qualitative and quantitative research methodologies - on the experimental innovative measures introduced in order to influence the family-work balance of co-operative workers.

2.6. Objective Measures of the Quality of Different Childcare Arrangements

In Italy childcare services at the workplace are scarce and there have been no known studies on them, to the author's knowledge. In this section we will refer exclusively to objective measures adopted in several research works (Ingrosso, 1988; Ferrari, 1994; Becchi et al., 1999; Cooperativa Sociale Koine, 2000) for evaluating the quality of crèches.

Relating to the global level of quality of the service means referring to the following three elements (Becchi et al., 1999): a) the "perceived" quality by operators and especially by users as recorded through an evaluation of several aspects of the service; b) the "organisational" quality and c) the "managerial" quality. The Svani scale is used for the evaluation of crèches. It is the Italian version of the American Infant-Toddler Environmental Rating Scale, particularly useful for evaluating the "educational" quality of crèches (Ferrari, 1994; Becchi et al., 1999).

Ghedini (1995) points to the importance of considering the "flexibility" of the service, its "continuity" and "visibility" as essential issues in relation to the quality of crèches.

CHAPTER 3

3. ATTITUDINAL STUDIES—SUBJECTIVE MEASURES

3.1.Attitudes of Men and Women as Workers and Parents towards:

3.1.1.Work-Life Balance

Issues of the different management strategies of daily life and the reconciliation between family and professional work for mothers and fathers are extensively studied in Italy.

At a national level, there are several pieces of research focusing on the different uses of time of men and women with specific reference to the Italian case (Istat, 1993; Sabbadini and Palomba, 1994; Sabbadini, 2001), or with a comparative perspective (Bimbi, 1995; Belloni, 1996; Pattaro, 2000). Such studies provide interesting information on the division of family labour and on the patterns of time-organisation within Italian households. Data used in this research is mainly collected through time-budget diaries and highlight profound differences between fathers and mothers in the organisation and sequence of daily time (i.e. time for oneself, market-oriented time, family-oriented time, etc.).

The analysis of female and male organisation of daily time is relevant as it not only identifies profound differences in the amount of time spent on different activities, but also allows for a definition of a range of activities which are socially attributed to different categories – in our case: "fathers" and "mothers" – (Belloni, 1995b). In this way it is possible to derive interesting information on the different strategies of the division of labour and on the gender asymmetries within Italian households.

Such time-studies include investigations on the "time of towns" (Belloni, 1984; Le Nove, 1990; Balbo, 1991; Bimbi, 1991b), examining the structure of urban space-time relations, by consequently referring to the issue of the reconciliation between different life spheres. It gives particular importance to the issue relating to "time economies" of the welfare state, by analysing the different strategies of the re-distribution of care-work between the public, the private, the family private (*privato familiare*) and the non-profit private spheres (Bimbi, 1995).

There is a group of localised studies (Balbo *et al.*, 1990; Bimbi and Castellano, 1990; Giovannini and Ventimiglia, 1994; Irer, 1998) that mainly use qualitative methods and focus on organisation and reconciliation strategies, and especially on the motivations, the visions and attitudes of the individuals towards the different strategies of daily life management. These studies highlight a wide gap between fathers and mothers not only in relation to daily life experiences and the different strategies adopted, but also the perception of the different time components and life spheres. These issues assume considerable importance in defining the strategies of family-work reconciliation and in determining the different levels of cooperation between the two partners (Bimbi and Castellano, 1990; Giovannini and Ventimiglia, 1994).

Some studies (Molinari, 1996; Nava, 1996; Giovannini, 1998), define different typologies of maternal and paternal involvement in family management, by pointing out the issues linked to different degrees of interchangeability (*interscambiabilità*) and cooperation between the partners for family work and childcare activities. Each typology refers to different strategies of family-work reconciliation and to different negotiation processes.

From all the studies we have considered, it emerges that in Italy, even though regional differences persist, there is a strong asymmetry between men and women as far as the division of family labour is concerned. Even when we consider cases where the two partners devote an equal amount of time to paid-labour, family work remains an exclusive female obligation (Sabbadini and Palomba, 1994; Palomba, 1997; Pattaro, 2000; Sabbadini, 2001). This implies a heavy "double burden" for women who have to try to reconcile work and family tasks or subordinate paid work to unpaid work, at least in some phases their life cycle (Belloni, 1996; Pattaro, 2000).

The problem of family-work reconciliation is of primary importance for today's women who - as it emerges from the research carried out by Irp (Menniti and Terracina, 1994), would like to harmonise their working careers and the realization of their personal and family life, in a less problematic way, by reaching a more equal division of family obligations with their partners. For fathers, as well as for men in general, the family-work reconciliation does not seem to be a pertinent problem, except in terms of a lack of spare time to spend together with their children (Bimbi, 1990; Ventimiglia, 1996). Paid work - even though it is no longer regarded, as in the past, as an exclusive sphere for the definition and self-realization of the male figure, continues however to be the priority on a day-to-day level. Fathers rarely reduce their paid working time after the birth of their children and in there is even a tendency to increase it in order to face additional economic needs (Bimbi and Castellano, 1990; Sabbadini and Palomba, 1994; Ventimiglia, 1996; Pattaro, 2000). Only a minority of fathers, moreover, opt to use parental leave, even though this is perceived by both fathers and mothers to be an optimal solution for favouring a good paternal involvement in childcare and for reaching a good family-work reconciliation more easily (Zanatta, 1999). It is also noteworthy that here the attitudes differ from behavioural practices. There are several reasons for this and they are linked to the presence of objective constraints, relating to the dominant structures and patterns at the workplace (Saitta, 1996; Irer, 1998).

As far as family work is concerned, fathers – even though they are aware of the existing asymmetry in the division of tasks and they do not approve of it on a theoretical level – seem to accept the existing situation for practical reasons (Bimbi and Castellano, 1990; Scisci, 1999). Paternal justifications refer to the stronger female aptitude, to their lack of time, to the fact of "not being" or "not feeling" qualified to do to certain tasks (Bimbi and Castellano, 1990; Giovannini and Ventimiglia, 1994; Goriup, 2001). Paternal involvement both in childcare and especially in domestic work, is very low and, where present, it is in terms of assistance offered to the mother and not in terms of an effective sharing of responsibilities (Bimbi and Castellano, 1990; Ventimiglia, 1996 and 1999). On the other hand, many mothers adjust their behaviour to this situation, through looking at the asymmetry as a normative-value model (Scisci, 1999). Sometimes it seems that the cost of negotiation to obtain greater equality is too high from a relationship point of view (Bimbi and Castellano, 1990). In actual fact, as noted by Ventimiglia (1996), in couples where the division of family labour is the result of a reciprocal pragmatism, conflicts do not arise nor are perceived. On the contrary, where a negotiation process is entered into in order to reach a greater sharing equality, the level of conflict is likely to be higher.

The issue of 'time for oneself' is particularly important for women (Balbo *et al.*, 1990; Piazza, 1993; Leccardi, 1994; Belloni, 1995a). A constant search by women for time for themselves has been recorded, not only in quantitative but also in qualitative terms. On the contrary, when studying men, the problem of a lack of time for oneself is less self-evident (Sabbadini and Palomba, 1994). This confirms the heavy imbalance in the management of family work that leaves the majority of tasks to women.

Several studies (Balbo *et al.*, 1990; Bimbi and Castellano, 1990; Balbo, 1991; Bernardi and Mancini, 1994; Palomba and Sabbadini, 1994; Ventimiglia, 1996 and 1999) identify not only differentiated timing for men and women on the basis of different daily-time rhythms, but also very different strategies of living in different spaces and times. A typically female managerial strategy for daily life emphasises time-crossing (*trasversalità*) and the co-management of different spaces, through a constant commuting - of a psychological nature – between family needs, children, and professional work tasks. This is quite different to the 'single-tasked' man (*monotematicità maschile*), who tends to divide his different life areas and to run the different spheres within "exclusive" and separated moments: working time, family time, time for oneself, time with children, and free time.

3.1.2. Flexible Working Patterns
The majority of forms of working flexibility on one hand relieve women from their "double burden" and on the other hand imply heavy consequences not only in terms of wages, but also in relation to future working developments and to possible career chances (Addis, 1997). For example, the choice of working part-time, even though it is considered by many women with senior professional positions (Irer, 1998) a possible strategy to meet the needs of childcare, especially for toddlers (Rossi, 1999; Scisci, 1999), creates some problems for subsequent re-entry into full-time jobs

(Addis, 1997). From an economic perspective, Cappellini (1999) points out that part-time work can be a "bridge" or a "trap" for subsequent full-time re-entry.

3.1.3. Childcare
In Italy the percentage of children in crèches is less than 6% of the total number of entitled children (Ascoli and Pavolini, 2001). The paucity of community childcare facilities, especially for infants, leads people to use informal and family networks. In Italy, this strategy is one of the most common (Censis, 1984; Musatti, 1992; Sabbadini, 2001) and is the consequence of the Italian model of welfare. This is characterised by a value system that sees the primary responsibility for the satisfaction of needs as the household and informal networks (Sgritta, 1988).

The various studies dealing with these issues highlight the different attitudes of parents towards different care-solutions for children up to three years old: in some cases crèches seem to be the preferred arrangement, but the real choice of the service can be subsequently affected by the small number of crèches or by access constraints (Ingrosso, 1988; Balbo *et al.*, 1990; Irer, 1998); in other cases, grandparents, especially maternal ones, seem to remain the preferred solution, even in the presence of a good number of childcare services (Musatti and D'Amico, 1996; Rossi, 1999; Scabini and Regalia, 1999; Ondina Greco, 2000). Private childcare services (baby-sitters, private crèches, etc.) are not widespread (Musatti, 1992) and are not much analysed in these studies.

Even though it is the most common arrangement, the family as the provider of childcare services is not always without problems. However, informal networks maintain a primary role, if not as a childcare strategy chosen by the family, at least as an important mediation figure between the family and services for children older than three years old (when kindergartens are little-used) (Balbo *et al.*, 1990).

The majority of parents consider the opportunities for women to use working-time reduction strategies without negative economic and professional consequences to be an optimal childcare solution (Rossi, 1999). According to parents, another solution is represented by the services for infancy that offer diversified and flexible strategies according to different needs (Musatti, 1992; Menniti, 1993; Irer, 1998; Scisci, 1999; Rossi, 1999). More generally, the need for widespread, accessible and efficient services is emphasised in a number of studies; in fact childcare services are considered as primary supporting-instruments for working parents and are preferred to other kinds of intervention such as economic subsidies (Menniti, 1993; Scisci, 1999).

Some studies carried out at a local level (Ingrosso, 1988; Balbo *et al.*, 1990; Musatti, 1992; Trifiletti and Turi, 1996; Arona, 1997; Irer, 1998) and at a national level (Sabbadini, 2001) record the different motivations of parents choosing a crèche over other childcare options. The decision to enrol a child in a crèche is not dictated only by the "need" or by the lack of alternatives, but by the importance assigned to a qualified and professional childcare approach, and especially to the fact that crèches are considered important from an educational point of view.

4. STUDIES ON GENDER ROLE ATTITUDES

The present section presents studies relating to the vision of gender roles within the Italian population and those on role changes over time. There is a dearth of studies at a national level on gender roles and an abundance of studies carried out at local and regional levels using smaller samples.

4.1. Studies on Women

Most Italian studies on the vision of gender roles focus on women and the changes that have modified the roles of women from the '60s onwards (Saraceno, 1987 and 1993a; Siebert, 1991; Bimbi, 1992; Ginatempo, 1994; Mauri and Billari, 1999; Di Vita and Mancuso, 2000). Other studies also focus on the consequences of changes of gender-based roles on the system of relationships and on the family dynamics affecting expression and development patterns (Scabini and Donati, 1991; Melchiorre, 1992; Donati, 1997).

By comparing several cohorts of women during the last three decades, substantial differences emerge (Saraceno, 1987). One can see a radical transformation of both the subjective experience of the "double burden" phenomenon and the management practices of daily life. In this manner different models of the "double burden" phenomenon are defined. These reflect the different strategies of family-work reconciliation, a different attitude towards professional work and a different interpretation of gender roles (Saraceno, 1987; Zanuso, 1986).

The most significant dimensions of the changes of women's behaviours and gender patterns can be found in the following three elements: the relevant increase in female labour force participation; the extended female education that is greater than for men (Barbagli and Saraceno, 1997) and grants women the possibility to aspire to superior employment in comparison to the past; and the modernization of reproduction work that has been accompanied by a re-definition of demographic choices (Bimbi, 1990; Saraceno, 1993b). Following such changes, a transition within the last three generations of women has taken place between different reconciliation patterns of roles as mothers, wives and workers (Saraceno, 1987).

The first typology of the "double burden" phenomenon refers to the first generation of women who have been actors of the changes of women's life models at the workplace and within the family. It shows a difficult reconciliation between work-oriented time and family-oriented time. These two dimensions present some discontinuities, particularly within the different phases of women's life cycles

(Bimbi, 1993b). The "double burden" phenomenon is characterised for these women as an issue that is problematic both at the level of personal identity – as a consequence of breaks implied in comparison to the acquired models and to the personal belongings – and in terms of possibilities to manage the daily life by reconciling different roles (Zanuso, 1987).

The second cohort of women, born during the '50s, elaborates a strategy that is based on the continuity of market-oriented work and, in a high number of cases, on the investment in professional work and in the working career. Biographical paths are more diversified in comparison to the past, the "double burden" pattern, although more problematic, is accepted and perceived as unavoidable.

Finally, the youngest women's generation experiences market-oriented work as a given part of adulthood. Exclusive mother and wife roles are no longer a part of the perspective of young women (Bimbi, 1993a). After childbirth, the "double burden" pattern is accepted as a natural characteristic of their female life, even though the subjective and objective costs of this double role can be heavy (Romito and Saurel Cubizzolles, 1997), especially as a consequence of the poor adjustment of the father to new family models (Saraceno, 1996).

During the past decade, women have experienced a strong pull towards self-achievement within professional careers and, even after having got married; they perceive their paid working activity as an important area of self-achievement. In particular, they consider paid work as an arena for social relationships, as a compensating factor in their mother-child relationship, as a dissociation from family obligations, and as a source of economic independence (Bimbi, 1993a, Scarazzati, 1994; Irer, 1998; Di Vita, Annino and Mancuso, 2000).

Moreover, the roles of 'mother' and 'wife' are no longer seen by women as the only way to access adult life, as they were in the past; but now such roles are a result of a subjective choice between different possible alternatives (Bimbi, 1993a). Certainly, the female identity is no more exclusively founded on such roles (Bimbi, 1993a; Ginatempo, 1994). Despite the fact that having a child is still considered one of the most important goals in life (Palomba, 1991), in reproduction-choices parental costs are taken into account, especially in relation to women's life paths (Saraceno, 1996; Romito and Saurel Cubizzolles, 1997).

Women over thirty are postponing maternity decisions and thereby dissociating themselves from the child-rearing practices that obliged past generations to experience mainly mother and wife roles (Bimbi, 1993a). In this context the choice of an only-child is also perceived as one of the solutions that allows for a better reconciliation of family and work life (Bimbi, 1996; Nava, 1996; Saraceno, 1996). Such a pattern, even though it does not reflect the ideal of the majority of couples (Palomba, 1987), results in being the least problematic for the reconciliation of the different life spheres, especially for women.

4.2. Studies on the Father Figure

Studies on the father figure include both theoretical works and empirical investigations. The image of "new fathers" emerging from the different studies is a contradictory one. Italian fathers of today seem dissociated from past models, especially with respect to the emotional, and relational component of the relationship with their children (Ventimiglia, 1994 and 1996; Giovannini, 1998). However, regarding other aspects mainly relating to the dimension of the sharing of childcare-work (Bimbi and Castellano, 1990), today's fathers maintain substantial continuities with past generations. The transformation of parental, maternal and especially paternal roles does not follow a linear path, but is very much inherited from the past, despite being integrated with new elements (Ventimiglia, 1996; Bimbi, 1996; Giovannini, 1998).

The considerable emotional involvement of fathers in the life of their children is emphasized particularly in the studies carried out in the Emilia-Romagna region by Bimbi and Castellano (1990) and by Giovannini and Ventimiglia (1994). The majority of the fathers interviewed expressed the desire to have more free time to spend with their own children. Moreover, the return home from work is perceived by individuals as the most important and rewarding moment of the day. Fathers interviewed by Giovannini and Ventimiglia (1994) also underline the importance of the time spent with children and express the reward they feel in playing with them, in being together, in being physically affectionate with them. The emotional proximity to the child and the participation in her/his growth are considered fundamental elements not only for the development and the growth of the child, but also for themselves (Badolato, 1993; Ventimiglia, 1994). Fathers seem to perceive them as moments for personal growth, enrichment and as a primary source of satisfaction and reward.

Bozzi and Cristiani (1996) present the findings of a study carried out in a hospital in Milan. The high emotional involvement of fathers as recorded in this study as well as others (Nordio *et al.*, 1983; Giovannini and Ventimiglia, 1994), is pointed out both during pregnancy and delivery. The majority of fathers recall the playing-expressive element of the relationship with the child, but instrumental and caring activities are not mentioned. The dimension of care, therefore, still does not seem to be part of the imaginations of fathers, nor in the mental construction of the paternal role (Badolato, 1993; Molinari, 1996; Ventimiglia, 1996; Giovannini, 1998).

The relationship between the couple and its relational and negotiation dynamics seem to be of fundamental importance in obtaining a good level of paternal involvement in relation to childcare (Badolato, 1993; Bestetti, 1996). From the study by Bimbi and Castellano (1990) it emerges that mothers often have an ambiguous attitude towards the involvement of the father in childcare. On the one hand, mothers ask for more active paternal cooperation which somewhat relieves their "double burden", on the other hand they seem to want to keep for themselves this sphere of exclusive and traditional control that remains for some women the primary source of recognition and identification (Bimbi, 1990 and 1992). We therefore find a family situation in which a significant emotional and relational symmetry is accompanied by a strong asymmetry in the division of labour. The gap between the ideal and actual behaviour can be understood by taking into account the ambivalences accompanying the re-definition of gender and parental roles (Molinari, 1991 and 1996; Giovannini, 1998). Bimbi (1996) points out that, in a period of transition both women and men appear to need some continuity with family tradition and the gender asymmetries that characterise it, especially in relation to the domestic work.

CHAPTER 4

DENMARK

This literature review is divided into five main sections. The first section includes statistics on working time in Denmark, gender segregation in the labour market, domestic working time divided according to gender and types of day care institutions. In the second section, rules of leave are presented. In the third section, important research is presented under two subheadings: "Leave and the labour market", "Gender, working life and work-place cultures", and finally we present a discussion of "Scandinavian equality model(s)".

The latest results available in each area are presented along with the most recent available statistical material. Some of the studies presented, however, go back to the beginning of the 1990's but they have been used, as they are exemplary and/or sometimes also constitute the latest research carried out in the area.

1. DENMARK BY NUMBERS

The Danish female participation rate is among the highest in the world. In 1998 it was 73.2 % where the male participation rate was 81.6 % (Ligestillingsrådet & Danmarks Statistik 1999). The female participation rate is characterised by a so-called "plateau-model", that is, working without interruption. Generally women keep their connection with the labour market while they have babies/small children (Bonke, 1995).

However, the labour market is segregated by gender in Denmark. Csonka (2000) carried out a survey among almost 3000 public and private companies and found that three quarters of the companies were gender segregated, where segregation was defined as a gender majority of 60% or above. Ligestillingsrådet and Danmarks Statistik (1999) examined the total Danish population to reveal the bigger picture. A glance at the gender composition at the level of *business* reveals that men make up a total of 68-90% of employees in crafts-trades, transportation, agriculture, the fishing industry and industry in general, while women outnumber men in public and personal service. Looking further at the category of *public employees* the statistics show that there is a majority of women within county councils and municipal offices (more than 75%), while men occupy close to 60% of the state-employed jobs.

Research conducted by the Ministry of Finance in 1999 shows that in 38% of the categories of jobs in the public sector, men total more than 80% while women total 13% of the categories.

Looking at the distribution of gender in *top leadership positions* in the Danish labour market men account for 88%. In the category of *assisting spouse,* women account for about 96%.

A 'gender-gap' in wages of about 12% on average, which cannot be explained by seniority or level of education, is another parameter of inequality in the Danish labour market. The life-income of women is, furthermore, between 10% and 35% less on average, than that of men in the same work categories.

1.1. Working Hours and Gender

The official working week for a full time employee is 37 hours. The actual working time, though, can be rather different and a study (Bonke & Meilbak, 1999) among full time employed women and men under 48 and 45 years of age respectively, revealed an average working week above 37 hours. The results show that women work 38.8 hours weekly while men work 41.4 hours. A comparison between women and men with children of *0-2 years of age,* and the rest of the group of women and men shows that the working hours of parents are higher than those of the rest of the group. Mothers of children of 0-2 years of age work 39.5 hours a week and fathers work 41.9 hours a week. *Men with children aged 3-6* work even more, namely 42.4 hours weekly on average, while women with children in that age bracket work less, only 37.6 hours a week. Adding the time spent on transportation back and forth from work, every third family reaches a total work-time for husband and wife of 80 hours or more per week. There are even 10% of families in the category '90 hours or more'.

1.2. Flexibility At Work

To what extent can the labour market in Denmark be characterised as flexible? Research (Csonka, 2000) shows that in the years 1990 to 1995 there has been no notable development in the extension of the flexible labour market. While 22% of Danish companies are characterised by flexible management methods, relatively few employees are actually included in this flexibility. There is a mixed group of companies (39%), which have a few characteristics of flexible-management. This can be both a sign that the enterprise is on the way towards a higher degree of flexible management, or it can be a sign of neo-traditional enterprise culture (*a la* MacDonald's). On the basis of her analysis, Csonka leans towards the latter hypothesis.

Bonke and Meilbak's (1999) study reveals that 79% of the full time employees had *fixed working hours*, 8.5% had the possibility of changing the time to start work after agreement with their line-manager and 12.5% could plan their working time themselves. A little more than 50% of families do not have any flexibility in their work life. In 44% families one of the parents has flexibility, and only in 8.2% of the families do both the parents have the possibility of flexibility. It was found that 16.6% can do some of their work from home (i.e. work shorter hours at the workplace and work the rest of the working hours from their homes). Half of these people, however, spend less than 10% of the total working time working from their homes. The majority of people who work from home for some part of their working hours are parents. One in four families with pre-school and school children has this possibility, and it is more common for mothers (26.9%) than fathers (18.8%) to do so.

Apart from formal agreements of flexibility there are also various forms of informal agreements at Danish workplaces, which are negotiated on a daily basis, and where working time can be flexible, or one can, against all formal rules, bring a child to the workplace in emergency situations, where there are no other possibilities of care-taking. In a study of the adaptation possibilities between family-life and working life (Holt 1994) it appears to be relevant to look at the level of daily and pragmatic flexibility during work which takes place between colleagues, where workers deal with each others' bank transactions, cover for each other against the management, eat at irregular hours in order to shop for the family dinner in the lunch break, leave early to go to the dentist with the child, etc. These were all practiced by the female workers in the study, which demonstrates the extent to which women are involved with family work during working hours. It shows that when both parents are working (and the daily 'overlap' is small) a relatively high degree of flexibility is needed in order to make family-life function successfully.

1.3.Domestic Responsibility

In Denmark it is still the women who have the main responsibility for the home when it comes to laundry, cooking, cleaning etc. (Hestbæk 1995; Andersen & Hestbaek 1999; Holt, 1994; Bonke 1995). The responsibility often leads to a certain role strain for the women between work life and family-life, an 'intersection-pressure' which doesn't hamper the fathers to the same degree. However, research shows that there is a tendency towards a relative softening of these gender-roles.

1.4. Patterns of Childbirth in Denmark

The average age of child-delivery has increased steadily in Denmark during the last 20 years. In 1978 the age was 26.6 years (and 24.4 for first time delivering), and in 1998 it was 29.4 years (27 years for first timers). The fertility rate is 1.8. The highest educated women have babies later and have fewer babies (Ligestillingsrådet & Danmarks Statistik, 1999).

1.5. Children and Families

In 1981, 81.8% children were living with both (biological) father and mother, compared to the year 2000 when the percentage was 75.1%. In 2000 13.8% of children were living with their mothers (compared to 10.1% in 1981). In 2000 7.2% of children were living with their mother and her partner, while in 1981 this family pattern applied to only 3.9% of families. The number of children living alone with their fathers increased from 1.4% in 1981 to 1.7% in the year 2000 (Danmarks Statistik 2000a).

1.6. Childcare

1.6.1. Danish Childcare Model
In Denmark, parents and the public have the primary *responsibility* for the reconciliation of work life and family-life. This division must be viewed in the light of the ways in which the Danish Welfare state has developed. From the middle of the last century, there was an increase in the demand for labour and simultaneously an enlargement of the universalistic Welfare State. Thereby it became the state which provided incentive legislation, in the form of tax reform and labour market policies, as well as policies directed to remove family-related obstacles to women's full participation on the labour market, such as government sponsored childcare provision and paid maternity leave (Højgaard, 1997). Thereby a division of responsibility between the state and families in relation to childcare and the education of children and young people came about. To hold the workplace responsible for this reconciliation is, on the contrary, seldom regarded as desirable. Families are generally not interested in companies assisting with childcare, laundry or other such matters (Holt and Thaulow, 1996). A study that included 3,000 public and private companies showed, for example, only 1% had day-care facilities on site (Holt, 1998).

1.6.2. Day-care.
Day-care for children is predominantly a public responsibility in Denmark and this lies with the municipalities that are obliged to facilitate day care for children. They are responsible for organizing and providing childcare and for the *sort* of childcare that is offered. Two types of childcare for preschool children currently predominate: day-care institutions and private care - registered childminders - where a person takes care of up to five children in his/her own home. In 2000, 81,000 children between 0-3 years were in private care, while around 20,000 children in the same age group were in public day-care (day-nursery institutions are primarily a larger-city phenomenon; fewer than 80 out of 275 municipalities have day nurseries). 112,000 children attend kindergarten and 120,000 children attend institutions, which integrate children of age 0-13. A total of 470,000 children between 4-13 years of age go to after-school care (some/every day after school). The share of children in day-care are 54% of the 0-2 year olds, 90% of the 3-5 year olds and 75% of the 6-9 year olds, who attend after school-care (Ligestillingsrådet & Danmarks Statistik, 1999).

The municipalities may also provide financial support per child for privately run day-care institutions (Damgaard, 1998). These can include: several private caretakers joining in the care of the children, parents can get a financial contribution to hire somebody to baby-sit at home, or one can get money for taking care of own children. Moreover support is given to privately run institutions. These possibilities however are very rarely used.

2. DANISH RULES OF LEAVE

2.1. Maternity Leave

At the time of this study a female employee in Denmark has the right to stop working four weeks before her estimated delivery time. After the delivery, the woman has 14 weeks of maternity leave. During these 14 weeks, the father has the right to *paternity leave* for up to two weeks, plus up to a further two weeks during weeks 25-26. After the 14th week there are 10 weeks of *parental leave*, which can be shared by the father and the mother. However, the right to leave of absence can only be used by one of the parents at a time. In addition the mother has the right to a leave of absence from work in connection with pregnancy examinations; this right does not include the future father.

According to the law, one is entitled to the maximum subsistence allowance during maternity leave, paternity and parental leave. Most employees in the public sector, employees in the industrial area and in the service sector, get full salary during these types of leaves. In the private labour market, the paid leave is subject to collective bargaining, or depending on the terms that the individual employee can negotiate at his/her workplace. However, women (but not men) covered by the civil-service code receive full salary during maternity leave. In a survey conducted in 1998 about the social responsibility of companies (including about 3,000 companies) (Holt, 1998), 92% of the public companies stated that they gave full or part-payment during maternity leave while this was the case for only 57% of the private companies (it is companies with fewer than 50 employees, in particular, who do not offer full/part-compensation). Moreover many public employees have the right to leave of absence on full salary from the time when it is estimated that there are eight weeks to delivery time.

2.2. Childcare Leave

This is leave to take care of one's own children while the children are between 0 - 8 years old. This leave was introduced in 1992. It was partly initiated as a way of increasing job rotation in the Danish labour market and to combat unemployment, and therefore it was a precondition for granting leave that a substitute be hired during the leave. Moreover the leave was a method of cutting down on the long waiting lists for day care institutions, which was a problem at the beginning of the 1990's.

At the beginning, the wage-compensation during childcare leave was at 80% of the maximum subsistence allowance. Getting access to childcare leave was a matter of *agreement* with the employer. In 1994 the rule of substitutes for the person on leave was cancelled. At the same time, childcare leave was turned into a *right* and it was expanded to include insuranced-unemployed people and people on welfare. But as a consequence of the popularity of this, the government feared a lack of labour power and the income rate during leave was cut down later the same year to 70% of the maximum subsistence allowance, and in 1997 it went down to 60%, which is the current rate.

At the present time, childcare leave is divided into two parts, namely one of *right* and one of *agreement*. Both parents can take leave and they can take the leave at the same time or separately. Wage earners have the *right* to leave for a continuous period of from eight to thirteen weeks. If the child is under one year old at the time the leave is started, one has the right to 26 weeks (and at least eight weeks). Apart from the right-based leave, one has the opportunity to *negotiate* for leave with one's employer (for leave of continuous periods of at least eight weeks). The childcare leave cannot be more than 52 weeks in total. For people who are self-employed, the minimum leave is 13 weeks. In total the leave cannot be more than 52 weeks (with continuous periods of at least 13 weeks). People who are unemployed have the right to leave for at least 13 weeks, and 26 weeks with children under one year. In the case of the unemployed, it is the employment office that grants an agreement-based leave.

Children of up to three years of age cannot use public day-care facilities during the leave, while children aged three to eight are allowed to attend half day at a public day-care facility during the leave period.

Public employees have the right to a day off at the child's first sick day. A number of *care-days* are given on the public labour market, whereas in the private labour market it is dependent on negotiations in the workplace. Employees in the municipality area have the right to two care-days per child per year up until the year in which the child becomes eight. Holt (1998) stated that 77% of public companies with more than 200 employees have care-days beyond the child's first sick day. Only 25% of private companies with more than 50 employees have this measure.

2.3. Statistics on Leave-Use

In 1991, 55% of fathers took advantage of the possibility of the first two weeks of paternity leave, while the percentage in 1999 had risen to 67%. The two weeks of leave possible in weeks 25-26 after the birth of the child was used by only 3% in 1999. In 1991 3% of fathers used some or all of the 10 weeks of *parental leave* and the same percentage was used in the year 2000 (Carlsen, 1994; Danmarks Statistik, 2000b). The mother's use of parental leave is relatively static at about 72-74%. Carlsen (1994) states that the length of the leave and the period in which it is situated, namely in week 15-24, is paradoxical since the Department of Health suggests a period of breast-feeding of six months in consideration of the health of the child. In Carlsen's investigation of fathers on leave, the consideration of breast-feeding was one of the barriers to taking leave, which were mentioned by the fathers.

3. LEAVE AND THE LABOUR MARKET

3.1. Employer Attitudes towards Childcare Leave

The attitudes of employers towards childcare leave and the opinions of the employees who take childcare leave about their employers' attitudes towards their use of leave have been investigated in a survey conducted in 1996 (Andersen, Appeldorn & Weise). The research shows that employers in the public sector are more positive towards leave than employers in the private sector: 42% of the employers in private companies with fewer than 50 employees state that the right to childcare leave means that they will, to some or even to a large extent be reluctant to employ women with younger children.

Over a third (38%) of the private companies in the research state as their *fundamental outlook* that it is more reasonable for women to take leave than it is for men to do so; this was also true of 12% of the public employers. Male managers hold different views of their female and male employees' wishes for childcare leave. They are more negative towards leave for the men. Eighteen per cent of the employers in the private sector were found to be less sympathetic towards a male leave applicant than a female applicant.

A substitute is more frequently employed when a woman takes leave compared to when a male employee is away on leave. The researchers explained this difference with recourse to gender segregation in the labour market. At workplaces with a large number of women there is a larger buffer in the budget for eventualities such as leave, while at male-dominated workplaces, leave is not budgeted for at all. It is estimated that the companies view leave as a staff benefit to give to employees which one wants to retain. More than 70% of the employers stated that employees who have been on leave are among those, which they wished to retain, and the people on leave were characterised as highly qualified and motivated.

3.2. Employees' View of the Attitudes of the Workplace towards Leave

Andersen *et al.* (*Ibid.*) showed that 60% of employees characterised the management as 'positive' towards the leave, 20% said 'neutral' and 10% found the attitude of the management to be 'negative'. These figures hide the fact that the male employees in 20% of the cases experienced the management as negative and 27% experienced it as neutral. Men experience more opposition from male managers than from female managers, and often the female managers are supportive of the leave. This issue is regarded as relevant as three out of four male employees taking leave have a male employer (only 45% of the women on leave have a male employer). The women do not view their male employers as negative to their leave-taking. Fully 80% of the female and 60% of the male-leavers experience their *colleagues* as positive towards their leave. Finally the male colleagues in the public sector are (experienced as) more positive than the colleagues in the private sector.

3.3. Contextual Barriers Towards Male Leave-Use?

In a qualitative investigation of workplace-attitudes towards fathers and paternity leave (Carlsen, 1994) it appeared to be the norm to use all 14 days of paternity leave. The research included interviews with 30 fathers. It was noteworthy at the workplace when a father did not use his paternity leave, and during the course of the research not a single father could be found who had had a child during the previous two years, who had not used his paternity leave. Half of those interviewed who had not used parental leave said that the reason they had not used it was that the mother preferred to take all the leave (the research was carried out before childcare leave was initiated).

3.4. Fatherhood and Work Life

According to Højgaard (1997, 1998), men's attitudes as (working) fathers can be viewed from a social-constructionist/poststructuralist perspective emphasising the existence of a (historically specific) symbolic universe of masculinity and femininity as cultural transpersonal archetype. Consequently the relationship between masculinity and fatherhood is seen as a result of deep-rooted symbolic universes of meaning of masculinity and femininity structured as (hierarchical) opposites: an opposition forming the basis of a symbolic order that permeates our entire culture, though in no singular way - but indeed transiently and ambiguously. The state of the symbolic order means that parenthood assumes a different significance in the lives of men and women respectively. Along with this asymmetry various other dichotomies participate in the constitution of this differentiated parenthood: masculinity and work are much more closely linked than masculinity and fatherhood, whereas femininity and work are much more loosely linked than femininity and motherhood. But ambiguity can currently be seen in the fact that on the one hand, people in their daily lives often transgress the boundaries of the symbolic universes of masculinity and femininity while at the same time accepting the symbolic order of gender.

This analysis results in a notion of a current ambiguity in the possibilities of 'doing fatherhood'. On the one hand *the Danish welfare state* gives out ambivalent signals towards fatherhood. Paternity leave has been established and thereby signals that 'working men are also fathers' and that those fathers have rights in relation to the possibility of caring for their child - on the one side. On the other side, the leave is very short (2 x 2 weeks), not always compensated by full pay and no part of the 10 week parental leave is exclusively reserved for the father. The roles have been blurred – granting both parents access to leave, but policies nevertheless *preserve* a *traditional* gender order in a time of social and political pressures towards gender equality. On the other hand the workplace grants possibilities for fatherhood but none of the three work cultures identified by Højgaard (1998) encourage men to take parental leave and none make it easier or commonplace to do so. 'Active Fathers' are viewed as non-career minded people.

3.5. Stabilizing the Male-Breadwinner Model

So how do male workers find a way to be fathers? What characterises career-minded men, is that they only work to meet the family needs up to a certain point; and not at the expense of their work, Højgaard concludes. Fathers combine paternity leave with vacation, and this way the absence from the workplace is not *technically* leave and not visible as leave (and this pattern does not only go for career minded fathers). Fathers attempt to co-ordinate their absence with the workplace culture, and this co-ordination involves taking leave at times, which inconvenience the workplace minimally. Carlsen (1994) draws similar conclusions in his investigation of working fathers and fatherhood: that a (large) part of the time spent with the family by the father is not recorded statistically because the fathers use time-off and holiday as a means for leave. The period of 'leave' can be from a few weeks to many months.

For the time being, negotiating these ambiguities into viable social practices in the Danish labour market is the responsibility of individual men, and at the moment, it seems like this means simultaneously a stabilisation of the 'male working man', Højgaard concludes, though simultaneously stressing the fact that these negotiations take place *at all* is an expression of changes in the symbolic order of gender.

4. GENDER AND WORKING LIFE IN WORKPLACE CULTURES

In the following studies, the main issue has been to document the differences in the premises of the genders at the labour market. The research shows various forms that the differences can take, and the kinds of barriers they can bring to women and men and to family-life. The perspective is the ambiguity between the wage earners' formal and informal possibilities of reconciling work and family-life.

In Holt's (1994) study "Parents at Work" employees' attitudes and behaviour are negotiated via the interactions amongst co-employees. It is via these interactions that you are given - and give yourself permission to do certain things, and via these interactions that you are punished, when you cross the line for what is *understood* and *practiced* as permitted. Thereby the space for reconciliation between work and family-life can be extended or reduced.

The influence of numerical gender-dominance on the reconciliation possibilities was another issue investigated by Holt (*Ibid.*), that is, whether a workplace dominated by women had more space for reconciliation than a workplace dominated by men. But a female numerical-dominance did not change the *structural* male dominance. Holt concludes instead that the *structural premises* are decisive for the possibilities of reconciliation, and it is structural premises that generally disadvantage women. The differences are a consequence of the hierarchical structures of the labour market where men are in a superior position to women. The organisation of work, the degree of autonomy at work, the degree that the job is fixed to one place, the ways payment-systems are organised, and so on, consistently offer better opportunities for men than for women in the study.

4.1. Gendered Attitudes and Practices in Relation to the Reconciliation of Work and Family Life

In principle, fathers have the space to attend to the practical needs of parenthood. But how is this space actually used? Holt's study discriminates between adaptation to general family needs and adaptation to child's needs. The division shows that *the space for reconciliation is used gender-specifically*: that women predominantly use the space for reconciliation towards child's needs while the men predominantly use the space for reconciliation towards general needs. The women helped each other to make family-life and work-life hang together. When leaving the workplace unofficially to do banking transactions, they were done for several colleagues. The women took care of each others' shopping lists, covered for each other if problems with childcare meant arriving late to work, and so on.

The men in the study tended to carry out car maintenance and DIY and also sometimes helped with other family activities. The fathers who could avail of flexi-time also took part in other practical work at home.

4.2. Gender and Career Cultures

It was stated earlier how certain dynamics can be at play in *career-minded* workplace cultures. Carlsen's investigation showed how a management's attitude towards leave and fatherhood was a critical factor in determining whether or not fathers take up parental responsibilities.

Højgaard's studies take a cultural-analytical perspective towards workplace dynamics, which influence the actual use of family-friendly opportunities. Højgaard (1998) analyses a bank and two professional companies - all companies with good and institutionalised family friendly initiatives, a positive attitude concerning employees' balance between family and work life and the official attitude that gender does not have a role to play in terms of job opportunities - that everybody has the possibility of career advancement according to their abilities and interest to do so. The companies' work and gender cultures are all under the sway of an egalitarian understanding of gender. At the same time, however, employees and work functions are considered through an understanding of 'gender-as-difference', and explanations such as "when women in this company have babies, they simply lose interest in their career", are predominant in the understanding of the relation between gender and career. As a result, women must work against conceptions of femininity that are active in the culture, if they desire to advance in the enterprise (conceptions which are active simultaneously with the egalitarian attitude of the enterprise). These opposing signals have various consequences to the effect that women positioned as extremely qualified and valued by the employer are able to take advantage of the family friendly possibilities of the enterprise. Women in other positions can either choose to *not* have babies and family responsibilities or they can have babies and *not* expect career opportunities.

4.3. Family Friendliness at Workplaces

Research shows that both formal barriers in terms of structural premises at workplaces and informal barriers in terms of workplace cultures and constructions of gendered identities, obstruct a gender-egalitarian reconciliation between work and family-life and act as obstacles for working fathers' access to equal opportunities in child raising. Another type of research examines the types of conflicts family members have, between the world of work and that of family, but before this is explored in further detail, some figures concerning family-friendliness in workplaces are due.

In a study of the social responsibility of companies (Holt, 1998) indicators of company-family-friendliness were produced. Generally the large companies had most to offer. In 35% of the public companies and 27% of the private companies, special working time for parents was possible. In 59% of the public companies with fewer than 50 employees, the employees were allowed to bring children to work (a large proportion of the workplaces in this category were day-care institutions). The percentage for the rest of the companies was around 30%. In around 12% of minor and middle public companies and in minor private companies, parents were able to work at home if the children required this. In the category of large public companies, the percentage was 20% and in middle and large private companies, 26% and 40% employees respectively were able to work at home if they wished.

4.4. Flexibility Based on a Gender-segregated Labour Market

It is often argued that flexibility is a top priority *model of solution* to difficulties concerning the reconciliation of work and family-life in various studies. But 'flexibility' can contain new pitfalls for women (and men) when the abstract concept of flexibility is mediated through concrete gendered employees' occupation and work- (and family) practices.

Problems can occur when an implicit expectation of increased efficiency and intensified involvement in work life is imbedded in new 'flexi-jobs'. Such expectations can be difficult to meet by mothers who have the main responsibility for their families. The effect can be reduced job-satisfaction, higher degree of stress etc. compared to men. Csonka (2000) has carried out research on the elaboration of flexible work and she highlights these patterns.

According to Csonka (2000), gender inequality in the labour market is reflected in the flexible labour market. The research shows that there are a number of *substantial* differences in the content and modes of operation of flexible work. There are fewer women than men who experience the work as varying, who experience control of their working situation, and who experience opportunities to learn new things - there are gendered versions of flexible work. The female version of flexible-work prioritises relationships outside work while the male version emphasises relations which have to do with the organisation of the work itself. In that way, men are better positioned in the most central elements in the definition of flexible work - namely, at the level of self-determination, the level of challenges and variation in the work. The gender differences are also expressed by the fact that *two thirds* of the male employees have a time-flexibility which goes beyond one hour daily, whereas this only goes for half of the female flexi-workers. As a consequence of these characteristics, Csonka concludes that it is far from certain that flexible work, if it becomes more widespread, will ease the reconciliation of work and family-life. Flexible work seems to have two versions and one is viewed as less healthy than the other.

5. SCANDINAVIAN EQUALITY MODEL(S)

To what extent have the Scandinavian countries replaced the traditional male-breadwinner model with a model of equality where both co-habitees contribute to the support of the family? Ellingsæter (1997) makes a comparison between Sweden, Denmark and Norway in three areas: a) the employment pattern of women, such as their participation rate and the extension of part-time working, for example, b) she analyses the norms which parents believe are being directed towards them, and c) the preferences of the parents concerning financial support.

In relation to how the national equality climate is estimated, differences are shown between the countries. The informants were asked to estimate what kind of 'model of support' one thought was the most *predominant* and the choice was between 'men are single breadwinners', 'women are junior supporters', 'we have an equal sharing'. In Sweden and Denmark the idea of the man as the breadwinner is as good as absent, while the two other models get more or less equal endorsement in the two countries. The Norwegian answers show a plurality of norms. All models get support, but the least support falls to the model of equal sharing. In Sweden there is large support for part-time working among women, and this is pervasive in spite of the fact that the most favourable conditions for working mothers are found in Sweden (*Ibid*, p.47). She points to the fact that the integration of mothers of pre-school children took place about 10 years later in Norway than it did in Sweden and Denmark (where it took place in the 1970's). In Sweden the possibility of women's occupational employment was supported by the state via a growing public service (like in Denmark during this period).

A differentiated picture appears when parents are asked about their ideal model of support. In Denmark 63% would prefer the equal-sharing model, 28% the junior-model and only 8% prefer the traditional-male-model. These preferences are gendered in that it is men who would prefer the latter model. Women are typically more interested in equality than men. In Sweden 55% would prefer the equal split, 36% the junior model and 11% the male-breadwinner model. In Sweden, also, it is the women who prefer the equal sharing model.

Almost 50% of the Norwegian men prefer the traditional breadwinner model. In total, including both male and female respondents, 16% prefer this model, but the support to the junior model is 26% while the equal-split model is supported by 56% of Norwegians. The most equality-oriented women in Norway are the highly educated women who work in gender-mixed organizations.

Ellingsæter concludes that the analysis indicates that "the idea of an equality-based Scandinavian model with combined parenthood and economic support is too simple (Ellingsaeter, 1997). The differences raise new questions about the relationship between politics, or the organisation from the state's 'hand' and the development in the practices and preferences of the support/maintenance of families. This may question the research about gender and the welfare state and thereby question the presumptions which are based on a too simple an understanding of the relationship between politics on the one side and individual practices, norms and preferences on the other side" (*Ibid,* p. 48).

CHAPTER 5

IRELAND

In this review we present first the statutory policies that exist in Ireland in relation to policies that may be considered "family-friendly". These include maternity leave, paternity leave, parental leave, childcare and flexible working patterns. Where no statutory policy exists, the current state of play in relation to policy in a given area is presented.

In the next section we present in greater detail the current status of family-friendly working arrangements in Ireland. We refer in particular to part-time work, job-sharing, flexible working hours, term-time working and tele-working, as well as other arrangements. We present results from case studies carried out in small, medium and large Irish firms with regard to the attitudes of management to those policies and their efficacy.

Childcare has been a particularly critical issue in Ireland in the whole policy debate surrounding the increasing labour force participation of married women. For this reason a separate section is devoted to a discussion of the history of this issue at national level going back to the early 1980s. Current policy is also discussed in terms of its strengths and weaknesses.

Finally, in the last section we present results of attitudinal studies, which have been carried out in Ireland concerning flexible working patterns, childcare, and gender roles generally. These provide a picture of public attitudes from the mid 1970s to more recent times in relation to public policy preferences in this area

1. NATIONAL SOCIAL POLICIES

1.1. Maternity Leave

The Maternity Protection Act of 1994 provides for a minimum of 14 weeks paid maternity leave, as well as an optional four additional unpaid weeks of leave. A minimum of four weeks must be taken before the birth and four weeks after the birth. This Act superseded the Maternity (Protection of Employees) Act of 1981, which had similar provisions. However, the later Act also incorporates health and safety provisions for pregnant women, new mothers and breastfeeding mothers as laid down in the EU Directive of 1992. The Act does not require an employer to pay the employee during her maternity leave. This is covered by social benefit, on the basis of the woman's social insurance contributions (Department of Justice, Equality and Law Reform, 2001).

Women employed in the public service are entitled to receive full pay during maternity leave. The employer recoups the amount of social welfare benefit due to the woman. Employers in the private sector may also opt to pay employees their full salary during this time.

More recently the Government extended the length of maternity leave. As of 2001 women are entitled to four additional weeks' paid leave plus four additional weeks' unpaid leave. This brings the total entitlement to 18 weeks paid and 8 weeks unpaid maternity leave, for a total of 26 weeks leave.

In addition to the extended maternity leave, other improvements include:

(1) The period of unpaid leave will count for accrual of annual leave
(2) Paid time-off will be provided for mothers to attend ante-natal classes
(3) Fathers will be entitled to paid time off to attend two ante-natal classes immediately prior to the birth
(4) Employers will now be required to provide either an adjustment of working hours or facilities in the workplace to facilitate breastfeeding for four months after the birth (O'Donoghue, 2001).

Since then the *Report of the Working Group on the Review of the Improvement of the Maternity Protection Legislation* (2001) recommended even further increases in maternity leave. It stated:

> "It is a widely held view, supported by leave arrangements in several other countries, that the best interests of infants under 12 months old are served by their remaining in the direct care of their parents. An increase in the length of maternity leave could contribute very positively to this goal (p. 51)."

In addition to supporting the view that parental care is best for infants, the Working Group also pointed out that:

> "One of the arguments for an increase in the length of maternity leave is the difficulty for parents to get access to high-quality, affordable childcare, particularly for babies under 1 year old. Access to childcare in this category is a particularly acute problem at present. There are few childcare places for children under 1 year due to the higher costs for childcare providers of providing childcare for this age group . . .Any increase in maternity leave would contribute towards the alleviation of this serious problem (*Ibid.* p. 50)."

1.2. Paternity Leave

In Ireland there is no statutory entitlement to paternity leave, that is, leave for a father at the time of the birth of his child. The Civil Service introduced three days' paid paternity leave per child from 1st January 2000. Some other employers also provide paternity leave (Dept. of Justice, Equality and Law Reform, *op.cit.*; National Framework Committee on Family-Friendly Policies, 2001).

1.3. Parental Leave

The Parental Leave Act, 1998 provides for an individual and non-transferable right of both parents to 14 weeks of unpaid leave to care for children under five years of age. The Act also entitles an employee to a number of paid days' leave to deal with family emergencies resulting from injury or illness of a family member (*force majeur*). This entitlement cannot exceed three working days in any 12 consecutive months and five days in any 36 consecutive months. The Act transposes an EU Directive into Irish Law. This Act is to be reviewed by a Government Working Group commencing in 2001 (O'Donoghue, *op. cit.*).

> "The leave may be taken either as a continuous block of 14 weeks or, by agreement between the employer and the employee, may be broken up over a period of time. An employee must give written notice to the employer of his or her intention to take parental leave, not later than six weeks before the employee proposes to commence the leave. The employer may decide to postpone the parental leave if he or she is satisfied that granting the leave would have a substantial adverse effect on the operation of his or her business. The postponement may be for a period not exceeding six months, to a date agreed on by both the employer and the employee" (Parental Leave Act 1998, in Equality Authority, 1998).

1.4. Childcare

There is, as yet, no statutory childcare policy in Ireland. Childcare provision has been left to parents to arrange for themselves (Expert Working Group on Childcare, 1999). The compulsory school age in Ireland is six. However, "junior and senior infant classes" are provided in national schools for four and five year olds. In 1993 there were 86,175 children in the age group 3 - 6 attending publicly funded early primary education; 52% of the total age-group. This constituted 1% of three year olds, 55% of all four year olds and nearly all five year olds (99%) (European Commission Network on Childcare, 1996). Thus, public provision in Ireland is extremely limited for the age group 0 - 3, but rises significantly at age four, when entry to junior infant classes is possible.

The Report on the National Forum for Early Childhood Education (1998) notes that based on OECD statistics on participation in early childhood education, rates for three and four year olds in Ireland are low compared to other EU and OECD countries.

> "Apart from Child Benefit and limited interventions for children at risk of social and educational advantage, there is virtually no State investment in the care of children before entry to primary school" (Commission on the Family, 1998).

Data based on a survey module on childcare included in the National Household Survey in late 2002 provides current information on patterns of childcare use in Ireland (CSO, 2003). Over 73,000 families, or 42.5% of all families with pre-school children relied on childcare provided by someone other than the parents during working hours. Not surprisingly, it was found that couples where both partners were at work had the greatest need for childcare. Over three-quarters (55,300) had some form of childcare arrangements for their preschool children. The type of care was distributed as follows:

Table 5.1. Non-Parental Childcare Arrangements for Pre-School Children of Employed Couples

Childcare Arrangement	Percentage
Unpaid relative	28.5%
Paid relative	12.6%
Paid carer	33.2%
Créche/Montessori	22.1%
Other	3.5%
Total	**100.0%**

Based on CSO (2003) Table 3

The average weekly cost of childcare for families with pre-school children only nationally was €105.36; the comparable cost in Dublin was over €131. The survey found that just under 20% of families with preschool children would welcome the availability of alternative childcare arrangements. Around half of these would like a crèche or Montessori, preferably work-based. Over 45% said they were not availing of their desired option due to the cost and 33.5% said the option was not available (*Ibid.*).

1.5. Current Childcare Strategy in Ireland

Current childcare strategy in Ireland is reflected in a speech by the Minister for Justice, Equality and Law Reform (O'Donoghue, 1999), in the Report of the Expert Working Group on Childcare (1999), the White Paper on Early Childhood

Education (Department of Education and Science, 1999) and in the last several Budgets by the Minister for Finance, beginning in December 1999.

The thrust of this strategy has been to subsidise existing childcare services in the community (private providers and employers) and to only directly provide services to the disadvantaged. There is a move toward greater co-ordination of government services (in which 11 different government departments are involved), to provide guidelines, information, advice and support to providers.

In addition, by reducing taxes in the budgets of 1999 and 2000, the Government increased the take-home pay of workers so that they would be better able to afford to pay for childcare. Individualisation in taxation was also introduced, thus increasing the take-home pay of employed married women, which in some cases gave couples more disposable income to pay for childcare.

While these budgetary measures could be seen to have been positive in the short term, the lack of a comprehensive, integrated long-term strategy still remains (Fine-Davis, 2001, 2003).

1.6. Flexible Working Patterns

Until recently there was little family-friendly flexibility in the Irish workplace (Mahon, 1998). However, more recently it has come higher on the political agenda. Given Ireland's current economic prosperity, the scenario has changed and employers are finding it more difficult to recruit and retain staff. As a result employers are increasingly realising that they need to implement more family-friendly policies. This is particularly so given the major potential for growth in female labour force participation.

In addition, Ireland, together with the other EU Member States was party to the Amsterdam Treaty. Reconciliation of work and family was a key theme addressed in the guidelines for Member States to implement in their employment policies. In Ireland this has been given expression in part by the establishment of a National Framework Committee for Family-Friendly Policies, which was part of the Programme for Prosperity and Fairness to which the Government and the social partners are party. "The Framework Agreement encourages management, unions and employees to come together to find out what the needs of the employee and the company are, and then to identify how they can, in their particular enterprise, meet these needs to the mutual benefit of both company and employee" (ICTU Statement in National Development Plan, 2001).

Reconciliation of work and family has traditionally focused on women and their dual role. More recently this has begun to shift and males' dual roles are also being considered (Fisher, 2000; Commission on the Family, 1998).

As of now none of the family-friendly working arrangements are available on a statutory basis. The philosophy seems to be one of working out individual arrangements at the level of each organisation or company. The one exception to this concerns part-time work, which has just recently become covered by legislation.

1.7. Part-Time Work

The Protection of Employees (Part-Time Work) Act, 2001 was recently passed by the Dail (Irish Parliament). The purpose of the Act was to implement the provisions of the Directive 97/81/EC of the Council of the European Union concerning the Framework Agreement on Part-Time Work. The Act provides for the removal of discrimination of part-time workers where such exists. Specifically, it provides that "a part-time employee shall not be treated less favourably than a comparable full-time employee in respect of his or her conditions of employment." The Act aims to "improve the quality of part-time work, to facilitate the development of part-time work on a voluntary basis and to contribute to the flexible organisation of working time in a manner which takes into account the needs of employers and workers." Benefit accorded to part-time employees shall be on the basis of the principle of *pro-rata temporis*, i.e. on a *pro-rata* basis according to the hours worked.

2. CURRENT STATUS OF FAMILY-FRIENDLY ARRANGEMENTS IN IRISH WORKPLACES

There are several modes of flexible working arrangements currently in practice to varying degrees in Irish workplaces. These include:

(1) Flexitime
(2) Part-time Working
(3) Job-Sharing
(4) Flexi-Place, Tele-working or e-working
(5) Term-Time Working
(6) Career Breaks

In this section we present data on the availability and take-up of family-friendly policies in Ireland, including results of studies, both case studies and quantitative studies, concerning the experience of Irish companies with family-friendly policies.

Research has been conducted on the prevalence of family-friendly policies in small and medium-sized enterprises (SMEs) by Fisher (2000) for the Equality Authority. This study (*Ibid.*) sent questionnaires to 500 SMEs throughout Ireland, 250 to small enterprises and 250 to medium-sized ones.

This study found that 49% of the organisations studied had part-time work available, 31% had flexi-time and 23% had job-sharing. Personalised/flexible hours were available in 28%, though they were more common the smaller companies, of which 39% had them. Tele-working/ working from home was available in 28% of the companies.

In summary, 53% of all the companies studied provided at least one family-friendly working arrangement. This was true of 49% of the small enterprises and 60% of the medium-sized ones. Childcare was the primary reason given by employees for requesting family-friendly working arrangements (FFWAs). The main reason for not implementing FFWAs was that there was no request for them by employees. The main problems associated with FFWAs were that they were perceived as open to abuse by employees and they placed additional demands on supervisors' time. In spite of these reservations, 100% of those firms operating FFWAs rated them as successful and 96% would recommend them to other companies (*Ibid*, p. 17).

The National Framework Committee on Family-Friendly Workplace Policies (2001) commissioned research into FFWAs in small, medium and large organisations. Studies of major corporations revealed a very high level of provision of FFWAs. This was true of companies such as Eircom, the Electricity Supply Board (ESB), Intel Ireland Ltd., IBM, Allied Irish Bank, Citigroup, and Royal and Sun Alliance. These companies frequently not only provided FFWAs in terms of arrangement of hours and leave time, etc., but also in many cases provided on-site childcare facilities, tele-work, paid paternity leave (usually three days), tuition refund schemes, etc.

IBM regards family-friendly programmes to be "a strategic business initiative, not a charitable endeavour" (*Ibid: IBM*, p. 2). Allied Irish Bank offers among other arrangements, Personalised Hours, in which staff currently working full-time (36.25 hours per week) can change to any combination of hours varying from 14.5 - 31.25. They also offer Special Short-Term Breaks for staff in various situations (*Ibid: AIB, p. 2*).

Research on medium-sized firms has also yielded positive results with FFWAs. Many schemes are available, including staggered start and finishing times, job sharing, working from home, parental leave, etc. Most of these arrangements were organised on an informal person-to-person basis. Benefits reported from FFWAs included higher productivity:

FFWAs were also found to be effective in small companies. One manager accepts that they cannot offer "the benefits of a large company", but feels that

> "...being flexible with the staff helps us with recruiting and holding on to people." (Ibid: Interviews with Small Firms Operating FFWAs, p. 2)

However, while the intention may be for FFWAs to be open to both sexes, it appears that employer expectations and employee behaviours are still largely traditional. For example, one manager in one of the small firms studied described FFWAs as:

> "...enabling women to look after their family and carry out other aspects of their lifestyle." (*Ibid*: Interviews with Small Firms Operating FFWAs, p. 2)

It was noted in the Report that this comment "reflected the view of a number of employers that such arrangements were specifically related to female employees and their childcare needs" (*Ibid*, p. 2).

More recent research by Drew and colleagues (2002) based on a survey of 912 employers in the public and private sector, as well as over 1,000 managers and employees in five selected companies found that flexible working was sought by men as well as women, however the take up of work life balance policies were "highly gendered". The options that implied no loss of pay, such as flexitime and tele-working tended to be more favoured by men, whereas women were more likely to opt for reduced hours, e.g. part-time work and job sharing. Drew asserts that "a major challenge will be to avoid a twin track in which men are in the *fast lane* involving continuous and often excessive hours in full-time employment . . . and women in the *"slow lane"*(pg. 138) working or seeking reduced hours and or opting for career breaks. If this occurs she believes it will support the belief that work-life balance is only for mothers of young children and not applicable to all. Drew et al. concludes that we need to think in terms of work-life balance for all groups, rather than merely in terms of "family friendly policies."

3. CHILDCARE IN IRELAND: AN HISTORICAL PERSPECTIVE AND CURRENT POLICY ISSUES

3.1. Background

As early as 1983 the Working Party on Childcare Facilities for Working Parents in its *Report to the Minister for Labour* recommended that there should be a national programme of community-based childcare facilities. Public attitudes, as examined in surveys, have also indicated a high level of public support for publicly provided childcare and family friendly policies. This has been apparent since 1983 (Fine-Davis, 1983a, 1983b). Ten years after the Working Party's Report, the Second Commission on the Status of Women (1993) recommended that:

> "...public policy and social partners policy should take on board the principles that:
> 1. work and domestic commitments have to be reconciled;
> 2. responsibility for children should be shared between father and mother;
> 3. childcare support is a public policy function."
> (Recommendation 4.18)

As noted above, since that time funds have been allocated by the Government for childcare, however, these have primarily been for administrative costs, e.g., establishing guidelines, stimulating the development of community childcare, providing information and liaising and monitoring. What provision of childcare there has been has been largely for children at risk and for the disadvantaged, who can also be seen to be 'at risk' (See *First and Second Progress Reports of the Monitoring Committee on the Implementation of the Recommendations of the Second Commission on the Status of Women*, 1994, 1996 respectively).

What has been most notable about the Government's response to childcare from the period 1983 to 1999 has been its focus on examining the issue rather than on directly dealing with it. The issue of childcare has been examined by a succession of subsequent Working Groups and Government reports over the 16-year period since the initial Working Party Report of 1983 (Working Party on Childcare Facilities for Working Parents, 1983). These have included:

- Working Group on Childcare Facilities for Working Parents, *Report to the Minister for Equality and Law Reform* (1994);
- *Strengthening Families for Life: Final Report to the Minister for Social, Community and Family Affairs* (Commission on the Family, 1998), which includes a chapter on childcare arrangements in Ireland, based on a commissioned study carried out by the ESRI;
- *The Economics of Childcare in Ireland* (Goodbody, 1998);
- *Report on the National Forum for Early Childhood Education* (1998);
- *Report of the Partnership 2000 Expert Working Group on Childcare* (1999); and
- *"Ready to Learn" - White Paper on Early Childhood Education*, (Department of Education and Science, 1999).

Many of these reports have repeated recommendations of earlier reports.

While economic barriers to providing childcare were highlighted in a 1985 Government report, *Irish Women: Agenda for Practical Action*, produced by the Working Party on Women's Affairs and Family Law Reform (1985), this argument can no longer hold. Ireland is a thriving buoyant economy and women's labour force participation, including that of married women, has contributed significantly to the "Celtic Tiger", as pointed out in the ESRI's *Medium Term Report* (Fahey and Fitzgerald, 1997). This admission is in contra-distinction to the widely held view of the 1970s and '80s that were married women to enter the labour force, this would take away jobs from men who needed them more (Fine-Davis, 1988a).

The labour force participation of married women in Ireland has increased significantly over the last 30 years, from 7.5% in 1971 to 46.4% in 2001 for all ages. In 2002, the participation rate for married women was almost the same as that of all women – 48% (CSO, 2002). Moreover, the participation rate for married women is markedly higher in the key childbearing/rearing age group (25-34): 64.7%. This figure has also increased dramatically over the last 12 years, rising from 39% in 1989 to 64.7% in 2001 *(CSO: Labour Force Surveys (1971 – 97), Quarterly National Household Surveys (1999 - 2001)).*

Table 5.2: Married Women's Labour Force Participation in Ireland (%)

	1971	1977	1981	1987	1989	1994	1997	1999	2000	2001
All Ages	7.5	14.4	16.7	23.4	23.7	32.4	37.3	45.3	45.9	46.4
Age 25-34					39.0	54.5	58.2	66.3	67.3	64.7

Sources: CSO: Labour Force Surveys (1971 - 97); Quarterly National Household Surveys (1999 - 2001)

The numbers in part-time employment also increased in the first quarter of 2002 and again most of the increase was accounted for by women, who account for over three-quarters of those in part-time employment in Ireland (CSO, 2002).

3.2. Labour Force Projections and the Need for Childcare:

In a projection of future childcare needs, it was estimated that:

> "The total labour force in 2011 is likely to be of the order of 1,899,000, an increase of about 25 per cent . . . over the 1997 level of 1,525,000. A large share of this increase is projected to come from growth in the number of women, and especially married women, in the labour force. The female labour force is projected to grow by 218,000 (from 589,000 in 1997 to 807,000 in 2011), an increase of 37 per cent, accounting for 58 per cent of the total increase" (Goodbody Economic Consultants, 1998, p ii)

On the basis of this, "the demand for childcare could increase by between 25 and 50 per cent over the period to the year 2011." (*Ibid, p. iii*). Since this projection was made in 1998, it will be noted that in the first quarter of 2002 the numbers of people in Ireland in full-time employment increased from the previous year by 2%; women accounted for over 80% of this increase (CSO, 2002).

3.3. Current and Projected Childcare Supply:

The Goodbody Report (*op.cit.*) pointed out that those at work tend to use childminders – this is supported by large-scale research (Commission on the Family, 1998; see also Langford, 1999), whereas those working in the home generally avail of playgroups; however, this situation is likely to alter rapidly: "...given the tightening labour market...an increase in the supply of childminders in unlikely to be forthcoming as potential childminders will find alternative employment. Accordingly there will be significant additional demand for use of group based facilities" (Goodbody, *op. cit.*). They concluded, "There is a strong case for state intervention on a temporary basis to support the development of childcare as a viable industry" (*Ibid.*).

Research published as part of the Government Working Party on Childcare Facilities for Working Parents (1983) found that while many mothers used untrained childminders, their preference was for trained personnel in a childcare facility (Fine-Davis, 1983a). Moreover, childminders watching three or fewer children are currently completely outside the regulatory system (Goodbody, *op. cit.*, p. 27). Because childminders are still, by and large, in the black economy, creative policies need to be put forward to address this group.

3.4. Child Development Arguments for Educational Childcare:

These are some of the demographic and economic reasons, which were recently put forward for State intervention in pre-school childcare prior to the last three Budgets, the first two of which contained childcare provisions. The child development arguments are also strong. These arguments were presented in the Goodbody Report, which also contained extensive reference to international psychological evidence. To summarise Goodbody on this key area:

> "Quality childcare has a beneficial impact on the development of children and especially on disadvantaged children. This impact is enhanced when the childcare provision includes an element of early education. The benefits to children persist through to adulthood and are garnered by both the child, the State and society as a whole" *(Ibid, p. iv)*.

Goodbody further pointed out "parents may not appreciate or take account of the full benefits to children and to society as a whole in reaching decisions on childcare..." This tends to "result in parents demanding lower quality care than could be optimum". This is true of parents generally, "but particularly true of parents with low incomes. The loss to the State...is greater in respect of children from the disadvantaged segment of society (*Ibid.*)".

They stated that "there are strong economic, as well as social reasons for supporting childcare for this group". In conclusion they asserted that:

> "Support from the State should be focused on ensuring that parents have access to high quality childcare provision which incorporates a strong element of early education. State support should extend to childcare generally, but there is a need for a particular focus on the less advantaged" (*Ibid.*).

The emphasis on the value of quality childcare was strongly reinforced by the Report on the National Forum for Early Childhood Education (1998) and by the Expert Working Group on Childcare (1999). The latter report asserted that "The rights and needs of each child must be the first and primary consideration in the delivery of childcare (Expert Group on Childcare, 1999, p.44)". More significantly, they stressed that:

> "The basic principle underlying the rights of children is that society has an obligation to meet the fundamental needs of children and to provide assistance to aid the development of the child's personality, talents and abilities. Therefore, a right of access for every child to quality childcare in a safe and secure environment where he/she is respected and accepted, should be guaranteed regardless of the status of the child" (*Ibid.*).

3.5. Social Returns - Cost Benefit Analysis

The Expert Working Group Report cited a widely reported longitudinal study from the U.S. which found that "children who attended a carefully designed programme, known as the High/Scope Programme, were more likely to stay on into third-level training and education, less likely to get into trouble with the law and more likely to be supporting themselves when compared to a control group who had not experienced the programme. When reviewed in terms of cost-benefit analysis, the researchers found that for every $1 invested in this type of early education programme, the State saved $7 per child by age 27 years" (Schweinhart & Weikart, 1993 as cited in Expert Working Group on Childcare, 1999, p. 53).

The cost savings to Governments was underscored also by the White Paper on Early Childhood Education (Department of Education and Science, 1999):

> "Significant benefits to society as a whole accrue to investment in education. Research has shown that the rate of return is greatest at lower levels of education. . . Social returns may also accrue in the form of measurable savings on Government expenditure. In particular, improved levels of education tend to lead to reductions in costs associated with unemployment, crime and healthcare." (p. 10)

In view of the strong child development arguments, not to mention the social returns, a national programme of high quality educational childcare of consistent quality throughout the country would appear to be the best solution to meeting Ireland's childcare needs.

3.6. Current Childcare Strategy in Ireland

In spite of the arguments put forward in numerous commissioned reports for a coherent, high quality childcare programme, the thrust of current childcare strategy in Ireland has been to subsidise existing childcare services in the community and to only directly provide services to the disadvantaged. Child Benefit Allowance has also been increased substantially in recent budgets, which, it is argued gives parents choice in terms of childcare, applies to all income groups and to both employed and non-employed mothers. However, Child Benefit is also a measure to reduce child poverty and in this sense it may be used for other life necessities rather than targeted at childcare costs.

In addition, by reducing taxes in the 1999 and 2000 Budgets, and to a lesser extent in the 2001 Budget, the Government increased the take-home pay of workers so that they would be better able to afford to pay for childcare. By introducing individualisation in taxation in 2000, some of the double allowances given to married couples in 1980 that were not, in many cases, being adequately targeted at childcare costs, were recouped. The result of individualisation meant that in effect the take-home pay of employed married women would be relatively increased in the higher income groups, giving many couples more disposable income to pay for childcare. To offset the loss of allowances for non-employed women who provided care in the home, a £3,000 carer's allowance was provided.

3.7. Deficiencies in Current Strategy

3.7.1. Issues of Consistent Quality
While the recent Budget measures have been helpful in the short term in terms of stimulating the provision of childcare places and in helping to subsidise childcare costs, they have not moved Ireland any closer to having the kind of comprehensive, integrated national programme of childcare facilities evident in some other European countries such as France and Denmark. The funding allocated in the recent budgets will go towards workplace childcare, private sector childcare, local childcare initiatives and community-based groups. The question remains: how consistent can the quality of such a diversity of childcare provision be?

Were there a national programme of public childcare facilities, consistent high quality could be guaranteed. Given the benefits of quality early childhood education, the lack of a centralised high quality programme is a serious social policy deficit with implications for children and their development, for working parents in meeting their childcare needs and for society in preventing later social problems.

3.7.2. Issues of Cost

In addition to the need for consistent quality through a coordinated national childcare strategy, the issue of cost still remains. Childcare costs in Ireland consume a higher proportion of working parents' earnings than in any other EU member state (Langford, 1999; *Irish Times*, 17th May 2001, p. 3). Childcare costs are so high that people, especially those on lower wages, have to spend a very significant proportion of their take-home pay on childcare. According to the Irish Congress of Trade Unions, childcare costs for working parents have more than doubled since 1998 (Yeates, *Irish Times*, 6 August 2001, p. 7). Moreover, tax relief for childcare expenses is still not available.

The Government is still grappling with the childcare issue. It was at the top of the political agenda in 2001 – 2002 during the height of the 'Celtic Tiger' when employers were short of labour. It is unfortunate, as well as instructive, that the economic buoyancy of the market was the critical catalyst which highlighted the childcare issue. The need had been there for decades, but women workers were not seen as sufficiently critical to the workplace before. Predictably, as the economic situation has down turned only somewhat, affecting the country's finances, childcare fell to a lower priority and any bold plans which might have been envisaged were shelved once again.

However in view of demographic trends, it is inevitable that Ireland will continue to face this issue and it is to be hoped that it will look to the more developed countries of Europe for models of excellence. With one of the lowest childcare provisions in Europe, Ireland is in a unique position to benefit from the wealth of knowledge and experience which has been gathered on childcare in Europe.

4. ATTITUDINAL STUDIES: CHANGING GENDER ROLES AND SOCIAL POLICIES IN IRELAND

4.1. Social Change in Ireland

Ireland is a society, which has undergone rapid social change over the last several decades. It went from a relatively isolated agrarian economy to an industrial economy beginning in the 1960s. A further important factor in shaping the cultural ethos and specifically the role and status of women has been the strong influence of the Catholic Church, to which 95% of the population belongs. This influence of Church teachings on the norms and values of the society have been in many cases complemented by laws of the State (although these are increasingly being modified to reflect social change) and are underpinned by passages in the Irish Constitution concerning the role of women.

2.1 In particular, the State recognises that by her life within the home, woman gives to the State a support, without which the common good cannot be achieved.
2.2 The State shall, therefore, endeavour to ensure that mothers should not be obliged by economic necessity to engage in labour to the neglect of their duties in the home.

(Article 41.2, Irish Constitution, 1937)

Barry (1998) believes that even today "Irish women continue to experience systematic disadvantage in economic, social and political life" (p. 355). She notes that "a critical barrier to accessing paid employment among mothers in Ireland is the lack of State support for childcare services" (*Ibid*, p. 364).

> "Despite the image Ireland cultivates as a child and family-oriented society, there is an abysmally low level of support in terms of back-up services for families where women wish to secure and maintain paid employment" (*Ibid.*).

The period of social change in gender roles which Ireland has been experiencing since the late 1970s has been related to several factors. These have included:

(1) The removal in 1973 of the marriage bar, which had required that women give up their jobs when they got married;

(2) The implementation in 1975 of the Anti-Discrimination (Pay) Act;

(3) The implementation of the Employment Equality Act in 1977 and the establishment of the Employment Equality Agency, whose role it was to enforce this legislature and to promote equality in the workforce;

(4) The Supreme Court decision of 1980 removing tax laws which discriminated against employed married women and acted as a deterrent to their employment;

(5) The legalisation of the sale of contraceptives in 1980.

(Fine-Davis, 1988a, pp. 16-17).

As a result of these legislative and administrative changes, the labour force participation of married women began to increase dramatically as noted earlier, and concurrent with the increased labour force participation came a decrease in fertility (Sexton and Dillon, 1984).

4.2. Changing Gender Role Attitudes

Relatively little research has been conducted on gender role attitudes in Ireland and that which has was primarily done in the 1970s and 1980s. Thus, until there are more current studies, we must rely on these earlier surveys. Fortunately, they were carried out at a period of maximum social change and were able to capture the concomitant changes in gender role attitudes.

Studies during this period documented that attitudes to gender roles in Ireland were very traditional (Fine-Davis, 1983c, 1988a). For example, in 1975 46.4% of a Dublin sample agreed that "Some equality in marriage is a good thing, but by and large the husband ought to have the main say in family matters." More than half (52.4%) believed that "A husband has the right to expect that his wife will be obliging and dutiful at all times." A large majority (70.1%) believed that "Being a wife and mother are the most fulfilling roles any woman could want" and slightly more than half (51.3%) said that "If equal job opportunities are opened to women, this will just take away jobs from men who need them more". Equally, there were ambivalent attitudes toward maternal employment. While 76.5% said that "A woman who has a job she enjoys is likely to be a better wife and mother because she has an interest and some fulfilment outside the home," equally 68.4% of the sample felt "It is bad for young children if their mothers go out and work, even if they are well taken care of by another adult." Moreover, 65% felt that "When there is high unemployment, married women should be discouraged from working" (*Ibid.*).

Attitudes toward the role of women were found to be significantly related to other social attitudes and beliefs, a key element of which was religiosity. For example, religiosity was found to be strongly correlated with disapproval of employment of married women, particularly mothers, and with holding traditional views about appropriate gender roles (Fine-Davis, 1989a). There was also a strong convergence of traditional sex-role ideology and perceptions of females as inferior. While men were significantly more likely to hold these views than women, it was found that even women were subject to these attitudes and perceptions.

Concurrent with changing legislation, increased labour force participation and decreasing fertility, there was a significant change in attitudes towards gender roles. In a study carried out in 1986 comparing attitudes in a Dublin sample comparable to that studied in 1975, significant shifts were found for all groups - male and female. Most people no longer believed that a woman's role should be that of wife and mother, with the male playing the dominant role both inside and outside the home (Fine-Davis, 1988a). There were also highly significant shifts for all groups concerning equal pay. There was now universal acceptance of this principle, which suggests that the passing of the Equal Pay Act in 1975 had had an effect on attitudes. Attitudes changed to become congruent with social norms and required behaviour The issue of maternal employment was controversial in 1975 and remained so in 1986. There were, nevertheless, major shifts in a more positive direction. The attitude change effects that were evident even extended to basic perceptions of female inferiority. This shift was particularly notable since such beliefs have been identified as a major root cause of inegalitarian gender roles.

Many of the same items were also included in a 1978 nationwide Irish sample and these were also compared with 1986 national Irish data (*Ibid.*). Similar attitude shifts were also found in the nationwide samples. However, rural respondents, while also shifting in a more egalitarian direction, nevertheless remained more traditional than their urban counterparts over time.

Whelan and Fahey (1994) observe that it is not overwhelmingly clear that Irish society was moving in an egalitarian direction in the 1980s, as evidenced by the failure of the abortion and divorce referenda of 1983 and 1986 respectively, in which public debate was "convulsed by controversy over the 'politics of the family'" (p. 45). However, those may have been hiccups in an otherwise overall trend, as evidenced in part by the subsequent passage of divorce legislation in 1995. The issue of abortion is a thornier one, but the decision in the 1992 X case was significant and public opinion polls show increasing public acceptance of abortion under certain circumstances (Fine-Davis, 1988b; Irish Times/ MRBI Poll, 1997; Lansdowne Market Research Poll, 2001). Given the dramatic changes in female labour force participation and gender role behaviour since these earlier studies of the '70s and '80s it is very likely that similar research carried out today would yield very different results.

4.3. Public Support for Family-Friendly Policies

In the context of changing social attitudes and increased labour force participation of married women, people have expressed consistent support for family-friendly policies. The relatively high level of support for such policies was in contrast to the still traditional attitudes to gender roles referred to above. Such discrepancies may reflect a lag effect between attitudes to social policies and more basic underlying attitudes.

Attitudes concerning potential social policies which could assist employed married women and women working in the home indicated a high level of support for potential policy changes in this area. For example, 71.7% favoured provision of tax relief to people who employed childcare workers and cleaners/home-helps in their homes (Fine-Davis, 1983a). Tax concessions for childcare and household help were also supported by mothers of dependent children (both employed and non-employed) (Fine-Davis, 1983b). The Working Party on Childcare Facilities for Working Parents (1983) taking cognisance of these views recommended in its Report to the Minister for Labour that "Fees and other related expenses incurred by working parents to have their children cared for at home, or otherwise, should be reckonable for income tax purposes (*Ibid*, p. 9). Public policy has still failed to act on these and subsequent similar recommendations.

There was widespread support for the provision of childcare centres expressed by a national sample of employed and non-employed mothers (Fine-Davis, 1983b), and indeed the attitudes of the population at large were very much in tune with those of mothers concerning responsibility for funding childcare facilities. The national survey of mothers also found a high degree of support for various changes in the community, including flexible hours (88.3%), greater availability of part-time jobs (96.4%), extended leave for childbirth/ child-rearing (73.9%), parental leave for child's illness (90.9%), flexibility for breastfeeding mothers (67.7%), and work-sharing (89.2%) (Fine-Davis, 1983b).

A subsequent nationwide study also examined attitudes to potential changes in the workplace and the community, which might be of assistance to working parents (Fine-Davis, 1988c). Similar questions were asked of a broader sample to those, which had been asked five years previously in the nationwide study of mothers (Fine-Davis, 1983b). In the more recent study, the most favourable attitudes to flexible hours were expressed by employed married women, but positive attitudes towards this policy were widespread among all groups, including men. A majority of women saw flexible hours as relevant to themselves. Employed married women saw them as most applicable with 32.5% saying they applied "a great deal" and a further 30% saying they applied "to some extent". Over 50% of non-employed married women and employed single women also felt that flexible hours could apply to them. A rather high proportion of married men (43.2%) also said flexible hours could apply to them (Fine-Davis, 1988c, pp.43-44).

A high level of support was also shown in the study for greater availability of part-time jobs. Non-employed married women were particularly supportive of this. Overall, 95% of them expressed approval, with 72.5% expressing strong approval. This is somewhat higher than previous Irish studies but very much in line with expressed preferences of non-employed women for part-time jobs (Fine-Davis, 1977, 1983a, 1983b). These results suggested that greater availability of part-time jobs would encourage more married women into the labour force.

Both paternity leave and parental leave were also strongly favoured. The need for parental leave was indicated by the fact that mothers reported that they commonly had to use their own annual leave, sick leave, or unpaid leave in case of a child's illness (Fine-Davis, 1983b).

There was also strong support for the extension of shopping and banking hours (Fine-Davis, 1988c). Both of these have occurred in Ireland since the study took place and ATM machines have also come into use, greatly facilitating banking. Other changes favoured by the sample included changing/ extending hours of public offices (e.g. post-office, revenue, social welfare); providing a national programme of childcare facilities for young children; providing short-term crèche facilities in shopping centres, hospital clinics, etc., and providing tax concessions for childcare costs (*Ibid*, pp. 46-47).

The results indicated that the high level of support for such changes, which was evident in the earlier study of mothers, was also widely shared by other groups. This was particularly true of married men, who clearly seemed to share the concerns of married women in these areas (*Ibid*, p. 63).

It is evident that public policy is only recently beginning to address the public preferences that were evident two decades ago. No doubt the changing economic situation in Ireland with decreased unemployment generally, the increasing labour force participation of married women, and the need to recruit female labour to the workforce have contributed to this policy response. It is also undoubtedly the result of changing gender role attitudes in Ireland (and elsewhere) and the increasing importance placed on the reconciliation of work and family.

4.4. Fathering

In contrast to other countries, there has been very little research on fathering in Ireland. One of the few studies in this area was conducted by McKeown et al. (1998), who carried out a literature review concerning fathering, referring to the Irish experience in an international context. One of the main conclusions was that:

> "There appears to be virtual unanimity among researchers that the more extensive a father's involvement with his children the more beneficial it is for them in terms of cognitive competence and performance at school as well as for empathy, self-esteem, self-control, life-skills and social competence; these children also have less sex-stereotyped beliefs and a more internal locus of control" (McKeown et al., 1998, p. 423).

These authors note that the international evidence on fathers' involvement suggests that there has been some increase in participation in childcare and domestic activities. However, fathers' behaviour has not kept pace with changing attitudes and cultural expectations in this area (*Ibid*, p. 425). They suggest that the implication of their analysis is that:

> "public policy should seek to create family-friendly measures, especially in the workplace, which maximises the choices men and women have to negotiate roles and responsibilities and will allow fathers as well as mothers the time and space for childcare" (Ibid, p. 427).

Ireland is likely to continue to follow the lead of other countries more advanced in the area of family policy, as well as to continue to be influenced by trends in other member countries of the EU. The significant shifts in gender role attitudes observed from 1975 to 1986 are likely to have continued as more women have entered the labour market and as social change has continued at a rapid pace. As a result the reconciliation of work and family for men and women is increasingly being seen as an important social and political issue.

CHAPTER 6

A COMPARISON OF THE FOUR COUNTRIES: AN OVERVIEW

As a prelude to our study, in order to place the comparative analyses in context, we have presented individual country literature reviews covering several common areas. We shall now briefly summarise the similarities and differences observed through a comparison and synthesis of these reviews, while also drawing upon comparative demographic data for the four countries, as well as for the EU as a whole.

1. WOMEN'S LABOUR FORCE PARTICIPATION

As a backdrop to the whole issue of reconciliation of work and family life, women's increasing participation in the labour market has been the critical factor. Over the last few decades, the overall trend in the EU has been for women's employment rates to have risen, while men's rates have either remained stable or declined. Participation rates of women (in the age group 15-64) increased from 45% in 1985 to 54% in 2001, whereas men's have declined during this period from 75% to 72.5% (Villa, 2002). As a result the gender gap in the employment rate in the EU has been reduced from 30% in 1985 to 18.5% in 2000 (*Ibid.*).

There is much greater variability in employment rates of women across the EU than there is of men. It may be seen that the highest rate of female labour force participation is in Denmark (71.6%), followed by Sweden (69.3%), and other Northern countries, such as the Netherlands, U.K. and Finland. The lowest rates tend to be found in the Southern Mediterranean countries, such as Italy (39.6%), Spain (40.3%) and Greece (41.2%). Portugal is an exception, with a relatively high rate of 60.3%.). The EU average is 54%.

Table 6.1. Employment Rates by Gender in the European Union (EU15), 2000

	MF %	M %	F %	Gender Gap %
Denmark	76.3	80.8	71.6	9.2
Netherlands	72.9	82.1	63.6	18.5
UK	71.5	78.1	64.8	13.3
Finland	70.8	70.2	64.3	5.9
Sweden	70.8	72.3	69.3	3.0
Portugal	68.3	76.5	60.3	16.2
Austria	68.2	76.9	59.5	17.4
Ireland	65.2	76.2	54.1	22.1
Germany	65.4	72.7	57.9	14.8
France	62.0	69.1	55.1	14.0
Luxembourg	62.7	75.0	50.1	25.9
Belgium	60.5	69.5	51.5	18.0
Greece	55.7	71.1	41.2	29.9
Spain	54.8	69.7	40.3	29.4
Italy	53.7	67.9	39.6	28.3
EU Total	**63.2**	**72.5**	**54.0**	**18.5**

Source: Eurostat, ELFS as cited in Villa (2002)

Thus, our sample of countries includes the EU country with the highest female labour force participation (Denmark), the country with the lowest rate (Italy), and two countries at about the EU average (France and Ireland).

The traditional male breadwinner model has undergone change and it is now common for both parents to be working, even when there are young children. Table 6.2. presents recent data compiled by the OECD (2001), which compares Italy, Ireland and France in terms of the labour force participation of men and women in couples with at least one child under six years of age. As these are three of the countries on which we are focusing in the present study, it is of interest to examine the prevalence of this pattern in these countries, as well as to examine trends in employment of this group over time.

Table 6.2. *Percentage of Couples Living Together with at least one Child Under Six, Where Woman Works Full or Part-Time and Man Works Full-time:*
Cross National Comparisons - 1984 & 1999

	Father working Full-time, Mother working Full-time (%)		Father working Full-time, Mother working Part-time (%)	
	1984	1999	1984	1999
Italy	33.3	32.6	3.7	9.5
Ireland*	11.4	29.6	3.6	11.4
France	35.9	31.3	11.9	19.7
Denmark	NA	NA	NA	NA

* 1997 instead of 1999   Source: OECD, Employment Outlook (2001),Table 4.2
NA = not available

It may be seen that in 1999 the pattern of both parents working full-time was more common in Italy (32.6%) and France (31.3%), than in Ireland (29.6%). However, while the Italian and French proportions were quite similar to those in 1984 (33.3% and 35.9% respectively), the Irish percentage had risen considerably since 1984, at which time it was only 11.4%.

It is interesting to observe that part-time employment of the mothers in these couples is much less common than full-time employment, given that full-time employment with one or more preschool children would be presumed to be more demanding. In 1999 only 9.5% of Italian women in this group worked part-time. In Ireland the figure was 11.4% and in France it was 19.7%. However, in all three countries the level of part-time employment rose from 1984 to 1999. This may be due to increasing availability of part-time work, which may be beneficial, in the sense that it can be a measure to facilitate work-life balance; alternatively, it could signal greater casualisation of the female work-force. By aggregating the percentages employed full and part-time, it may be seen that in 1999 42.1% of Italian women in this category (i.e., in couples where the partner was employed full-time and there was at least one child under six) were employed. The comparable figure for France was 51% and in Ireland it was 41%.

There is, unfortunately, no comparable data available for Denmark. However, on the basis of other data available for Denmark, it is apparent that the rates of labour force participation of Danish women in this group are even higher than those of Italian, French or Irish women. In 1999 in Denmark 86% of all children had both parents working full-time and 6% part-time. Aggregating these figures, it can be seen that 92% of Danish children had both parents working (Danmarks Statistik, 2002, Table 3.2.1, p. 66).

Among the 2-8 year old group, over 90% of the children had parents working full-time in 1999 *(Ibid, p. 67)*. Danish data for 1989 indicated that 65% of all children had both parents working full-time and 17% part-time. This indicates that from 1989 to 1999 full-time employment increased and part-time decreased. The decrease in part-time employment differs from the pattern seen in the other three countries.

2. RELATIONSHIPS BETWEEN FERTILITY AND EMPLOYMENT

Of the four countries we are examining, Ireland traditionally has had the highest birth rate. It will be seen in Table 6.3. below, that in 1980 the crude birth rate in Ireland was 21.8 births per 1,000 people. This compared with 14.9 for France, 11.3 for Italy, 11.2 for Denmark, and an overall EU average of 13.0. It may be seen that in three of the four countries, as well as in the EU as a whole, the birth rate fell from 1980 to 2001, with the greatest drop being seen in Ireland – going from 21.8 to 15.0; though the Irish rate is still well above the current EU average of 10.6. In contrast to the trend seen in the other countries, in Denmark, the birth rate rose slightly, from 11.2 to 12.2.

Table 6.3. Crude Birth Rates 1980 – 2001 (per 1000 population)

	1980	2001
France	14.9	13.1^p
Italy	11.3	9.4e
Denmark	11.2	12.2
Ireland	21.8	15.0^e
EU	13.0	10.6^e

<u>Crude Birth Rate:</u> *The ratio of number of births to mean population in a given year.*
Source: Eurostat (2002)

The relationship between female employment rates and fertility rates is complex and has been referred to as the 'participation-fertility puzzle' (Bettio and Villa, 1998; see Villa, 2002). On the one hand, most EU countries demonstrate increasing rates of female labour force participation and decreasing fertility. On the other hand,

A COMPARISON OF THE FOUR COUNTRIES: AN OVERVIEW

and counter-intuitively, those countries with the highest rates of female participation also show the highest fertility (*Ibid;* see also Fagnani, 2000, 2002a). For example, as may be seen below, while the total fertility (TFR) in Denmark is among the highest in the EU (1.74), the Danish female participation rate is also among the highest (71.6%). This trend is apparent in other Scandinavian countries. France has an ever higher total fertility rate than Denmark, together with high labour force participation of women with young children.

Table 6.4. Total Fertility Rates 1980 – 2001

	1980	2001
France	2.0	1.90^p
Italy	1.6	1.24^e
Denmark	1.6	1.74
Ireland	3.3	1.98^p
EU	1.8	1.42^e

p=provisional data   e=Eurostat estimate
(Total Fertility Rate: The average number of children that would be born alive to a woman during her lifetime if current age specific fertility rates were to continue)
Source: Eurostat (2002)

In contrast, Italy has a low total fertility rate (1.24) and a low female participation rate (39.6%). Villa (*op .cit.*) points our that "Among other factors, the increasing burden on women, having to continue paid work with family responsibilities, has played a major role in lowering fertility" (p. 16). Yet "those countries which have been able to develop the supply of social services (all personal services, in particular childcare services) and to move towards a more equal sharing of family responsibilities (between men and women) have not only successfully expanded female employment, but they also managed to halt the declining trend in fertility" (*Ibid. pp.* 16-17).

3. COMPARATIVE SOCIAL POLICIES

The literature reviews for each of the four countries presented a detailed picture of the policies available in each in relation to assisting working parents. It was evident that policies relating to maternity, paternity, parental and other leave varied greatly by country (See Table 6.5. for a comparison of policies in each of the countries). In particular, it was notable that paid paternity leave was available in Denmark and in France. In Denmark it is available to fathers for four weeks – two weeks during the first 14 weeks and two weeks during weeks 25-26. In France it is available for two weeks. In Italy it is only available under very specific circumstances, such as in the case of the mother's death or severe incapacitation. In Ireland there is no legal entitlement to paternity leave; it is at the discretion of the employer. However, in the civil service three days paid leave are given. The introduction of paternity leave in France is seen as a turning point in French family policy in the sense that this marks the first time that the father's role has been symbolically acknowledged. This may have an impact on the workplace by underscoring men's roles as fathers as well as workers. It would not be surprising if other countries followed suit by introducing paternity leave.

While it is laudable that 67% of Danish fathers used their paternity leave in 1999 and this was an increase over the 55% who took it in 1991, nevertheless, we must not forget that even in Denmark it was pointed out that men often take this leave in such a way as to minimise its impact on the organisation, i.e. to merge it with leave time. Hence, it is still not quite acceptable for men to publicly acknowledge their right to take time off at this critical personal time. The reason for this may be, as pointed out in the Danish literature review, that the Danish welfare state is giving out "mixed messages", i.e. ambivalent signals to men regarding fatherhood. On the one hand, paternity leave has been statutorily provided; on the other hand it is short and not always compensated and no part is exclusively for men.

The length of time that parental leave is available differs enormously among the four countries. In France it is up to three years, i.e. for children aged 0-3. While this is unpaid, there are provisions for payment (Allocation Parentale d'Education – APE), and also options for part time work. In Italy, parental leave (known as optional leave) can be taken for six months by mothers and seven months by those fathers who have taken three months of paternity leave, up until the child is eight years old. In Denmark parental leave may be taken for 10 weeks following the 14th week of maternity leave and it can only be taken by one parent at a time. Payment is negotiable with the employer. It is fully paid in the public sector and sometimes less in the private sector. In Ireland there is provision of 14 weeks of parental leave per parent, which can be taken up until the child is five years of age. However, it is unpaid.

Other forms of leave are also available in varying ways in each of the four countries. For example, in Denmark additional generous leave is available to parents for childcare. This is over and above the allowance for parental leave. Danish social policy also allows for parents to take fully paid time off to care for sick children. Provisions for leave to care for sick children are also available in

A COMPARISON OF THE FOUR COUNTRIES: AN OVERVIEW

Italy. In France time off to care for sick children is available, but it is unpaid. In Ireland, there is paid *force majeur* leave; however, this is only three days in one year or five days within a three-year period.

Thus it is clear that the policies in the four countries differ substantially, to some extent in scope (i.e. type of policy available) and in extent of provision. In addition, we have seen that the provision of childcare also differs significantly between the four countries, with well-developed public programmes in France and in Denmark, and with lesser public provision in Italy and Ireland. In France 36% of two year olds and 98% of three year olds attend écoles maternelles. This care is state provided and open 35 hours a week. In Denmark 54% of children 0 – 2 are in day care and this applies to 90% of 3 – 5 year olds. In Italy informal networks play a primary role in childcare, as is the case in Ireland. In Italy the family can be seen as the "implicit partner" of Italian social policies. While public crèches have been introduced since 1991 for children up to three and are run by municipalities at local level, they are not universal services and there has been no organic development at national level since the 1970s. However, for children from the age of 3 – 5, kindergartens are seen as providing universal educational rights for children. This is in contrast to Ireland, where public provision does not begin until age four. Thus, as of 1993 only 1% of Irish three year olds were in public childcare, 55% of four year olds and nearly all five year olds (99%) (European Commission Network on Childcare, 1996). While these figures may have increased since these statistics were collected, it is nevertheless clear that public provision in Ireland is extremely limited for the age group 0 - 3, but rises significantly at age four, when entry to junior infant classes is possible.

TABLE 6.5. STATUTORY AND OTHER LEAVE PROVISIONS: CROSS-NATIONAL COMPARISONS

MATERNITY & RELATED LEAVE	FRANCE	ITALY	DENMARK	IRELAND
Paid Leave	16 weeks (26 weeks in case of a third child or a higher rank order)	20 weeks (8 weeks to be taken before the birth)	18 weeks (4 weeks to be taken before the birth). Sometimes more, particularly in public sector.	18 consecutive weeks (4 weeks to be taken before birth)
Rate of Pay for Paid Leave	Full pay with an upper limit - of €2,352 per month by 2002	(a) 80% pay or (b) Full pay	Negotiable with employer. Often at full pay, particularly in public sector; sometimes at reduced pay.	70 % of weekly pay – minimum payment of €141.60 and a maximum payment of €232.40 per week.
Other leave	None (unpaid parental leave takes over)	Daily Leave for breastfeeding until child is 1 year old. 1-2 hours per day, 100% paid.	Time off to attend pregnancy-related medical examinations. Additional 10 weeks Parental Leave can be taken by either parent following the last week of Maternity Leave (pay is negotiable with employer—full pay in public sector)	Optional further 8 weeks unpaid to be taken immediately after maternity leave. Paid time off to attend ante-natal or post-natal medical visits.
Leave paid for by	Her health insurance, which is funded by statutory contributions from both employer and employee	(a) Social insurance contributions (b) Top-up to full pay (optional) by mother's employer if provided in the labour contract (i.e. in public sector)	Mother's employer	Maternity benefit available from the Dept. of Social, Community and Family Affairs. There is no obligation for employers to top up the benefit.

TABLE 6.5 (cont). STATUTORY AND OTHER LEAVE PROVISIONS: CROSS-NATIONAL COMPARISONS

PATERNITY & RELATED LEAVE	FRANCE	ITALY	DENMARK	IRELAND
Statutory Paid Leave	2 weeks (21 days if multiple births)	12 weeks after the birth, under certain conditions: • Mother's death or severe incapacitation • Child left by mother • Child entrusted solely to the father	4 weeks total – 2 weeks during first 14 weeks + 2 weeks during weeks 25-26.	There is no legal requirement – it is at the discretion of the employer The civil service gives 3 days paid leave, and some employers provide some days leave
Rate of Pay for Paid Leave	Full pay with an upper limit - of €2,352 per month by 2002	(a) 80% pay (b) Full pay	Negotiable with employer. Often at full-pay, particularly in public sector; sometimes at reduced pay.	Non-applicable
Other leave	None (unpaid parental leave takes over)	In addition to maternity leave, 24 weeks at 30% pay, to be taken by mother or father, by social insurance contributions.	10 weeks Parental Leave can be taken by either parent following the last week of maternity leave. Pay is negotiable with employer, full pay in public sector.	None
Leave paid for by	His health insurance	a) Social insurance contributions b) Top-up to full pay (optional) by father's employer if provided in the labour contract (i.e. in public sector.	Father's employer	Employer, if at all

TABLE 6.5 (cont). STATUTORY AND OTHER LEAVE PROVISIONS: CROSS-NATIONAL COMPARISONS

PARENTAL & RELATED LEAVE	FRANCE	ITALY	DENMARK	IRELAND
Known as	Parental Leave (Congé Parental d'Education CPE)	Optional leave	Childcare Leave	Parental Leave
Paid/unpaid	Unpaid although economically active parents having *at least two* children may receive Allocation parentale d'Education paid by Social Security (flat-rate benefit). (From 2004 onwards, this will be provided to parents with only one child for a period of 6 months)	Child under 3 years - 30% pay. In the public sector, the first 30 days of optional leave are fully paid. Child 3-8 years – unpaid. For those with salaries less than approximately €13,000, 30% is paid	60% of Salary Paid	Unpaid
Paid for by	Unpaid (see above)	Social insurance contributions	Employer	Non-applicable
Time	All employees, male or female, who have worked for one year in company before child born can work part time 16-32 hours per week or cease employment.	6 months for Mothers 7 months for Fathers who have taken 3 months of paternity leave	Statutory 8-13 Weeks. More is negotiable with Employer up to 52 Weeks. This leave can be taken by both parents at the same time or separately.	14 weeks per parent. This can be taken consecutively or with the agreement of employer, broken up over a period of time
Age of child by which leave must be taken	0-3 years old	0-8 years old (can be split up between years)	0-8 Years Old	0-5 years old

TABLE 6.5 (cont). STATUTORY AND OTHER LEAVE PROVISIONS: CROSS-NATIONAL COMPARISONS

LEAVE FOR CHILD'S ILLNESS	FRANCE	ITALY	DENMARK	IRELAND
Known as	Sick Child leave	Leave for caring of a sick child.	Child Sick Days	Force Majeur (for family illness or emergencies)
Paid/unpaid	Paid	Child under 3 - unpaid, but working parents are entitled to figurative contributions for a max of 30 days per year (*contributi figurativi*). Child between 3-8, unpaid, but entitled to a reduced coverage of contributions (*copertura contributiva ridotta*)	Full Pay	Full Pay
Paid for by	Health Insurance	Social insurance contributions	Employer	Employer
Time	6 or more days per year (depending on company agreement)	Sick Child Leave - Child under 3 – limitless. Child between 3-8 – 5 days a year for each parent	Public sector –Day off on child's first sick day. 2 days off per child/per year in municipality area. Private sector – negotiable.	≤ 3 working days in any 12 consecutive months and 5 days in any 36 consecutive months
Age of child by which leave must be taken	0-12 years old	Sick Child Leave–0-8 years old	0-8 years old	Any Age

Note: The Statutory Provisions outlined in this table were current as of the date of the survey and do not necessarily reflect any changes made since that time.

4. FLEXIBLE WORKING

While flexible working has been introduced in all of the countries to some extent, drawbacks are evident. For example, in France flexibility has been introduced in crèche opening hours. Some crèches are now open until late in the evening. Yet this can bring problems to those staff for whom this impinges on their own work-life balance. The 35-hour week was a search for better work-life balance. However, to date, only larger companies have been required to implement the law, it is too early to assess.

In Italy job sharing (*contratti di solidarieta*) has primarily been in response to redistribute work in economic crises. Tele-work is regulated by collective agreements and appears to have interesting implications for work time issues. Flexible working for women may relieve women of the "double burden," but it often has the negative consequences of lower wages and negative impact on future working and career mobility.

In Denmark 22% of companies are characterised by flexible management; however, it was noted that relatively few employees are actually involved in this flexibility (Csonka, 2000). Much of the flexibility found was of the informal kind in which female colleagues supported each other (Holt, 1994). It was quite clear from this research that when both parents are working, a high degree of flexibility is necessary in order to make family life function (*Ibid.*).

In Ireland flexible arrangements are not available on a statutory basis; the philosophy is one of working out individual arrangements at the level of each organisation between employer and union and/or employees, as the case may be. The larger companies are more likely to provide a greater range of flexible working options than are smaller companies. However, it is clear that women are the main ones to take up flexible working options (National Framework Committee on Family-Friendly Workplace Policies, 2001; Drew *et al*, 2002) and there is the fear that men and women will operate on a two track system (*Ibid.*).

5. GENDER ROLES AND ATTITUDES

While policies are gradually being developed to accommodate the needs of dual breadwinner couples, it is clear that attitudes have not kept pace with the social changes which constitute the reality of people's live. This is true of employers, it is true of fathers and, to some extent, it is also true of women themselves. For example, in Italy it was noted that even though fathers are aware of the "existing asymmetry" in the division of labour and they do not approve of it "theoretically," they seem to accept the *status quo* for "practical reasons" (Bimbi and Castellano, 1990; Scisci, 1999). Paternal involvement in childcare and domestic work is very low and is primarily given in the form of "assistance" to the mother (Bimbi and

Castellano, 1990; Ventimiglia, 1996, 1999). On the other hand, many mothers accept this and adjust to the asymmetry, as the cost of negotiating greater equality is too high (Scisci, 1999). Moreover, there is evidence of female "ambivalence" towards greater involvement on the part of the father (Bimbi and Castellano, 1990). While on one level women request more paternal cooperation, at another level they may want to keep certain spheres of activity for themselves, partly as a means to retain control in certain areas (Bimbi, 1990, 1992). It was concluded by Bimbi (1996) that in a period of transition both men and women may need to retain some continuity in gender asymmetries, especially in relation to domestic work. This notion is echoed in Højgaard's (1997, 1998) analysis to the effect that the relationship between masculinity and fatherhood is the result of a deep-rooted symbolic universe of meaning pertaining to masculinity and femininity, which are structured as (hierarchical) opposites. This symbolic order dictates that parenthood has different meanings for men and women. For men, masculinity and work are more closely linked, whereas for women femininity and work less so, while femininity and motherhood are more strongly linked. This thus helps to support the *status quo*.

Attitudinal research in Ireland has shown that there have been significant shifts in a more egalitarian direction during a period of rapid social change during the mid 1970s through the 1980s. These shifts showed more support for egalitarian gender roles, greater support for maternal employment, etc. However, lingering ambivalence toward maternal employment remained to some extent (Fine-Davis, 1988a), though this may have been largely related to the times of economic crisis when unemployment was high. In contrast, Irish attitudes to social policies that would support working parents, such as attitudes to flexible working and public provision of childcare were very progressive, even two decades ago (Fine-Davis, 1983a, 1983b, 1988c).

6. RESEARCH ON FATHERING

Relatively little research on fathering has been carried out in the context of the plethora of studies in other related areas. Italy stands out as one of the very few countries where innovative studies have been conducted. Some of this research has indicated that new fathers show a great emotional/ relational involvement with their children and that contact with their children greatly contributes to their own sense of well-being and quality of life; however, this involvement mainly revolves around play and does not extend to care-giving (Bimbi and Castellano, 1990; Giovannini and Ventimiglia, 1994; Badolato, 1993).

Other findings on fathering indicate that fathers, while wishing to spend more time with their families (Bimbi, 1990; Ventimiglia, 1996), often actually increase their working hours after the birth of children as they face additional economic pressures (Bimbi and Castellano, 1990; Sabbadini and Palomba, 1994; Ventimiglia, 1996; Pattaro, 2000).

An Irish review of research on fathering in an international context concluded that the more extensive involvement fathers have with their children, the better it is for them in terms of cognitive development and performance at school as well as in terms of the development of critical personal traits, such as self-esteem, empathy, social skills and non-stereotyped beliefs (McKeown *et al*, 1998).

7. CONCLUSION

The individual country reviews as well as this brief overview and synthesis confirm that we are in a state of social transition in gender roles and have not sufficiently adapted to the transition we are experiencing. Individual countries are responding with varying levels of social support. Employers are also responding with partial, but not sufficient workplace flexibility. Gender role attitudes are changing, but in some cases women are reluctant to relinquish the power they have traditionally retained in the home and men are not easily responding to female requests for domestic sharing; the latter phenomenon is in part related both to men's *perceived* as well as *actual* demands of the workplace and their perception of the male role.

There is clearly a need for more information in all of these areas so as to gain greater understanding of the processes operating as well as to help inform developing social policy, both at the workplace and at governmental level. We hope through the collection and analysis of comparative data in the present study to add to this understanding.

CHAPTER 7

METHODOLOGY

1. METHOD

1.1. Research Design and Sampling

The sample of the study consisted of 100 men and women in each country for a total of 400 respondents. Each of the respondents was: 1) employed. 2) living in a couple with a partner/spouse who was also employed; and 3) had at least one child under six.

The sample was stratified by sex, socio-economic status and employment in the public *vs.* the private sector. These sampling parameters held for all of the four countries participating in the study and hence the samples are comparable. All of the Irish respondents were from Dublin and the samples from the other three countries were also from major cities, i.e., Paris, Copenhagen and Bologna.

Respondents were located for the research through employers in the public and private sector; through community agencies and through childcare centres.

The stratification design for the total sample is illustrated in Table 7.1. and that for each of the four individual countries is illustrated in Table 7.2.

Table 7.1: Sample Design: 4 Countries (N=400)

		Public Sector	Private Sector		
Male	Low SES	50	50	100	
	High SES	50	50	100	200
Female	Low SES	50	50	100	
	High SES	50	50	100	200
	Total	200	200	400	

Table 7. 2: The Individual Country Samples (N=100)

		Public Sector	**Private Sector**		
Male	Low SES	12-13	12-13	25	
	High SES	12-13	12-13	25	50
Female	Low SES	12-13	12-13	25	
	High SES	12-13	12-13	25	50
	Total	50	50	100	

The schema used for measuring socio-economic status was that of the Hall-Jones classification of occupational status (Hall & Jones, 1950; Hutchinson, 1969). This has eight levels of occupational status, ranging from unskilled manual to professionally qualified/high administrative, as illustrated below:

Hall-Jones Categorisation of Socio-Economic Status (SES)
- (1) Manual Routine
- (2) Semi-Skilled
- (3) Skilled-Manual
- (4) Clerical White-Collar
- (5) Supervisory (Lower Grade)
- (6) Supervisory (Higher Grade)
- (7) Managerial and Executive
- (8) Professionally Qualified/ High Administrative

1.2. Questionnaire

The questionnaire was designed to explore people's attitudes and experiences in coping with balancing work and family, with particular reference to the different perspectives of men and women. Attitudes towards and experience of different workplace social policies were also explored. In developing the questionnaire an extensive review of the literature in the four countries was carried out. There was, in addition an international search for relevant items. The authors actively collaborated in the development of the questionnaire and the final set of items includes some replicated from other studies by the authors and others, as well as the adaptation of some previous items and the creation of some new items. The sources for the items from Italy were: Bimbi & Castellano (1990), Di Vita *et al.* (2000), Giovannini & Ventimiglia (1994), Ingrosso (1988), Musatti (1992), and Zanatta (1999). The items from Denmark were from Højgaard (1990, 1996b), and Holt (1994). Items from

France were from Fagnani & Letablier (2000). Items from Ireland were from Fine-Davis (1983b, 1988c), Davis & Fine-Davis (1991), Fine-Davis et al (1981). Other items were included from Sweden (Haas, 1993). The questionnaire contained several sections, as follows:

- Demographics
- You and Your Children
- Childcare Arrangements
- The Workplace
- Combining Work and Family
- Well-Being

1.2.1. Demographics
The section on Demographics covered sex, age, marital /cohabitation status, education, partner's education, occupation, partner's occupation, employment in public *vs.* private sector, sex of supervisor, length of own and partner's commuting time, mode of transport to work, length of own and partner's work week, and whether on works typical or atypical hours.

1.2.2. You and Your Children
This section obtained data on the number of children and the ages of the youngest and next youngest child. It also asked whether the birth of the youngest child caused any significant changes for the respondent in a number of areas, and if so, to what extent. Questions were included concerning whether or not the respondent or his/her partner modified their working time after the birth of the youngest child and whether or not they or their partner temporarily interrupted their work activity following the birth. Extensive data was collected concerning who usually carried out various household and childcare tasks in the home – the respondent, his/her partner, both of them, or someone else. Three questions were included concerning desires about time: 1) the extent to which the respondent would like to spend more or less time with the family; 2) whether they would like their partner to spend more or less time with the family; and 3) the extent to which they would like more or less personal time.

Detailed information was collected on childcare arrangements, including what arrangements were used when usual arrangements fell through. The cost of childcare was obtained as well as overall satisfaction with childcare arrangements.

1.2.3. The Workplace
Several sets of attitudinal items were included in this section. These were designed to ascertain the attitudes in the workplace towards working parents and the possible barriers to reconciling work and family. Respondents were also asked about the extent of potential flexibility in the workplace and then the actual flexibility they took advantage of at work.

1.2.4. Combining Work and Family
In this section respondents were asked a series of questions concerning combining work and family. They were asked about their working hours in relation to their childcare arrangements and how easy or difficult they found combining work and family. The measure of ease *vs.* difficulty in combining work and family was a key dependent measure in the study.

Finally, they were asked about 14 different social policies to help working parents (e.g., maternity leave, paternity leave, part-time working, job sharing, career breaks, flexible hours, tele-working, parental leave, etc.). Firstly, they were asked if each of the policies was available at their workplace, second, whether or not respondents used the policy themselves and thirdly, what their attitude to the policy was – favourable or unfavourable.

1.2.5. Well-Being
The final section of the questionnaire concerned respondents' overall well-being in several key life domains. These included satisfaction with health, work, family life, relationship with spouse/partner and satisfaction with life in general. These items were designed to be key dependent measures of well-being.

1.2.6. Translation of the Questionnaire into Four Languages
The questionnaire was translated from the English into the languages of the other three participating countries – French, Danish and Italian and the interviews were conducted in the native language of respondents by native speakers. The English version of the questionnaire may be found in Appendix B. The translated versions may be found in (Fine-Davis *et al.*, 2002).

1.3. Data Collection

1.3.1. Interviews
Interviews were carried out by interviewers on a one-to-one basis. Each interview took approximately 45 minutes. Interviews were generally carried out in the

workplace, although some were carried out in the respondents' homes and a few were carried out in the workplace of the interviewer, i.e., at the university.

1.3.2. Data Analysis
The approach taken in the study was to examine percentage results first, by country and sex. Where applicable, Chi-Square tests were carried out. The next main set of analyses carried out were analyses of variance. The stratification design of the sample, with the systematic variation of the key independent variables of 1) country, 2) sex, 3) socio-economic status, and 4) public *vs.* private sector, enabled us to carry out both three and four-way analyses of variance using various combinations of these variables. This allowed us to examine the main effects of each of these variables, while controlling for the effects of the other variables. It also allowed us to examine any significant interaction effects between these independent variables in determining the dependent variables. Where there were significant main effects or interaction effects, we have presented the relevant cell means in text, together with the F-ratio, df and level of significance. We have not included the full ANOVA tables in the report for reasons of space; however, they are available upon request from the authors.

In order to examine the relationships between variables, correlational analyses were carried out, as well as multiple regressions. These tools were primarily used to examine the relationship of a wide range of potential "predictor" variables to key dependent measures, including, Ease *vs.* Difficulty in Combining Work and Family, and five global measures of well-being: Satisfaction with Health, Satisfaction with Work, Satisfaction with Family Life, Satisfaction with Relationship with Spouse/Partner and Life Satisfaction.

Because of the extensive amount of data generated, we have decided to include the more powerful ANOVA results in text and to place the corresponding percentage tables in the Appendix. The latter are presented by country and in many cases also by sex. Because of their importance in revealing relationships between measures, correlational analyses and multiple regressions are also included in the main body of the text.

Data entry and analysis were carried out by the Survey Unit of the Economic and Social Research Institute, Dublin.

1.3.3. Generalisability of the Findings to the Larger Population
It should be borne in mind that the samples, while systematically stratified and comparable from country to country, were nevertheless small. Furthermore, they were of city populations – Paris, Bologna, Copenhagen and Dublin. Thus, while we can be confident of the differences and relationships found in our sample, where these were statistically significant, we cannot generalise to the larger population

with samples of this size. Thus, the results hold for our sample and they are suggestive of trends, which are likely to occur in larger samples. Data would need to be collected on larger representative samples in order to generalise to whole countries. However, where possible, we have compared the data obtained in the present study with comparable data obtained on larger, more representative samples.

It was the purpose of this study to develop and pilot an instrument in the area of reconciliation of work and family life which could be used in larger, more representative samples. We hope that further work both in national and cross-national contexts will take place, benefiting from the developmental work, which has taken place in this study.

2. CHARACTERISTICS OF THE SAMPLE

Most respondents were in their mid-30s, ranging from a mean of 33 years in France to 37 years in Ireland, with an overall mean age of 35 years for all countries (Appendix Table A1).

Approximately three-quarters of the respondents were married (73%), and one-quarter were co-habiting (27%). The highest percentage of co-habiting couples was in France[1] (42%), the next highest in Denmark (32%), the next in Ireland (22%) and the lowest in Italy (11%) (Appendix Table A2). This corroborates Eurostat (2001) data indicating that there is a much higher proportion of births outside of marriage in Denmark and France (approximately 40%), whereas in Italy it was 8.7% in 1998.

We operationalised socio-economic status (SES) by using the Hall-Jones Classification system of Occupational Status (Hall & Jones, 1950; Hutchinson, 1969). While this is not the most recently developed system of classification, it is quite useful because of its number of categories (eight) and the fact that it is an ordinal scale. This makes it very amenable to bi-variate and multi-variate analyses, as opposed to some other systems of classification which combine ordinal and nominal categories in one scale and are thus virtually useless for analysis with other variables.

The socio-economic status of the respondents was one of the stratification variables in the sampling design. Thus 50% of the sample fell into the categories 1 – 4 (lower SES) and 50% into categories 5 – 8 (higher SES). The full distribution on the Hall-Jones categories, ranging from manual-routine, through to professionally

---

[1] It is to be noted that when we refer to our data from "France", we are referring to our sample from Paris; similarly when we refer to "Denmark", we are referring to our sample from Copenhagen; "Italy" refers to our sample from Bologna, and "Ireland" refers to our Dublin sample.

qualified/high administrative is contained for each of the countries in Appendix Table A3.

The respondents were well distributed along the educational continuum, reflecting a wide variety of educational backgrounds, with some having only completed primary school and others having completed postgraduate studies. The vast majority of respondents (approximately three-quarters) had either completed some level of secondary education or had a university degree. The French sample had a higher proportion of respondents who had completed higher education than did the other countries, however, their distribution in terms of occupational status or SES, as described above, did not differ from those in the other countries (Appendix Table A4).

Sector of employment was one of the key independent variables in the stratification design. Thus, we systematically sampled half of respondents from the public sector and half from the private sector (Appendix Table A5).

Most respondents interviewed (86%) had either one or two children; approximately half of this group (45.5%) had one child and 40.5% had two children. Only 10.5% of the sample had three children, 3 % had four, and 0.5% had five children. Irish respondents were much more likely to have three children or more children (27%) than were respondents from any of the other countries (8% of French, 9% of Italian and 12% of Danish) . The overall mean number of children was 1.7, with Irish respondents having the highest mean (2.0 children), and the French respondents having the lowest (1.5). The mean number of children among the Italian respondents was 1.7 and it was 1.8 in Denmark (Appendix Table A6).

It was specified in the sample design that the youngest child should be less than six years of age. The mean age of the youngest child was 2.6 years overall, ranging from a mean of 2.3 years in Italy, to 2.7 years in Denmark and France. It was specified in the sample design that only second youngest children aged 12 or younger would be considered in the study. The mean age of the second youngest child was 6.3 years overall, and ranged from 5.9 years in Italy to 6.6 years in France (Appendix Table A7).

CHAPTER 8

CHILDREN AND FAMILY LIFE

1. THE EFFECT OF THE BIRTH OF THE YOUNGEST CHILD ON WORK AND FAMILY LIFE

The birth of the first child represents an event with several consequences in terms of the adjustment and the re-definition of life patterns of the parents at different levels. Firstly, it profoundly modifies the couple's relationship, together with the dynamics and interaction mechanisms established between the partners. We considered in the design of the study whether to focus in particular on the birth of the first child or the youngest child, as some couples in the sample would have more than one child. We decided to focus on the youngest child since that was the most recent event the parents had experienced and hence it would be fresher in their memory, and perhaps still having ongoing effects.

Structured methods are particularly useful in throwing light on transformations which have affected the partners' daily habits and relationship with each other as well as with their wider networks. The question chosen to tap into this area was taken from a study by Giovannini and Ventimiglia (1994).

"Did the birth of your youngest child cause any significant changes for you in relation to:
- The way you organised your day?
- Your life habits?
- Your professional tasks?
- The amount of domestic chores?
- Your friendships?
- Your free time?
- Your relationship with your partner?"

Respondents were asked to respond on a scale ranging from "none" (1), "a little" (2), "quite a lot" (3) to "very much" (4).

We shall discuss in text percentage responses to each of the items in this set; actual percentage tables can be found in Appendix A. We shall also present in this section, results of a series of three-way analyses of variance (ANOVA), examining the effects of country, sex and socio-economic status (SES) on each of the individual items referring to different areas of life as dependent variables.

Table 8.1. below presents the mean scores by country for each of the individual dependent variables listed above. Where there was a significant effect of country in the 3-way ANOVA this is indicated. We shall also discuss significant effects of sex and SES as well as any significant interaction effects in connection with each of the variables.

As may be seen in this Table, the area of life most disrupted by the birth of the youngest child is the respondents' free time. The mean score of 3.2 falls slightly above 'a fair amount' (3). The area next most affected was the amount of domestic chores (3.0) and the way the respondents organised their day (3.0). Life habits and relationship with partner were next most affected by the birth (2.9 and 2.7 respectively). Those areas least affected by the birth of the youngest child were the respondents' professional tasks (2.0) and their friendships (2.2) with 2 = "a little"

Table 8.1. Effect of the Birth of the Youngest Child on Work and Family Life: Mean Scores by Country (N=400).

	France	Italy	Denmark	Ireland	All Countries	Significance
The way you organised your day	3.0	3.1	3.0	3.0	3.0	n.s.
Your life habits	2.9	3.0	2.7	3.0	2.9	n.s.
Your professional tasks	1.6	2.3	1.8	2.2	2.0	***
The amount of domestic chores	3.0	3.1	2.6	3.1	3.0	**
Your friendships	2.0	2.3	2.4	2.1	2.2	*
Your free time	3.5	3.2	2.8	3.4	3.2	***
Your relationship with your partner	2.5	2.8	2.7	2.8	2.7	**

(1 = none: 4 = very much)

* $p \leq 0.05$ ** $p \leq 0.01$ *** $p \leq 0.001$

1.1. The Way Respondents Organise Their Day

In all countries, 71% of respondents reported that the way they organised their day had changed either "a fair amount" (31%) or "very much" (40%) when their youngest child was born; only 7.5% said that it had not changed at all (Appendix Table A8).

There were no significant differences between male and female respondents or between countries. There was, however, a significant difference between respondents in lower vs. higher SES jobs. For those in higher SES jobs the birth of the youngest child had a significantly greater effect on the way they organised their day (3.2) than it did for those in lower SES occupations (2.9) ($F = 9.53$, $df = 1$; $p \leq 0.005$). This may be due to the fact that higher SES occupations make more time demands on employees. It also may be that people in lower SES occupations have greater access to a wider family network, which may provide support. We will examine these hypotheses in subsequent sections.

1.2. Life Habits

A third of all respondents said that their life habits had changed "very much" when their youngest child was born. In Denmark the figure was somewhat lower – 22%, compared to 32-34% for the other countries. A further third of respondents said that their life habits changed "a fair amount" (Appendix Table A9).

There were no significant differences between males and females, nor between countries. There was, however, a moderately significant effect of social class indicating that the life habits of those of higher SES changed more than those of lower SES (3.0 vs. 2.8; $F = 4.89$, $df = 1$; $p \leq 0.05$). This effect of SES reinforces that found above in relation to the way respondents organised their day.

1.3. Professional Tasks

There was a great diversity of responses concerning the effect of the birth of the youngest child on respondents' professional tasks. The greatest effect was reported by Italian parents, only 26% of whom said that there was no effect. This is in contrast to French parents of whom 62% reported that there was no effect on their professional tasks. Irish and Danish parents fell in between, with 37% of Irish parents reporting no effect and 51% of Danish parents (Appendix Table A10).

This is confirmed by the ANOVA results, shown below, indicating a significant country effect. There was also a significant effect of sex showing that female respondents reported that their professional tasks had changed more following the birth of their youngest child than did male respondent (2.3 female vs. 1.8 male). A significant interaction effect of sex by country, illustrated below shows that this effect was particularly pronounced in Italy (1.9 for males *vs.* 2.8 for females), was there, but to a lesser extent in France and Denmark, and was totally absent in Ireland (2.2 for males *vs.* 2.2 for females). The greatest effect on professional tasks was perceived by Italian women, and the least effect by French men. The reason for the lack of sex difference in Ireland is not immediately apparent, however, it could relate to the relative lack of childcare facilities in Ireland and hence the greater intrusion of childcare responsibilities on both parents' working life. The high score manifested by the Italian women may reflect the traditional culture of Italy in which it is the social norm for women to more totally embrace the mothering role and hence they may be more reluctant to relinquish control over home and children. The widespread availability of public childcare in Denmark and France may help to explain the relatively lower levels of intrusion of the birth on the respondents' professional tasks.

Table 8.2. Effect of the Birth of the Youngest Child: Changes in the Professional Tasks of Respondents: Mean Scores by Country and Sex (N=400)

	France	Italy	Denmark	Ireland	All countries
Male	1.3	1.9	1.6	2.2	**1.8**
Female	2.0	2.8	2.0	2.2	**2.3**
Total	**1.7**	**2.3**	**1.9**	**2.2**	**2.0**

(1 = none, 4 = very much)
Country: $F = 10.07$, $df = 3$; $p \leq 0.001$
Sex: $F = 27.36$, $df = 1$; $p \leq 0.001$
Sex x Country: $F = 3.58$, $df = 3$; $p = 0014$

1.4. Domestic Chores

A majority of respondents overall (64%) said that there was a significant change in the amount of domestic chores they faced; 37% said "a fair amount" and 27% said "very much". Danish parents were noteworthy in that a full 18% said that the amount of domestic chores that they did had not changed at all following the birth of the youngest child; whereas in the other countries, the percentage saying "none" ranged from 1 - 9% (Appendix Table A11).

The noteworthy difference for Denmark in comparison with the other countries is reflected in a significant main effect for country ($F = 11.51$, $df = 3$; $p \leq 0.005$).

1.5. Friendships

Looking at the all country data, most respondents replied that their friendships had either not changed at all, or had changed only a little following the birth of their youngest child. Ireland had the highest number of respondents who said that their friendships had not changed at all (44%) compared with the other countries (France 34%, Italy 25%, Denmark 23%) (Appendix Table A12).

There was a low but significant effect of country, with the effect of the birth on parents' friendships changing more in Denmark and Italy, and less so in Ireland and France (F = 2.65, df = 3; p≤0.05).

1.5. Free-Time

Respondents agreed across all countries that their free time had changed significantly following the birth of their youngest child, with only 7% reporting that it had not changed at all. However, only 19% of Danish respondents reported that it had changed very much compared to 51% of the French, 42% of the Irish and 39% of the Italians. Similarly, a full 13% of Danish respondents said that their free time had not changed at all compared to 4 -5% in the other countries (see Table A13).

There was a highly significant difference between countries (F = 6.40, df = 3; p≤0.001), with Danish parents reporting that the birth of the youngest child had affected their free time significantly less than it had done for parents in any of the other countries. This may be related to the greater family-friendly nature of the Danish workplace and society in general. This will be explored in greater detail in a subsequent section.

1.6. Relationship with Partner

Respondents' answers concerning the effect of the birth on their relationship with their partner varied quite a lot. A quarter indicated that the birth had had no effect on their relationship with their partner, a third said that that it had "a little " effect and 41% said that it had had either "a fair amount" or "very much" effect on the relationship (Table A14)

There was a significant difference between countries: the birth of the youngest child had affected relationship with the partner least in France (2.5), whereas it had had a greater effect on respondents' relationships in the other three countries, who did not differ greatly from each other (means = 2.7 - 2.8).

A low but significant interaction effect by country and sex, illustrated below reveals that in Denmark and in Ireland, the effect of the birth on the relationship with the partner was greater for males than for females, whereas in France, the effect was greater for females. In Italy there was essentially no difference between the sexes.

Table 8.3. Effect of the Birth of the Youngest Child: Changes in the Respondents' Relationship with their Partner: Mean Scores by Country and Sex (N=400).

	France	Italy	Denmark	Ireland
Male	2.3	2.8	2.8	3.0
Female	2.6	2.9	2.5	2.7
Total	2.5	2.8	2.7	2.8

(1 = none, 4 = very much)
Country: $F = 4.71$, $df = 3$; $p \leq 0.005$
Country x Sex: $F = 3.23$, $df = 3$; $p \leq 0.05$

An examination of the all-country data shows that 74% of respondents said that the birth had affected their relationships with their partners positively (27%, "somewhat positively", 33% "positively" and 14% "very positively"). Only 26% said that the birth affected the relationship negatively, with the vast majority of these (23%) saying that it affected the relationship "somewhat negatively". Less than 3% reported that the birth had affected the relationship "negatively" or "very negatively" (Appendix Table A15).

These responses may, of course, reflect in some part, a social desirability response set. This is evidenced by the fact that 25% of the Danish respondents who said that their relationship with their partner had changed did not answer this question, and it may be inferred that this masks a negative response, since it may be presumed that they would have answered the question had the change been in a positive direction. An analysis of the 25 Danish respondents who failed to answer this question, showed that they were equally divided by sex (12 women, 13 men); thus, there was no sex-bias in the lack of response.

Analysis of variance revealed a significant effect of country, with Danish respondents more likely to report a positive effect on the relationship (4.8 out of 6); the means for the other countries ranged from 4.1 – 4.3. However, in light of the fact that a quarter of the Danish respondents did not answer this question, the results for Denmark may be suspect.

It may be seen in the table below that men were more likely than women to feel the relationship had changed in a positive direction. This is true in France, Italy and Ireland. In Denmark this trend is not apparent; in fact there is a slight tendency for Danish women to be more likely to see the change as positive, though the sex differences are slight. Many of the male respondents anecdotally reported that the birth brought them closer to their partner. To the extent that women were somewhat less likely to report a positive effect than men, may reflect the greater amount of work women have in connection with a birth, particularly if they are also working.

Table 8.4. *Effect of the Birth of the Youngest Child: How the Respondents' Relationship with their Partner Changed: Mean Scores by Country and Sex (N<400).*

	France	Italy	Denmark	Ireland	All countries
Male	4.3	4.5	4.7	4.4	**4.4**
Female	4.0	4.0	4.9	3.9	**4.2**
Total	**4.2**	**4.3**	**4.8**	**4.1**	**4.3**

(1 = very negatively, 6 = very positively)
Country: $F = 4.94$, $df = 3$; $p \leq 0.005$
Sex: $F = 5.13$, $df = 1$; $p \leq 0.05$

2. DIVISION OF LABOUR WITHIN THE HOUSEHOLD

2.1. Individual Domestic and Childcare Activities in the Home

One of the main areas of the study was an examination of domestic and childcare activities and a comparison of mothers and fathers in terms of who did what and in terms of the reciprocal perceptions of who carried out which activities. One of the methods that has been used to study this area is to collect information about the frequency of the different activities concerning childcare and domestic chores (Giovannini and Ventimiglia, 1994). Another way to study the division of labour in the family is to present a list of activities to which the respondent is asked to indicate the person who usually carries them out. In this way one can obtain information about the availability of family and/or other networks in supporting the household management (Zanatta, 1999). Both methods are useful in comparing activity areas of parents in their everyday life. Questions usually refer to activities carried out during the week in order to emphasise problems of reconciliation of work and family life and underline the differences between females and males in daily organisation. In designing the items in this area, we drew upon the work of Giovannini and Ventimiglia (1994), Zanatta (1999) and Haas (1993).

Respondents were asked to indicate who *usually* carried out 12 different domestic and childcare activities during weekdays, including, "Shopping for food", "Preparing meals", "Cleaning", "Playing with the child/ren", etc. The responses could be: "Me", "My Partner", "Both of Us" or "Other". The last option was chosen so infrequently on all but two of the measures (washing/ironing and cleaning) that it is not included in the analyses except in those two cases. It should be borne in mind that, as we did not interview couples, the male and female responses do not reflect reciprocal perceptions in couples. We are merely examining male and female respondents about themselves and their partner; their actual partners did not take part in this study.

We present below percentage responses for each of the items by country and sex. As the response categories are nominal, we carried out Chi-square analyses by sex for each country and for all countries together.

2.1.1. Shopping for Food

The most common response to the question of who usually goes shopping for food in the household was 'me' for women (49%) and 'both of us' for men (52%). Overall more women than men usually did the shopping for food, as evidenced by the fact that 49% of women reported that they usually did the shopping compared to 17% of men who said that they usually did so.

There seemed to be "over-reporting" on this measure, whereby male respondents appeared to overestimate their shopping activity – there was a discrepancy between the proportion of women who said that they alone did the shopping (49%) and the proportion of men who said that their partners did the shopping (31%). Men conversely were more likely to report that both partners did it together (52%) than were women (41%). There was a significant difference between male and female responses for all countries. The disparity in male and female perceptions was greatest in Denmark and Ireland, followed by Italy. While sex differences in France were still apparent, they were smaller, suggesting greater congruity of perceptions among French men and women on this item.

There were significant differences for each country between the male and female responses, with a similar pattern as described above for all countries.

In summary, the following two trends can be seen:

(1) Women do more of each domestic activity;
(2) Men tend to over-report the amount of each domestic activity they do.

The same trends were also seen for the majority of the other variables, with the main exceptions being bathing and playing with the children.

*Table 8.5. Who Usually does the Shopping for Food:
Percentage Distributions by Country and Sex (N=400).*

	France %		Italy %		Denmark %		Ireland %		All Countries %	
	M	F	M	F	M	F	M	F	M	F
Me	18.4	42.0	12.0	36.7	20.0	58.0	16.0	60.0	16.6	48.7
My partner	26.5	14.0	26.0	6.1	36.0	6.0	36.0	12.0	31.2	10.1
Both of us	55.1	44.0	62.0	57.1	44.0	36.0	48.0	28.0	52.3	41.2
Total	100.0	100.0	100.0	100.0	100.0	100.0	100.0	100.0	100.0	100.0
	$\chi^2 = 7.10$ df = 2 $p \leq 0.05$		$\chi^2 = 12.39$ df = 2 $p \leq 0.005$		$\chi^2 = 20.37$ df = 2 $p \leq 0.001$		$\chi^2 = 21.37$ df = 2 $p \leq 0.001$		$\chi^2 = 55.62$ df = 2 $p \leq 0.001$	

2.1.2. Preparing Meals

Concerning the preparation of meals, there was a highly significant difference between male and female responses for all countries. The most common response to the question of who usually prepares meals in the household was 'me' for women (60%) and 'my partner' for men (43%), so overall more women than men usually prepare the meals. There was evidence of " over-reporting", or at very least discrepant perceptions - on this measure also. There was a discrepancy between the number of women who said that they alone prepared meals (60%) and the number of men who said that their partners usually prepared the meals (43%). Men conversely were more likely to report that both partners did it (40%) than were women (30%).

There were significant differences for each country between the male and female responses, with a similar pattern as described above for all countries.

Table 8.6. Who Usually Prepares Meals:
Percentage Distributions by Country and Sex (N=400)

	France %		Italy %		Denmark %		Ireland %		All Countries %	
	M	F	M	F	M	F	M	F	M	F
Me	12.5	51.0	2.0	63.3	34.0	72.0	18.0	54.2	16.7	60.2
My partner	54.2	16.3	49.0	4.1	32.0	10.0	38.0	8.3	42.9	9.7
Both of us	33.3	32.7	49.0	32.7	34.0	18.0	44.0	37.5	40.4	30.1
Total	100.0	100.0	100.0	100.0	100.0	100.0	100.0	100.0	100.0	100.0
	$\chi^2 = 21.17$ df = 2 $p \leq 0.001$		$X^2 = 48.34$ df = 2 $p \leq 0.001$		$\chi^2 = 15.04$ df = 2 $p \leq 0.001$		$\chi^2 = 18.41$ df = 2 $p \leq 0.001$		$\chi^2 = 92.90$ df = 2 $p \leq 0.001$	

2.1.3. Washing Up
The differences between male and female responses were not so different in relation to who does the washing up. The differences were highly significant in the all-country data, but in the individual country data, only Italy showed significant differences between male and female respondents.

The most common response to the question of who usually does the washing up in the household was 'both of us' for both male (58%) and female (46%) respondents. There was some over-reporting on this measure also – there was a discrepancy between the number of men who said that their partner usually did the washing up (22%) compared to the number of women who said that they usually did the washing up (38%) and the number of women who said that their partners did the washing up (16%). Men were also more likely to report that both partners did it (58%) than women were (46%). On the other hand, women were more likely to give estimates of partners' participation that more closely corresponded to men's own assessment of their participation when it came to men with prime responsibility for washing up (16% estimate by women and 20% estimate by men).

Table 8.7. Who Usually does the Washing Up:
Percentage Distributions by Country and Sex (N=400)

	France %		Italy %		Denmark %		Ireland %		All Countries %	
	M	F	M	F	M	F	M	F	M	F
Me	20.5	31.9	13.6	63.8	15.9	24.5	29.2	32.7	20.0	38.0
My partner	25.0	21.3	38.6	6.4	13.6	20.4	10.4	16.3	21.7	16.1
Both of us	54.5	46.8	47.7	29.8	70.5	55.1	60.4	51.0	58.3	45.8
Total	100.0	100.0	100.0	100.0	100.0	100.0	100.0	100.0	100.0	100.0
	$\chi^2 = 1.54$ df = 2 n.s.		$\chi^2 = 27.13$ df = 2 $p \leq 0.001$		$\chi^2 = 2.33$ DF = 2 n.s.		$\chi^2 = 1.11$ df = 2 n.s.		$\chi^2 = 14.60$ df = 2 $p \leq 0.001$	

2.1.4. Managing Home-Life

In relation to who has most responsibility for "managing home life", there were again highly significant differences between perceptions of male and female respondents in all countries. The most common response to the question of who usually manages/ organises/plans family tasks and home life was 'me' for women (60%) and 'both of us' for men (55%). Only 4% of men said that they were responsible. There was a tendency toward over-reporting on this measure also – there was a discrepancy between the number of women who said that they alone managed home life (60%) and the number of men who said that their partners managed the home life (41%). Men conversely were more likely to report that both partners did it together (55%) than were women (38%). This suggests that both men and women either over-report the extent to which they themselves manage home life, or under-report the amount that their partners do.

There were highly significant differences for each country between the male and female responses, with a similar pattern as described above for all countries. As in the case of meal preparation, there tended not to be over-reporting, but rather congruity in the male and female perceptions of who did what.

Table 8.8. Who Usually Manages Home Life:
Percentage Distributions by Country and Sex (N=400)

	France %		Italy %		Denmark %		Ireland %		All Countries %	
	M	F	M	F	M	F	M	F	M	F
Me	0.0	46.0	6.0	60.0	0.0	70.0	10.0	60.0	4.0	59.8
My partner	48.0	4.0	32.0	0.0	50.0	0.0	30.0	6.0	40.5	2.0
Both of us	52.0	50.0	62.0	40.0	50.0	30.0	60.0	34.0	55.5	38.2
Total	100.0	100.0	100.0	100.0	100.0	100.0	100.0	100.0	100.0	100.0
	$\chi^2=41.64$ df = 2 p≤0.001		$\chi^2=40.46$ df = 2 P≤0.001		$\chi^2=62.50$ df = 2 p≤0.001		$\chi^2=29.45$ df = 2 p≤0.001		$\chi^2=173.32$ df = 2 p≤0.001	

2.1.5. Washing and Ironing

As with the previous measures, there were highly significant sex differences, in the all country data and for each country separately concerning who did the washing and ironing. In approximately two-thirds of households it is the women who do the washing and ironing, and there is a high level of agreement between the male and female respondents about this: 65% of women said that they did, and 60% of men said that their partners did it themselves. It is noteworthy that there was no visible over-reporting on this measure. There is clear agreement.

It is interesting to note that whereas on most other measures of domestic activity, the option of having another person, other than the partner, do the chore was little used, in the case of washing and ironing, this option was more common. Over all countries, between 9-12% reported that another person did the washing and ironing. In Italy and France this trend was even stronger: 24% of French male respondents said that they had outside help in to do the ironing, and not a single male respondent said that they themselves usually did it. In Ireland and Denmark using outside help for washing and ironing was relatively rare. After washing and ironing, cleaning was the only other domestic activity where more than 10% of respondents reported "other" (see below).

Table 8.9. Who Usually does the Washing/Ironing Clothes:
Percentage Distributions by Country and Sex (N=400)

	France %		Italy %		Denmark %		Ireland %		All Countries %	
	M	F	M	F	M	F	M	F	M	F
Me	0.0	61.2	4.0	66.0	9.8	62.0	6.0	70.0	5.0	64.8
My partner	62.0	4.1	64.0	4.0	52.9	6.0	60.0	2.0	59.5	4.0
Both of us	14.0	18.4	14.0	14.0	33.3	32.0	34.0	24.0	24.0	22.1
Other	24.0	16.3	18.0	16.0	3.9	0.0	0.0	4.0	11.5	9.0
Total	100.0	100.0	100.0	100.0	100.0	100.0	100.0	100.0	100.0	100.0
	$\chi^2=56.53$ df = 2 p≤0.001		$\chi^2=53.99$ df = 2 p≤0.001		$\chi^2=40.00$ df = 2 p≤0.001		$\chi^2=56.94$ df = 2 p≤0.001		$\chi^2=199.68$ df = 2 p≤0.001	

2.1.6. Cleaning

In relation to cleaning, there were highly significant differences between reponses of male and female respondents in all countries. The most common answer to the question of who usually does the cleaning was 'me' for women (42%) and 'both of us' for men (51%). Looking at the 'me' responses for both men and women, 2-12% of the men said they usually do the cleaning compared to 40-46% of the women, so it is clear that overall more women than men usually do the cleaning. There was evidence of some over-reporting on this measure also – there was a discrepancy between the number of women who said that they alone did the cleaning (42%) and the number of men who said that their partners did (27%). Men conversely were more likely to report that both partners did it together (51%) than were women (36%). This suggests that both men and women either over-report the extent to which they themselves do the cleaning, or under-report the amount that their partners do.

There were also highly significant differences between male and female responses within in each country. As with many of the other measures, the French respondents showed less of over-reporting than respondents from the other countries.

As with washing/ironing, respondents reported using 'other' help with cleaning more often than they did in relation to most household and child-care tasks - about 15% of the total sample. As with the washing/ironing, this figure is far greater than the proportion of men with usual responsibility (8%). When comparing countries we can see again that the French respondents were the group most likely to have outside help for cleaning (24%). Irish respondents were the least likely to do so (6%).

Table 8.10. Who Usually does the Cleaning:
Percentage Distributions by Country and Sex (N=400)

	France %		Italy %		Denmark %		Ireland %		All Countries %	
	M	F	M	F	M	F	M	F	M	F
Me	2.0	42.0	12.0	46.0	10.0	40.0	10.0	42.0	8.5	42.2
My partner	34.0	6.0	26.0	6.0	26.0	6.0	22.0	8.0	26.5	6.5
Both of us	36.0	32.0	48.0	32.0	52.0	36.0	64.0	42.0	50.5	35.7
Other	28.0	20.0	14.0	16.0	12.0	18.0	4.0	8.0	14.5	15.6
Total	100.0	100.0	100.0	100.0	100.0	100.0	100.0	100.0	100.0	100.0
	$\chi^2=28.77$ df = 2 $p \leq 0.001$		$\chi^2=17.88$ df = 2 $p \leq 0.001$		$\chi^2=17.31$ df = 2 $p \leq 0.001$		$\chi^2=16.06$ df = 2 $p \leq 0.001$		$\chi^2=73.99$ df = 2 $p \leq 0.001$	

2.1.7. Taking the Children to School/Crèche

Taking the children to school was a rather different kind of activity to the others previously listed. The sex differences were not so pronounced for this variable – there were significant differences for the all-country data ($p \leq 0.01$) but in the French and Danish data the differences were non-significant and in the Italian and Irish data the sex differences were only moderately significant.

For the all-country data, the majority of both men and women reported that they both shared in taking the children to school, crèche, etc. (59% men, 54% women). Female respondents were more likely to respond that they themselves usually took the children (32%) than were men (18%). There was the same discrepancy between male and female reporting as on other variables, with 23% of men saying their partner usually took the children to the crèche/school, whereas 32% of women said that they actually did.

Table 8.11. *Who Usually Takes the Children to Crèche: Percentage Distributions by Country and Sex (N=400)*

	France %		Italy %		Denmark %		Ireland %		All Countries %	
	M	F	M	F	M	F	M	F	M	F
Me	14.6	22.9	17.8	41.9	19.1	20.4	19.6	42.6	18.3	31.6
My partner	14.6	16.7	24.4	11.6	21.3	14.3	32.6	14.9	22.6	14.4
Both of us	70.8	60.4	57.8	46.5	59.6	65.3	47.8	42.6	59.1	54.0
Total	100.0	100.0	100.0	100.0	100.0	100.0	100.0	100.0	100.0	100.0
	$\chi^2 = 1.35$ df = 2 n.s.		$\chi^2 = 6.84$ df = 2 $p \leq 0.05$		$\chi^2 = 0.81$ df = 2 n.s.		$\chi^2 = 7.17$ df = 2 $p \leq 0.05$		$\chi^2 = 10.36$ df = 2 $p \leq 0.01$	

2.1.8. Playing with the Children

The sex differences were not so pronounced on the variable "Playing with children" as they were on the housework-related variables. For the all-country data the differences were significant at the $p \leq .0.01$ level, but for the individual countries, Denmark was the only one with a significant sex difference; Danish women were more likely to see this as a male activity.

Nearly all the respondents said that both partners played with the children – 86% of both men and women questioned reported 'both of us'. There was no over-reporting here, unlike with the other variables: 9% of women said that their partner usually did the playing, compared to 10.5% of men who said that they primarily did the playing; 4.5% of women said that they usually played with the children, and 4% of men said that their partners usually did the playing.

*Table 8.12. Who Usually Plays with the Children:
Percentage Distributions by Country and Sex (N=400)*

	France %		Italy %		Denmark %		Ireland %		All Countries %	
	M	F	M	F	M	F	M	F	M	F
Me	4.0	4.1	22.0	12.0	8.2	0.0	6.0	2.0	10.5	4.5
My partner	4.0	4.1	2.0	6.0	6.1	20.4	4.0	5.9	4.0	9.0
Both of us	92.0	91.8	76.0	82.0	85.7	79.6	90.0	92.2	85.5	86.4
Total	100.0	100.0	100.0	100.0	100.0	100.0	100.0	100.0	100.0	100.0
	$\chi^2 = 0.00$ df = 2 n.s.		$\chi^2 = 2.59$ df = 2 n.s.		$\chi^2 = 7.88$ df = 2 $p \leq 0.05$		$\chi^2 = 1.23$ df = 2 n.s.		$\chi^2 = 8.65$ df = 2 $p \leq 0.01$	

2.1.9. Feeding the Children

In relation to who had primary responsibility for feeding the children, there were highly significant sex differences for all countries together and separately. Whilst the majority of respondents answered that both partners usually fed the children (70-80%), very few men reported that they were the sole one who usually did it. Italian men were least likely to say they were the ones who usually fed the children (0%) and Danish men were the most likely (6%). Two to four per cent of French and Irish men said they were primarily responsible for feeding the children. A fair proportion of women, on the other hand, said that they were primarily responsible for feeding the children. This ranged from 26% in Denmark to 37% in Italy, a complete mirror of the male responses in these countries. There was the usual over-reporting evident here, with 29% of female respondents saying that they usually fed the children, and only 18% of male respondents saying that their partners usually did so.

Table 8.13. Who Usually Feeds the Children:
Percentage Distributions by Country and Sex (N=400)

	France %		Italy %		Denmark %		Ireland %		All Countries %	
	M	F	M	F	M	F	M	F	M	F
Me	2.0	30.0	0.0	36.7	6.0	26.0	4.0	27.1	3.0	29.4
My partner	14.0	0.0	22.0	0.0	14.0	0.0	20.0	4.2	17.5	1.0
Both of us	84.0	70.0	78.0	63.3	80.0	74.0	76.0	68.8	79.5	69.5
Total	100.0	100.0	100.0	100.0	100.0	100.0	100.0	100.0	100.0	100.0
	$\chi^2 = 19.89$ df = 2 $p \leq 0.001$		$\chi^2 = 29.91$ df = 2 $p \leq 0.001$		$\chi^2 = 13.37$ df = 2 $p \leq 0.001$		$\chi^2 = 13.72$ df = 2 $p \leq 0.001$		$\chi^2 = 73.30$ df = 2 $p \leq 0.001$	

2.1.10. Changing Nappies/ Dressing theChildren

In relation to who changed the nappies/ dressed the children, there were again highly significant sex differences in every country. As with the previous measure, the majority of respondents in every country reported that both partners usually carried out these activities (68-81%), the second most common answer was that the woman of the house did so (31% of women said they were primarily responsible) and there was the usual reporting bias in every country (although less so in France), whereby only 17% of men reported that their partners usually changed the nappies/dressed the children.

Table 8.14. Who Usually Changes Nappies/ Dresses the Children:
Percentage Distributions by Country and Sex (N=400)

	France %		Italy %		Denmark %		Ireland %		All Countries %	
	M	F	M	F	M	F	M	F	M	F
Me	0.0	30.6	2.0	36.2	0.0	24.0	6.0	34.0	2.0	31.0
My partner	26.0	2.0	12.2	0.0	16.0	0.0	14.0	0.0	17.1	0.5
Both of us	74.0	67.3	85.7	63.8	84.0	76.0	80.0	66.0	80.9	68.5
Total	100.0	100.0	100.0	100.0	100.0	100.0	100.0	100.0	100.0	100.0
	$\chi^2 = 25.51$ df = 2 $p \leq 0.001$		$\chi^2 = 22.19$ df = 2 $p \leq 0.001$		$\chi^2 = 20.20$ df = 2 $p \leq 0.001$		$\chi^2 = 17.47$ df = 2 $p \leq 0.001$		$\chi^2 = 83.38$ DF = 2 $p \leq 0.001$	

2.1.11. Bathing the Children

There were highly significant sex differences on bathing children for every country. Both partners most commonly bathe the children, but overall, mothers do it more often alone than fathers do. There is no over-reporting bias, unlike for the majority of measures.

Table 8.15. Who Usually Bathes the Children:
Percentage Distributions by Country and Sex (N=400)

	France %		Italy %		Denmark %		Ireland %		All Countries %	
	M	F	M	F	M	F	M	F	M	F
Me	4.1	41.7	4.1	38.8	4.1	28.0	8.0	36.0	5.1	36.2
My partner	38.8	2.1	32.7	10.2	26.5	6.0	40.0	10.0	34.5	6.6
Both of us	57.1	56.3	63.3	51.0	69.4	66.0	52.0	54.0	60.4	57.1
Total	100.0	100.0	100.0	100.0	100.0	100.0	100.0	100.0	100.0	100.0
	$\chi^2 = 30.94$ df = 2 $p \leq 0.001$		$\chi^2 = 20.17$ df = 2 $p \leq 0.001$		$\chi^2 = 15.26$ df = 2 $p \leq 0.001$		$\chi^2 = 17.93$ df = 2 $p \leq 0.001$		$\chi^2 = 83.49$ df = 2 $p \leq 0.001$	

2.1.12. Picking the Children up When they Cry at Night

Picking up the children when they cry at night can interrupt a working parent's precious sleeping time. As in the case of most of the other domestic and childcare activities, there were highly significant sex differences for this question for the all-country data, but the differences were less pronounced in Ireland and Denmark and not significant at all in France. "Both of us" was the most common response for both men and women in the all-country data (60% men, 50% women). The next most common response for female respondents was "Me" (42%) and for male respondents, "My partner " (24%). Hence, although there is an over-reporting bias here, both male and female respondents agree that where both partners do not see to the children at night, it is more often the mother who does. Only 16% men said that they are the ones who pick up the children when they cry at night compared to 42% women.

Table 8.16. Who Usually Picks up the Children when they Cry at Night:
Percentage Distributions by Country and Sex (N=400)

	France %		Italy %		Denmark %		Ireland %		All Countries %	
	M	F	M	F	M	F	M	F	M	F
Me	14.0	32.7	16.3	53.1	16.0	44.0	18.0	38.8	16.1	42.2
My partner	22.0	16.3	32.7	0.0	24.0	10.0	18.0	4.1	24.1	8.0
Both of us	64.0	51.0	51.0	46.9	60.0	46.0	64.0	57.1	59.8	49.7
Total	100.0	100.0	100.0	100.0	100.0	100.0	100.0	100.0	100.0	100.0
	$\chi^2 = 4.85$ df = 2 n.s.		$\chi^2 = 25.61$ df = 2 $p \leq 0.001$		$\chi^2 = 10.34$ df = 2 $p \leq 0.01$		$\chi^2 = 8.28$ df = 2 $p \leq 0.05$		$\chi^2 = 41.15$ df = 2 $p \leq 0.001$	

2.2. Global Measures of Domestic and Childcare Activities in the Home

2.2.1. Sum of 'Me', Sum of 'My Partner and Sum of 'Both of Us'

We created three global measures for all of the domestic activities and child-care activities, summing the number of times respondents responded "Me", the number of times "My Partner", and the number of times "Both of Us". Given that we examined 12 different activities, the potential scale ranged from 1 – 12.

When looking at these global measures for all four countries together, there were no significant differences between the countries, or between high and low socio-economic status. There were, however, highly significant sex effects across countries on each of three measures.

Female respondents were significantly more likely to respond "Me", than were male respondents. That is, the female respondents reported that they did domestic activities themselves significantly more often (mean = 4.8) than did the male respondents (mean = 1.2). Conversely, male respondents were significantly more likely to respond "My partner" than were female respondents. Hence male respondents reported that their partners did the domestic activities alone significantly more often (mean =3.4) than did the female respondents reported their partner did (0.8). Male respondents were also significantly more likely to respond "Both of us" (mean = 6.9) than were female respondents (mean = 5.9), as discussed above.

The individual results presented above, together with these confirmatory summary measures, suggest that women in the four countries, are carrying out significantly more of the domestic and child-care activities than men.

Table 8.17. Summary Table Showing Who Usually Carries out Domestic and Childcare Activities: Mean Scores by Country and Sex (N=400)

	France		Italy		Denmark		Ireland		All countries	
	M	F	M	F	M	F	M	F	M	F
Sum of "Me"	0.8	4.3	1.1	5.4	1.4	4.7	1.5	4.9	1.2	4.8
Sum of "Partner"	3.6	1.1	3.6	0.5	3.2	1.0	3.2	0.9	3.4	0.8
Sum of "Both of Us"	6.7	6.1	6.7	5.4	7.1	6.1	7.2	5.9	6.9	5.9

(1 = minimum, 12 = maximum)
Sum of "Me" Sex: $F=291.4$, $df = 1$; $p \leq 0.001$
Sum of "Partner" Sex: $F=221.8$, $df = 1$; $p \leq 0.001$
Sum of "Both of us" Sex: $F=18.3$, $df = 1$; $p \leq 0.001$

2.2.2. HelpIndex

We also created a second type of global measure that showed how much help respondents receive with all the domestic activities put together. We called this 'HELPINDEX' and it was created by giving all the 'Me' responses a value of 1 (indicating no help), giving all the 'Both of us' responses a value of 2 (indicating a medium amount of help) and giving all the 'Partner' and 'Other' responses a value of 3 (indicating a lot of help). These were then summed to produce the HELPINDEX.

There were significant differences by country, sex and SES on the HELPINDEX and also a moderately significant interaction effect between those three variables. French respondents appeared to receive the most help with domestic activities and Irish respondents the least. Male respondents received significantly more help than female respondents. Those in high SES jobs received significantly more help than those in low SES jobs. Overall the group receiving least help was low SES, female respondents from all countries, as well as high SES, Italian women.

Table 8.18. Summary Table Showing How Much Help Respondents Receive with the Domestic & Childcare Activities (HELPINDEX): Mean Scores by Country, Sex and SES (N=400)

		France	Italy	Denmark	Ireland	Total Sex	Total SES
Male	Lo	27.5	26.4	25.1	25.8	26.6	low = 23.1
	Hi	27.5	27.7	27.1	25.6		
Female	Lo	19.9	19.9	19.8	19.7	20.3	high = 24.0
	Hi	22.5	18.8	21.3	20.5		
Total Country		24.4	23.4	23.3	22.9	23.5	23.5

(12 = minimum, 36 = maximum)
Country $F=4.49$, $df = 3$; $p \leq 0.005$ Sex $F=409.73$, $df = 1$; $p \leq 0.001$
SES $F=8.05$, $df = 1$; $p \leq 0.005$
Country x Sex x SES $F=2.85$, $df = 3$; $p \leq 0.05$

3. CHILDCARE

3.1. Usual Childcare Arrangements for the Youngest Child

As childcare is one of the most important factors in the whole equation of successfully reconciling work and family life, it constituted a major area of our study.

We asked respondents what their usual childcare arrangements were for their youngest child (aged under 6) when they themselves were at work – the most often used option, the next most often and the third most often.

In France the most common childcare option was the école maternelle. In the other three countries the most common was the childcare center, nursery or non-workplace crèche. Grandparents and partners were also a common first option in Italy and Ireland, as were unregistered child minders in Ireland.

The second most used option was the one parents usually used to bridge the gap between for example, when the childcare center closed and the respondent returned from work. Approximately 80% of parents used more than one childcare option, the second one usually being partners (32%) or grandparents (see Appendix Table A16).

Table 8.19. Childcare Arrangement for Youngest Child when Parent is at Work (Most Often): Percentage Distributions by Country (N=400)

	France %	Italy %	Denmark %	Ireland %	All Countries %
Self	2.0	0.0	0.0	0.0	0.5
Partner	1.0	13.0	3.0	15.2	8.0
Grandparent	5.0	21.0	2.0	17.2	11.5
Other relative	1.0	2.0	1.0	1.0	1.3
Work crèche /childcare ctr/ nursery	6.0	1.0	3.0	11.1	5.3
Other crèche /childcare ctr/ nursery	18.0	56.0	79.0	28.3	45.0
School/ école maternelle	46.0	0.0	1.0	12.1	14.8
Childminder (registered)	13.0	1.0	9.0	3.0	6.5
Childminder(unreg)/ babysitter/neighbour	6.0	2.0	2.0	12.1	5.8
Other/ N.A.	2.0	4.0	0.0	0.0	1.6
Total	100.0	100.0	100.0	100.0	100.0

Approximately half of the respondents interviewed used a third childcare option during the week, and again the majority of people used partners and grandparents as their third option. Irish respondents were least likely to use a third childcare arrangement during the week – 37% as compared to over 50% of the respondents from the other countries (see Appendix Table A17).

The histogram below shows a summary of the distribution of most used childcare options, grouped by type of care. The most notable finding is that group care is the most commonly used form of child-care for the young child, being used by 66% over all countries. It is also noteworthy that this form of care is much more common in Denmark in France than in Ireland or in Italy. In Ireland and Italy, while group care is also the most common mode of childcare, working parents in these two countries are much more likely to rely on their partners and grandparents, or other relatives (33% in Ireland and 36% in Italy) than are parents in France or Denmark, in which only 6-7% use relatives as the primary mode of childcare for the young child.

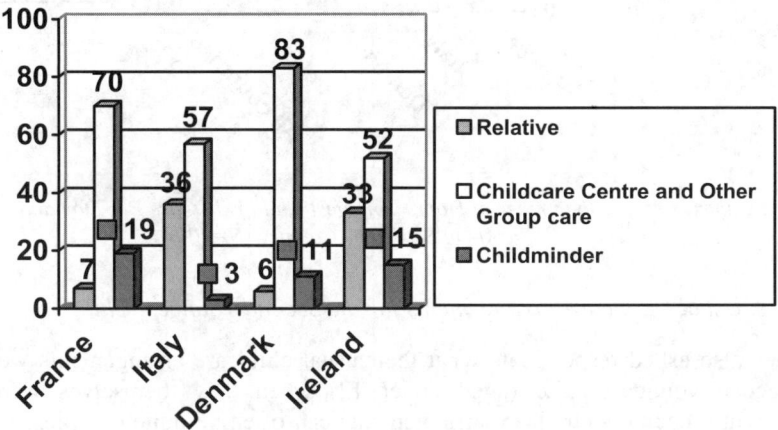

Figure 8.1: Summary Figure Showing Percentage of Respondents using Different Grouped Types of Childcare: Percentage Distributions by Country (N=400)

3.1.1. Hours Youngest Child is in Care

We found that on average the youngest child spent 33.4 hours per week, during weekdays, in care other than by their parents; this averages 7.3 hours per day (Appendix Table A18). Children were found to be in non-parental care for the longest time per day and per week in France – 37 hours per week on average. Children in Italy and Ireland were in non-parental childcare for the shortest time – 30-32 hours per week on average. The youngest child in the Danish and French samples were being cared for by someone other than their parents for a significantly longer time per day than the children in Italy and Ireland. There was a significant difference by country (per day: $F = 6.61$, $df = 3$; $p \leq 0.001$; per week: $F = 5.73$, $df = 3$; $p \leq 0.001$). The longer time spent in childcare by French and Danish children reflects the greater availability of childcare facilities for young children in these countries, and indirectly, the attitudes toward childcare.

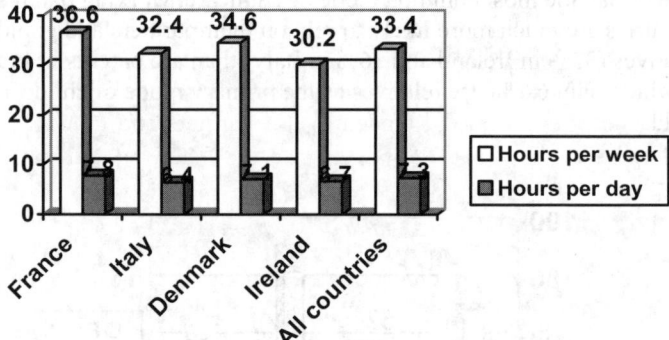

Figure 8.2: Mean number of Hours Youngest Child is in Care Per Day and Per Week: Mean Scores by Country (N=400)

3.2. Usual Childcare Arrangements for the Second Youngest Child

We also asked respondents what their usual childcare arrangements were for their second youngest child (aged under 12) when they themselves were at work. Because people's childcare arrangements can often be quite complex, we asked, as in the case of the youngest child (under six), about the care arrangement used most often, next most often and third most often.

It was found that most of the children attended either school or an école maternelle. This applied to 57% of the children. The next most common arrangement was for the child to be in a childcare center, nursery or other crèche. This applied to 33% of the children. The remaining 10% of children were cared for by a variety of other methods, including partner, grandparent, workplace childcare center, child minder, etc. School or école maternelle was most common in France (80%), followed by Ireland (72.4%). It will be recalled that in Ireland children are eligible, though not required, to attend "infant" classes from the age of four in publicly supported national schools. Four year olds attend "junior infant classes" and five year olds attend "senior infant classes." In Italy only 35.4% were in school and in Denmark the figure was 44%. In Italy and Denmark it was more common for the second youngest child to be in a childcare center, crèche or nursery (58% Italy; 51% Denmark). These results may be seen in Appendix Table A19.

For this group of children, parents and grandparents were the next most often form of childcare, providing a total of 58% of the secondary care (28% each). Grandparents were particularly involved in childcare in Italy (49%) and in Denmark (35%) and to a lesser extent in Ireland (16%) and in France (15%). Partners of the respondent were also very involved in secondary childcare. This was true for 34%

of Irish respondents, 32% of Italian, 28% of Danish and 22% of French. In France 22% of parents used child minders (unregistered), neighbours or babysitters (see Appendix Table A20).

Half of those interviewed did not use a third childcare option in their working week, but those who did tended to use partners and grandparents most often (see Appendix Table A21).

3.3. Reasons for Choosing Childcare Options

Childcare centres and crèches were among the most commonly used childcare arrangements in all of the countries. We asked those respondents who used this option their main reason for using it, and those who chose an alternative why they had done so. The most common reasons for having chosen a childcare centre/ crèche were that both parents were working (45%) and in order to stimulate the child intellectually and socially (45%). The stimulation of the child was seen as particularly important in Denmark, where it was cited by 73% of the parents, as well as in Italy, where 56% of the parents gave it priority. This aspect was given less emphasis by Irish parents, of whom 28% mentioned it, and among French parents, among whom it was cited by 21%. Given that the écoles maternelles are considered "schools", it may be that the French parents, in responding to this item were not considering them as "childcare centres".

The relatively low percentage of Irish parents citing "stimulation of the child" as an important reason for having chosen a childcare centre may reflect the relative recency of the introduction of formalised childcare centres in Ireland and the fact that the debate about childcare has only been occurring over the last few years (Fine-Davis, 2001, 2003). While the importance of high quality educational childcare has been highlighted in numerous commissioned Government reports (e.g., Report on the National Forum for Early Childhood Education, 1998; Goodbody, 1998; Expert Working Group on Childcare, 1999) it may be that this awareness has not yet reached the majority of Irish parents availing of childcare. For the Italians, relieving the grandparents of their burden of care was also important, and for the Danish respondents the professional skills of the staff were important (Appendix Table A22).

For those respondents who had not chosen a childcare centre, a variety of reasons was given and these varied quite a bit by country. For example, a shortage of places was cited by 25% of the French parents. Among the Italian parents, 15% said the child was too young to go to a crèche or childcare center. In Ireland, 23% said they favoured crèches, but only for part-time care; 15% of Irish parents said they felt relatives were better. The issue of cost was cited by 11% of Irish parents, a 7% of French and 4% of Italian; it was not an issue for Danish parents (1%) (see Appendix Table A23).

3.4. Cost of Childcare

At the time of the survey (late 2001-early 2002) the average amount spent by the respondents on childcare was €76 per week. This figure includes both those families in which grandparents or other relatives/partner were minding the children for nothing as well as those who were in the higher-priced centres. There was a significant difference between countries: Irish participants spent the most on childcare and Italian participants the least. There was also a significant difference between participants in high SES jobs and those in low SES jobs: those in high SES jobs spent €40 per week more on childcare on average. When examining the groups more closely, it appears that SES does not make a difference in how much participants spend in Italy or Denmark, but in France and Ireland the gaps are enormous: low SES French participants spend on average €40 per week; high SES participants spend €128. In Ireland, those in low SES jobs spend €57 and those in high SES jobs €116.

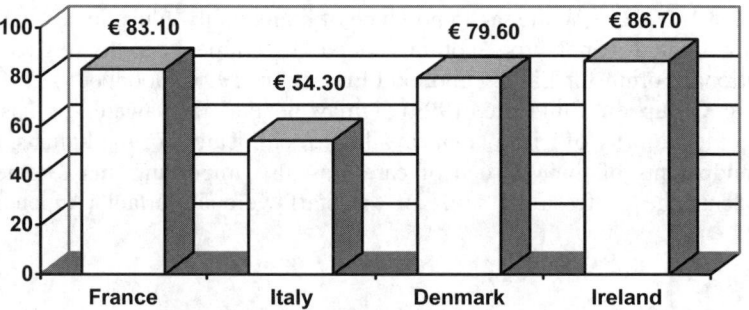

Figure 8.3: Mean Cost of Childcare per Week by Country (In Euros)

However, to really understand and interpret the gap in expenses devoted to childcare, it is important to take into account such issues as tax rebates and government subsidies: French working parents, for example, declared the amount of their expenses *before* tax rebates and childcare allowances which reduce very much the genuine costs of formal childcare. In Ireland, families receive child benefit payments, which have been increased in recent budgets. These too could theoretically offset childcare costs, although they were not taken into account in these self-report measures.

Table 8.20. Mean Cost of Childcare per Week:
Mean Scores by Country and SES (In Euros) (N=400)

	France	Italy	Denmark	Ireland	All countries
Low SES	€39.70	€52.30	€75.90	€56.90	€56.30
High SES	€128.30	€56.30	€84.70	€116.40	€96.70
Total	€83.10	€54.30	€79.60	€86.70	€75.90

Country F = 4.39, df = 3; p≤0.005
SES F = 30.22, df = 1; p≤0.001
Country x SES F = 4.39, df = 3; p≤0.001

As was noted earlier in Chapter 5 the current amount spent on childcare has increased since the time these data were collected (see for example, CSO, 2002).

3.5. Satisfaction with Childcare Arrangements

The majority of respondents reported that they were satisfied with their childcare arrangements. There was a significant difference between countries, with Italian participants reporting the least and Irish the most satisfaction (F = 4.49, df = 3; p≤0.005) with their childcare arrangements.

Table 8.21. Satisfaction with Childcare: Mean Scores by Country (N=400)

France	Italy	Denmark	Ireland	All countries
5.2	4.9	5.1	5.4	5.2

(1 = very dissatisfied, 6 = very satisfied)
Country: F = 4.49, df = 3; p≤0.005

The minority of respondents who were dissatisfied with their childcare arrangements reported a variety of reasons. In France the main reason for dissatisfaction among the mothers was that it was too expensive – as born out by the cost of childcare figures above which show that French participants in high SES jobs spent more than any other group interviewed on their childcare arrangements. In Italy and Denmark fathers expressed a lack of sufficient confidence in the personnel and in Ireland this view was held equally by mothers and fathers. French and Danish mothers expressed the view that the hours were too rigid and Irish fathers expressed dissatisfaction at the complexity of having several modes of childcare (see Table A24).

3.6. Alternative, "Back-Up" Childcare Arrangements

Even in the case of good childcare arrangements, emergencies can occur, breakdowns in arrangements can occur, etc. and alternative arrangements need to be found. We asked respondents what options they used when their usual childcare arrangements become unavailable, such as during holidays, when the crèche was closed, grandparents unavailable or the child was sick. We presented respondents with various possibilities: using their own/partner's sick leave, annual leave, flexi-time, parental leave, or an informal arrangement between their employer and themselves. We asked if they or their partner ever used any of these alternative back-up arrangements, and if so, how often.

In Italy, France and in Denmark there is provision for leave to care for sick children, which is a specific category of leave (e.g., "child sick days"). This is paid in Denmark and unpaid in France; in Italy, it is unpaid, but working parents are entitled to figurative contributions (*contributi figurativi*) in the case of children under three. For children 3 – 8 years of age it is also unpaid, but parents are entitled to reduced contributions. In Ireland the concept of child sick days does not exist, although *force majeur* leave, which is quite limited in scope, can be used for serious illness. The provisions available in each of the countries are discussed in greater detail in an earlier chapter. Because of the lack of availability of child sick leave over the four countries we did not include this as an option here.

3.6.1. Respondent's Own or Partner's Sick Leave

The majority of respondents (72%) never used their own sick leave when their usual childcare arrangements became unavailable (Appendix Table A25). However, 28% of the parents in the sample on occasion did have to use their own sick leave as a "back-up" arrangement and the majority of these were women ($F = 9.86$, $df = 1$; $p \leq 0.01$) (Appendix Table A26). Lower SES respondents were also more likely to use their own sick leave when their childcare arrangements broke down ($F = 5.68$, $df = 1$; $p \leq 0.05$). The group most likely to use their own sick leave in this situation was low SES females and the least likely was high SES males.

Respondents' partners tended not to use their sick leave when their usual childcare arrangements became unavailable either – 73% never used this option (Appendix Table A27). The mean response over all countries for partners' use of sick leave when their usual childcare arrangements broke down was 1.5 (rarely to never) (Appendix Table A28). There was a significant difference between male and female respondents on this measure (F = 7.07, df = 1; p≤0.01): males were more likely to report that their partners would take sick leave. This corroborates the finding in the earlier table that women are more likely to use sick leave in this situation than men are. There was also a moderately significant interaction effect of country and sex (F = 2.71, df = 3; p≤0.05). There was little or no difference between the sexes on this measure for Italian, Danish and Irish parents, but the French parents showed by far the greatest sex effect: French men were much more likely to report that their partners use their sick leave when their usual childcare arrangements become unavailable than were French women or any of the other groups.

3.6.2. Annual Leave

Annual leave was more commonly taken than sick leave when the usual childcare arrangements became unavailable. Approximately 42% of all parents in all countries used their own annual leave sometimes, often or always in this situation (Appendix A29). The mean response was 2.3 (rarely to sometimes). There was a significant country effect (F = 4.40, df = 3; p≤0.005). Danish respondents were least likely to take annual leave when their childcare arrangements became unavailable, and the Irish respondents were the most likely to do so. There was also a significant sex effect (F = 7.11, df = 1; p≤0.01) illustrating that mothers were more likely to take annual leave in this situation than were working fathers (Appendix Table A30).

Respondents' partners were also more likely to use their annual leave rather than sick leave when their usual childcare arrangements became unavailable, which backs up the previous set of findings. Half of respondents' partners used this as an option and 34% did so sometimes, often or always (Appendix Table A31). There were significant country differences (F=5.19, df = 3; p≤0.005) (Appendix Table A32). Danish respondents were the least likely to report that their partners would take annual leave when their usual childcare arrangements became unavailable (mean = 1.6, never to rarely) and Italian and Irish respondents were the most likely to do so (mean = 2.2, rarely to sometimes). The Danish responses are likely to reflect the fact that the public child-care facilities are so excellent that such back up arrangements are rarely necessary, and if a child is ill one can take paid child sick days.

There were also significant interaction effects of country and sector (F =3.14, df = 3; p≤0.05) and of country, sector and sex (F = 3.82, df = 3; p≤0.01). These effects related primarily to Ireland. Of all of the groups, it was most common for Irish males working in the public sector to say that their partner's would sometimes take their own annual leave if childcare arrangements broke down (mean = 3.2, sometimes) (Appendix Table A32). This is a surprising finding, given that the public sector is known for being advanced in terms of family friendly policies, and one would have thought that males would not have to rely on their partners for this. One certainly would not have expected public sector males to have to rely on partners more than private sector males. While this is an unexpected and interesting finding, it should be interpreted with caution given the relatively small numbers in the respective cells in the individual countries.

3.6.3. Flexi-time
Only a third of respondents used flexi-time when their usual childcare arrangement became unavailable – most of these being the Danish and, to a lesser extent, the French (Appendix Table A33). There was a significant effect of country, indicating that Italian and Irish parents were significantly less likely to use flexi-time as a back-up childcare arrangement in comparison with Danish and French parents ($F = 6.26$, $df = 3$; $p \leq 0.001$)). In addition to this highly significant country difference, there was also a significant effect of socio-economic status ($F = 8.81$, $df = 1$; $p \leq 0.005$). Respondents in high SES jobs were significantly more likely to use flexi-time than were respondents in low SES jobs, when their usual childcare arrangements became unavailable (Appendix Table A34). This suggests a greater degree of flexibility available to employees in higher SES occupations.

There was a significant interaction effect between SES, public/ private sector and sex ($F = 6.36$, $df = 1$; $p \leq 0.01$) (Appendix, Table A35). Male respondents in high SES jobs in the public sector were much more likely to use flexi-time when their usual childcare arrangements became unavailable than were any of the other groups. Those least likely to use flexi-time in this situation were male, low SES respondents, in both the private and the public sector, and female lows SES respondents in the private sector. Again this suggests less flexibility available to lower SES employees in general, especially those in the private sector. In fact it appears that where flexibility exists in the private sector it is more likely to be available to higher SES employees.

There was also a moderately significant interaction effect between the four variables of country, sex, SES and sector ($F = 3.08$, $df = 3$; $p \leq 0.05$) (Appendix, Table A36). The groups most likely to use flexi-time when their usual childcare arrangements become unavailable are: French female and Danish male high SES respondents working in the public sector and Danish female high SES respondents working in the private sector (rarely-sometimes). The group least likely to use flexi-time in this situation are Italian male low SES respondents working in the public sector (never).

A similar pattern was shown for the partners' use of flexi-time as an alternative childcare arrangement as for the respondents themselves: only a quarter of respondents ever used it, and most were Danish, and to a lesser extent, French (Appendix Table A37). The mean total response for partners' use of flexi-time as an alternative childcare arrangement was 1.6 (never-rarely). There was a significant difference between countries on this measure ($F = 6.62$, $df = 3$; $p \leq 0.001$)(Appendix

Table A38). The Italians and the Irish were the respondents least likely to report that their partners used flexi-leave when their usual childcare arrangements became unavailable, and the Danish and the French were the groups most likely to report that their partners did so. There was also a moderately significant difference between high and low SES (F = 8.9, df = 1; $p \leq 0.01$): respondents in high SES jobs were more likely to report that their partners took flexi-leave than were respondents in low SES jobs.

3.6.4. Parental Leave

Only 10% of respondents ever used parental leave as an alternative childcare option (Appendix Table A39). The reason for this is very likely the fact that parental leave is unpaid in Ireland and generally has to be taken in a block or in other ways by prior arrangement with the employer. In Denmark and France this type of leave is generally taken following maternity leave, as it is sometimes in Ireland, though in Ireland and in France it is unpaid. In Italy a modest payment is made; (see individual country Chapters 2 - 5 for more detail, as well as the comparative chart in Chapter 6

Italian parents were most likely to report using parental leave when their usual childcare arrangements were unavailable (17% did so to some extent) and French and Danish respondents were least likely to do so (only 3-5% reported doing so). This effect for country was modest, but significant (F = 2.90, df = 3; $p \leq 0.05$) (Appendix Table A40). There was a more significant effect for sector (F = 9.73, df = 1; $p \leq 0.005$) – respondents in the public sector were significantly more likely to report that they used parental leave when their usual childcare arrangements were unavailable than were respondents working in the private sector. There was also a moderately significant effect for sex (F = 5.13, df = 1; $p \leq 0.05$): women were more likely to report using parental leave when their usual childcare arrangements became unavailable than were male respondents.

This pattern was corroborated in the question asked about partners: only 4% of females said that their partners used parental leave when childcare arrangements broke down, whereas 13% of males said that *their* partners did (see Appendix tables A41-43).

3.6.5. Informal Arrangements

Informal arrangements were more commonly used than taking sick leave, annual leave or parental leave – 44% of respondents used this option to some extent. The Danish and Irish respondents were most likely to do so – a third of Danish respondents and a quarter of Irish respondents used it 'sometimes', while the Italians were least likely with only a quarter ever using it (Appendix Tables A44-45). There was also a significant interaction effect of country and SES (F = 4.55, df = 3;

p≤0.005): in Italy, Denmark and Ireland, respondents with high SES jobs were more likely to use informal arrangements in this situation, but in France, respondents in low SES jobs were much more likely to do so than their high SES counterparts.

There was a significant interaction effect between all four variables, country, sex, SES and sector (F = 4.13, df = 3; p≤0.01) (Appendix Table A46). The group most likely to use informal arrangements when their usual childcare arrangements were unavailable were Danish high SES parents in the private sector. The groups least likely to be able to avail of informal arrangements in this situation were low SES Italian parents: male public sector workers, and female private sector workers. Among low SES workers, French females in the private sector were relatively advantaged in this regard, having a relatively high degree of informal flexibility.

Data for partners largely corroborates results obtained *vis-a-vis* respondents: 40% of respondents said their partners sometimes used informal arrangements with their employers when childcare arrangements broke down. There were no significant country differences (Appendix Table A47).

3.6.6. Other Arrangements
The use of another relative as an alternative childcare arrangement was extremely common – 58% relied on other relatives "sometimes", "often" or "always", and only a quarter never relied on relatives. (Appendix Table A48).

The French were more likely than parents from the other three countries to rely on a neighbour or a babysitter when their usual childcare arrangements broke down (Appendix Table A49); 55% of French parents used this mode on occasion as compared with only 12% of Irish parents and approximately 22% of Danish and Italian parents.

3.6.7. Summary of Alternative Childcare Arrangements
As may be seen in the summary histogram below, the most common option for when the usual childcare arrangements become unavailable was the use of another relative. Over 80% of Danish, French and Italians used this to some extent, but only half the Irish respondents did. The Irish were, however, much more inclined to use annual leave than any of the other countries, although this was the second most common option for all the other respondents. Informal arrangements were the third most used arrangement, though less so in Italy. Flexi-time was important in France and France was the only country to really use neighbours/babysitters. Parental leave was the least used option in every country, even though it is specifically designed for parents' leave for child-care reasons. One would think that it should be the ideal policy to use in this situation. The fact that it is rarely used is presumably because it cannot be used flexibly and it is very often unpaid. It is clear that parents have to resort to a wide variety of *ad hoc* arrangements when their usual childcare

arrangements break down. Not only is this likely to lead to stress for parents, but in many cases it deprives them of their own entitlement to sick leave and annual leave. The fact that social class differences were detected in relation to informal arrangements, indicates that there are unequal conditions accruing to parents in different social circumstances.

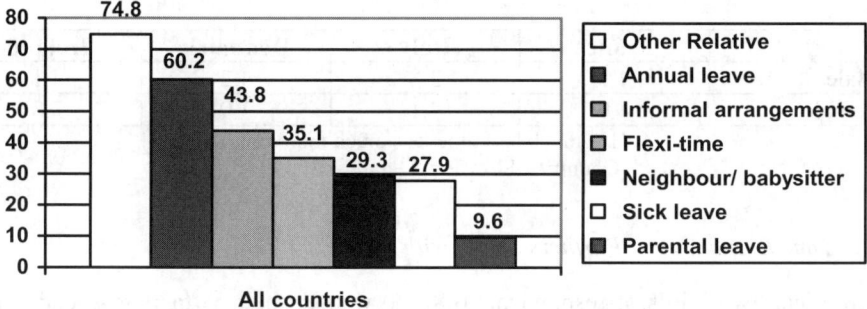

Figure 8.4: Percentage of People that Use Different Alternative Childcare Arrangements.

4. TIME PREFERENCES

The issue of working time and working time preferences are increasingly be examined by researchers and policy makers (e.g., Bielenski et al., 2002; Dutch Ministry of Social Affairs and Employment, 2002) We asked respondents whether they would like to have more or less time with their families, whether they would like their partners to spend more or less time with their families and whether they would like more or less personal time.

4.1. Time Respondents Spend with their Families

The majority of respondents from all countries wanted to spend "more time" (52%) with their families, with a further quarter wanting to spend " much more time" (23%). Only about a quarter (24%) wanted to spend "about the same" with their families as they were currently spending. This pattern appeared to be roughly the same across all countries (Appendix Table A50), and there were no significant differences between countries, sexes or SES groups.

There was, however, a moderately significant interaction effect between country and sex. In Denmark and Ireland, male respondents wanted to spend more time with their families than female respondents did. In Italy, the trend was reversed – female respondents wanted to spend more time with their families than male respondents did. In France both male and female respondents equally wanted to spend more time with their families.

Table 8.22. How much Time Respondents Would Like to Spend with their Family: Mean Scores by Country and Sex (N=400)

	France	Italy	Denmark	Ireland
Male	4.1	3.8	4.2	4.1
Female	4.0	4.1	3.9	3.8

(1 = much less time, 5 = much more time)
Country x Sex: $F = 2.94$, $df = 3$; $p \leq 0.05$

4.2. Time Respondents' Partners Spend with their Families

More than two thirds of respondents (68.5%) wanted their partners to spend either 'more time' (50%) or 'much more' time (18.5%) with the family; 29% were satisfied with the amount of time they currently spent. A negligible amount (2.6%) wanted their partner to spend less or much less time with the family. The pattern was consistent across countries (Appendix Table A51).

However, as was the case in the previous item, regarding respondents' own wish for more time with the family, there was a significant difference between male and female respondents on this measure: female respondents wanted their partners to spend more time with their families than male respondents did. This probably relates to the fact that men work longer hours than women and, as we have seen, women spend more time on domestic and childcare activities in the home.

There was also a moderately significant interaction effect between country and sex. Although female respondents in all countries wanted their partners to spend more time with their families than male respondents wanted their partners to do so, this result was most prominent for Italy and least prominent for Denmark.

Table 8.23. How much Time Respondents Would Like their Partner to Spend with their Family: Mean Scores by Country and Sex (N=400)

	France	Italy	Denmark	Ireland	All Countries
Male	3.7	3.5	3.8	3.6	3.6
Female	4.1	4.2	4.0	4.0	4.1

(1 = much less time, 5 = much more time)
Sex: $F = 33.96$, $df = 1$; $p \leq 0.001$
Country x Sex: $F = 3.72$, $df = 3$; $p \leq 0.05$

4.3. Personal Time

The need for 'personal time' (as opposed to time spent with the family) was also assessed. The most common response of working parents in the sample was for 'more time' (59%) and 16.5% expressed the wish for "much more time" (Appendix Table A52). Thus more than three-quarters of the sample would like more personal time. Less than a quarter were satisfied with the amount of personal time they currently had and only a tiny minority (less than 1%) wanted somewhat less personal time.

There was a significant difference between countries: French parents expressed the greatest wish for more personal time, followed by the Irish and the Italians, whereas Danish respondents were, on average the most content with the amount of personal time that they had. There was also a moderately significant difference between male and female parents, with mothers tending to express a wish for more personal time did fathers. There was a moderately significant interaction effect between country and sex, indicating that Italian and Danish mothers expressed a wish for more personal time than their male counterparts, whereas French and Irish parents, male and female, expressed roughly the same needs.

Table 8.24. How much Personal Time Respondents Would Like to Have: Mean Score by Country (N=400)

	France	Italy	Denmark	Ireland	All Countries
Male	4.1	3.7	3.6	4.0	3.8
Female	4.1	4.1	3.9	3.9	4.0
Total	4.1	3.9	3.7	4.0	3.9

(1 = much less time, 5 = much more time)
Country: $F = 5.18$, $df = 3$; $p \leq 0.005$, Sex: $F = 6.41$, $df = 1$; $p \leq 0.05$
Country x Sex: $F = 3.36$, $df = 3$; $p \leq 0.0$

CHAPTER 9

THE WORKPLACE

The previous chapter focused on the family part of the work-life balance. In this chapter we focus on the other half of the equation – namely the workplace. We begin with descriptive information, covering such issues as working time, commuting, etc. In the context of time and working arrangements, we examine the effect the birth of the youngest child had, if any, on the working arrangements of the parents. We then examine the nature of the workplace in terms of its potential and actual flexibility for working parents. Next, attitudes in the workplace are examined. These include perceived attitudes of colleagues, supervisor and employer concerning one's childcare responsibilities. We are particularly interested in the extent to which the attitude is supportive and flexible or rigid and inflexible.

A key set of questions in this section concerned attitudes in the workplace toward people who avail of "family friendly" policies, such as extended leave for care for newborn children, part-time working, job sharing, etc. Our purpose here is to see if such individuals are perceived in a less favourable light, for example, are they seen as "less serious" about their career? Similarly, attitudes towards the "long-hours culture" were explored as potential barriers to work-life balance. Finally, we examine results concerning workplace policies. Here we look at respondents' reports concerning the existence of a range of family friendly workplace policies, the extent to which respondents availed of these, as well as their attitudes towards the policies.

1. WORKPLACE DEMOGRAPHICS

As already noted, the sample was stratified by socio-economic status and sector of employment. Thus, half of all respondents were in jobs of lower socio-economic status and half in higher; half of all respondents were working in the public sector and half in the private sector. In this initial section on workplace demographics we examine variables relating to commuting, hours at work and related variables.

1.1. Commuting

Respondents were asked how long it took, on average, for them to get to work (in minutes) and also how long it took their partner to get to work. The average for all countries was just about a half hour (32 minutes). Commuting times were longest for Irish respondents (39 minutes on average) and for French respondents (38 minutes). Italian respondents had significantly shorter commuting times (24 minutes), as did Danes (26 minutes).

Table 9.1. Commuting Time: Mean Times by Country in Minutes (N=400)

France	Italy	Denmark	Ireland	All Countries
38	24	26	39	32

$F = 15.48$, $df = 3$; $p \leq 0.001$

In all countries, the car was the most common form of transport to work (58% in all countries). This figure was the highest for Ireland – 70%, and lowest for France, at 47%. The French were even more likely to use the Metro (train) to get to work. Approximately 50% used this form of transport.

In Italy, after the car, which was used by 64.5%, the next most common form of transport was a motorbike (15.6%) – none of the other countries showed this pattern. In Denmark, the bicycle was the next most common form of transport after the car; in the Danish sample a full 43.7% reported cycling to work. In Ireland using the bus was the next most common (13%) after using a car (70%). However, walking to work was more common in Ireland (13%) than in the other countries, though it was also popular amongst 9.5% of the French.

The Irish results are quite similar to results obtained in a recent nationwide Irish study (CSO, 2000). This study found that over half of Irish people in employment drove a car to work in the first quarter of 2000. Two thirds of these car journeys were of less than 10 miles duration. This implies that many people are using the car for short journeys which could potentially be done using other forms of transport such as bus, train or bike. Indeed, recent research has found that commuting by bus in Dublin is significantly faster than by car, according to a new survey of the effectiveness of quality bus corridors in the capital (Dublin Transportation Office, 2002). Thus, the dependence on the car may, in part, be meeting psychological needs and may not always be the most efficient way to get to work.

Table 9.2. Mode of Transport Usually Used:
Percentage Distributions by Country (N=400)

	France %	Italy %	Denmark %	Ireland %	All Countries %
Car	46.6	64.5	49.0	70.1	57.5
Train	49.8	2.1	9.1	7.0	17.1
Bus	9.3	10.0	6.2	13.4	9.7
Bicycle	1.5	4.9	43.7	2.4	13.2
Motorcycle	4.8	15.6	1.8	0.8	5.7
Walking	9.5	5.0	3.0	12.8	7.6
Other	0.0	1.0	1.2	0.0	0.5

Note: The totals in the table come to more than 100% as respondents often used more than one form of transport, and hence ticked more than one mode of transport.

1.2. Hours at Work

Respondents in the four countries spent, on average, 38 hours per week at work, however, men had a significantly longer working week than women (42 hours on average for men and 34 hours for women). This compares with Eurostat figures for the 15 member countries in 1998 of an average working week of 40 hours (Eurostat, 2001). Among the men in the present study, Danish men had the shortest working week (40 hours) and Irish men the longest (45 hours). French and Italian men fell in between with an average working week of 41 hours. Among women, the Irish had the shortest working week (32 hours) and the French and Danish women the longest working week (35 hours); Italian women fell in between with 34 hours.

The women in the four participating countries of this study thus work pretty similar hours, with only three hours difference between the highest and the lowest. The difference between the men is much larger - five hours, with the Irish men working the most (45 hours) and the Danish men working the least (40 hours). From a family perspective, it takes fewer working hours to support a family in Italy and Denmark -around 75 hours a week - a little more in France, 76 hours, and somewhat more in Ireland, namely, 77 hours.

There are not only differences within the sexes but also between the sexes: In all countries women worked significantly fewer hours (34) than men (42). The gap between men and women is smallest in Denmark – only five hours, as compared to 13 in Ireland, where Irish men had the longest working week (45 hours) and Irish women the shortest (32 hours). These figures may be compared with those obtained in the Quarterly National Household Survey (CSO, 2002), Ireland, which found that the average working week for Irish people in the first quarter of 2002 was 38 hours. For male workers it was 42 hours and for female workers, 32 hours. The relatively small gap between Danish men and women is not due to the fact that Danish women work so much more than the other women but rather, because the Danish men work less. So the Danish men get a lot of help from the women in the economic support of the family – or put in another way - there is greater equality between the sexes with respect to labour market participation.

The figure below shows clearly the trend that in every country female respondents worked shorter hours than men. It also illustrates the fact that Irish men work longer hours than any of the other groups, and that Irish women work shorter hours than any other group.

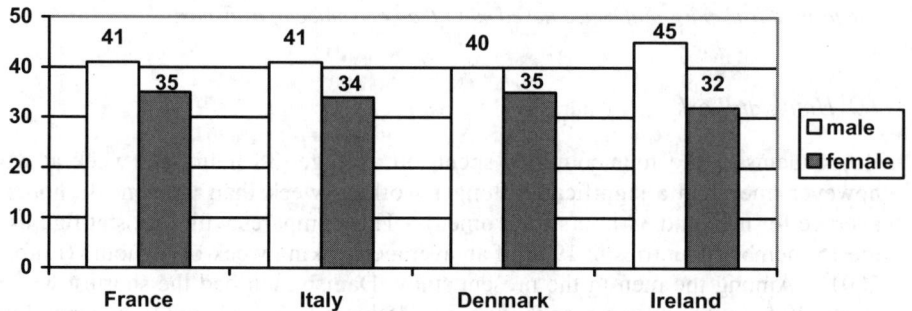

Figure 9.1. Hours Respondent Works per Week: Mean Scores by Country and Sex

The means illustrating these differences are presented below. In addition there was a significant interaction effect of country, sex and SES, indicating that Irish male low SES respondents worked the longest of all the groups – 49 hours per week, and Irish female low SES respondents worked the shortest number of hours in a week - 29 hours.

The hours worked by the respondent's partners, shows a similar pattern to the ones illustrated above: the partners of female respondents (i.e., men) work longer hours than do the partners of male respondents, and the gaps between countries are also similar. This adds validity to the responses given in the previous table (Appendix Table A53).

In all countries, seven out of ten respondents worked typical hours, i.e. approximately 9:00 a.m. to 5:30 p.m. (69%). This figure rose to eight out of ten in Ireland (80%), and dropped to six out of ten (60%) in Italy (Appendix Table A54).

Table 9.3. Hours Respondent Works per Week:
Mean Scores by Country, Sex and SES (N=400)

		France	Italy	Denmark	Ireland	All Countries
Male	Low SES	39	41	38	49	42
	High SES	42	41	42	41	42
	Total	41	41	40	45	42
Female	Low SES	32	34	35	29	33
	High SES	37	34	34	36	35
	Total	35	34	35	32	34

Sex: $F = 91.57$, $df = 1$; $p \leq 0.001$
Country x Sex: $F = 4.86$, $df = 3$; $p \leq 0.005$
Country x Sex x SES: $F = 6.70$, $df = 3$; $p \leq 0.001$

1.3. Sex of Supervisor

Approximately two-thirds of respondents (62%) had a male supervisor, and one third (34%) a female supervisor. This data reflects the widespread and well-known phenomenon that men tend to be more represented than women in managerial positions. Those who did not fall in these two categories were self-employed, for the most part. Denmark had the highest percentage of respondents with female supervisors – 41% compared with the lowest percentage, 29%, for Italy. The higher representation of female supervisors in Denmark is consistent with its longer tradition of equality, reflected also in its greater representation of women in politics.

When we examine the sex of supervisor in relation to the sex of respondent, we see that males are more likely to have a male boss (71%) and only 25% a female boss, whereas among female respondents, only 53% had a male boss and 43% had a female boss. This pattern was quite consistent across the countries. It may reflect the fact that many jobs are sex-segregated (e.g., nursing is primarily a female occupation, construction work is primarily a male occupation, etc.).

Table 9.4. *Sex of Supervisor: Percentage Distributions by Country and Sex (N=400)*

	France %	Italy %	Denmark %	Ireland %	All countries %		
	All	All	All	All	M	F	All
Male	64.4	61.0	58.0	65.0	71.5	52.7	62.1
Female	31.7	29.0	41.0	34.0	25.0	42.8	33.9
Both	1.0	1.0	1.0	0.0	0.0	1.5	0.7
N/A	3.0	9.0	0.0	1.0	3.5	3.0	3.2
Total	100.0	100.0	100.0	100.0	100.0	100.0	100.0

2. CHANGES IN WORK FOLLOWING THE BIRTH OF THE YOUNGEST CHILD

In the previous Chapter on Children and Family Life we examined the effect of the birth of the youngest child on the adjustment of the couple in terms of: 1) the way they organised their day; 2) their life habits; 3) their professional tasks; 4) the extent of their domestic chores; 5) their friendships; and 6) their free time.

In this section we now examine the effects the birth of the couple's youngest child had on their working time and that of their partner. Respondents were asked whether or not they or their partners had modified their working time following the birth of the youngest child, and if so, whether they had increased or decreased it, and finally whether or not they or their partners had temporarily given up their working activity apart from the period of paid maternity/ paternity leave.

2.1. Modified Working Time

The majority of male respondents (73%) said that they had not modified their working time following the birth of their youngest child, with only 27% saying that they had. This contrasts with the female respondents of whom half had changed their working time. On examining the data by country, it is apparent that there is great variability here. While only 8% of French fathers modified their working time, a full 46% of Irish fathers had. Danish and Italian men fell somewhere in between with 30% of Danish fathers saying that they had modified their working time and 24% of Italian fathers. There was much less variability among the mothers in the sample, in fact there was virtually no difference among Irish, French and Italian mothers, of whom slightly more than half modified their working time upon the birth of their youngest child. Only the Danish women differed: only 34% of them had modified their working time, whereas 66% had not.

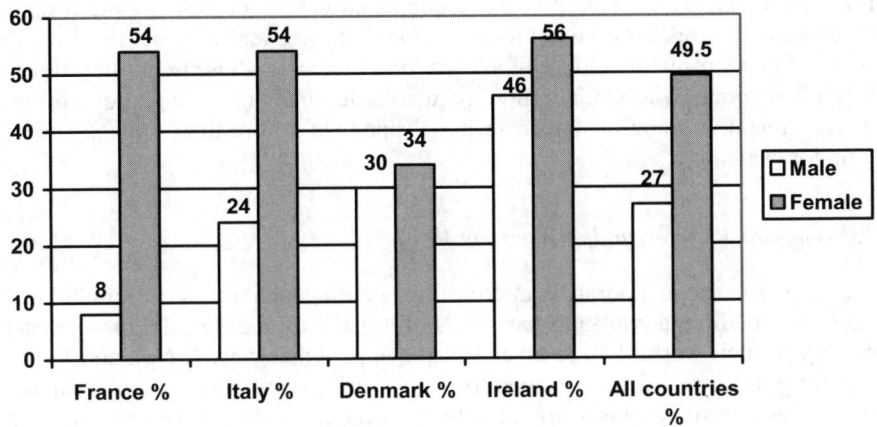

Figure 9.2. Whether Respondents Modified Their Working Time: Percentage Distributions by Country and Sex (N=400)

Approximately half (46.5%) of all males said their partners had modified their working time after the birth of the youngest child, whereas only 15% of the women said that *their* partners had modified their working time. In the case of the male data we see that it quite closely conforms to the percentage of females in the sample saying that they modified their working time (49.5%) thus tending to reinforce the results for the respondents. On the other hand, there is a greater discrepancy between the percentage of males reporting that they had changed their working time (27%) compared with the percentage of females who said their partner had changed his working time (15%). While we have seen many other instances of a correspondence in the data relating to partners which reinforces the data obtained in our own sample, we must bear in mind that the males in our sample are not the same people as the partners of the females in our sample and *vice versa*, so we should not expect a 1:1 correspondence (see Appendix Table A55).

2.2. Increased or Decreased Working Time

Of those respondents who had changed their working time (27% of male respondents and 50% female respondents), the majority had decreased rather than increased it (see Appendix Table A56). This was particularly true for female respondents, of whom 84% of those who changed their working time decreased it. It was less true for male respondents, of whom 59% of those who had changed their working time had decreased it. Eleven percent of men over all four countries increased their working time. However, it is noteworthy that whereas no French or Italian male respondents increased their working time at all, 20% of Danish men and 17% of Irish men did so. Those respondents who modified their working time, but whose hours stayed the same were often people who worked more regular hours than before, e.g., not working late or over-time and going on fewer business trips than before their youngest child was born, for example.

2.3. Temporarily Interrupting Working Activity

The responses on temporarily interrupting working activity were similar to those regarding modifying working time. Half (50%) of the female respondents had interrupted their working time (over and above paid maternity leave), and 21% of the male respondents had (see Appendix Table A57). In France not a single male respondent interrupted his working activity, whereas in Denmark only 38% of men did *not* do so. In Denmark there was also the highest proportion of women who did so – 92% interrupted their working activity, compared to 21% of French females, 38% of Italian females and 46% of Irish females.

Only 17% of women said that their partner had interrupted his working activity following the birth of the youngest child, whereas 41% of men said their partners had done so. This closely mirrors the responses of the respondents about their own behaviour, i.e. 50% of women said they had interrupted their working and 21% of men said they themselves had; this close mirroring of responses held up within countries.

It is interesting to note that whereas Danes were less likely than parents in other countries to modify their working time, they – both men and women - were much more likely to temporarily interrupt their working life after the birth of a child. This *modus vivendi* is made possible by the generous leave time available to working parents. In other countries, it would seem that reducing working hours is a more standard mechanism for coping.

3. POTENTIAL FOR FLEXIBILITY

3.1. Potential and Actual Flexibility in the Workplace

One of the key ways in which workplaces are experienced as family-friendly or not is in terms of the possibility for flexibility on a day-today basis. This can include, for example, the ability to make private phone calls, e.g. to doctors, handymen, etc., run private errands during working time, to owe work time or swap shifts.

Respondents in the study were asked about the *potential* flexibility in their workplaces (i.e., could they do certain things) and then asked about their *actual* flexibility, i.e. did they ever *do* certain things in the workplace. The items in this set are adaptations of items developed by Holt (1994).

The following table presents the responses by country concerning potential flexibility in the workplace.

Table 9.5. Potential Flexibility: Percentage "Yes" by Country (N=400)

	France %	Italy %	Denmark %	Ireland %	All Countries %		
					Males	Females	Total
Acceptability of Making Private Calls	92.9	84.0	100.0	90.1	95.0	88.5	91.7
Acceptability of Running private errands	31.0	28.0	69.0	54.5	53.7	37.3	45.5
Possibility of Owing Work-Time	43.0	50.0	80.0	50.0	52.5	59.0	55.8
Formal Agreement of Flexible Time	54.5	18.2	24.0	21.0	28.0	31.0	29.5
Informal Agreement of Flexible Time	52.0	20.8	52.0	60.0	43.5	49.2	46.3
Possibility of Swapping Shifts	35.0	49.5	47.0	31.0	39.5	41.7	40.6

It was acceptable for the majority of participants to make private calls during work time, with it being most acceptable in Denmark (100% of participants said it was acceptable) and least so in Italy (84%).

A high proportion of the Danish participants as compared to the participants of other countries, said that it was acceptable to run private errands during working hours (69% against the all country average of 46%), that it was possible to owe work time (80% against the all country average of 56%) and that it was acceptable to make private phone-calls during working hours (100% against the all country average of 92%).

In relation to being able to run private errands at work, the Danish high of 69% contrasts with the figure of 28% in Italy. The French also did not have much latitude in this area (only 31% said that it was acceptable). The Irish had more flexibility (55%), but less than the Danes.

In relation to owing work time, a similar pattern was apparent, with the French having least flexibility (43%), the Italians and the Irish having somewhat more (50%), and the Danes having the most (80%).

French participants, however, were more likely to have a formal agreement of flexible working time than any other country; 55% did so, whereas only 18-24% of those in the other countries did.

Informal agreements of flexible time were more common, being available to 52-60% of the respondents in France, Denmark and Ireland, but to only 21% of the Italians.

There appears to be more shift-swapping possible in Italy and Denmark than the other countries where almost half the participants could do so; in France and Ireland only 31-35% reported that they could do this.

There were virtually no sex differences on any of these measures except for running private errands where it was found that men were more likely to be able to do so (54% vs. 37%). Given that women were found to have greater responsibility for domestic and childcare, their lesser ability to run private errands during working time must add to their pressure in balancing work and family life.

3.2. Actual Flexibility

In addition to tapping potential flexibility we also examined the respondents' *actual* flexibility in the workplace. To some extent, these questions overlapped with the previous set (with regard to making private phone calls and running private errands) and to some extent, they overlapped with attitudinal questions asked in another section, i.e. concerning whether the respondent ever leaves early or arrives late due to problems regarding childcare and whether the respondent ever brings a child to work due to problems with childcare. In relation to making private phone calls and running private errands during work, the actual occurrence of these things almost perfectly mirrored the potential flexibility in these areas: 92% of respondents said that it was acceptable to make private calls at work, and 92% also said that they did make private calls at work. Similarly, 46% said that it was acceptable to run private errands at work, and 45% said that they actually did run private errands.

The sex difference that was apparent concerning the potential to run private errands with males being more likely to be able to do so was confirmed in the actual flexibility data. Twenty percent more men than women (54.5% vs. 34.5%) carried out private errands at work. Three-quarters of respondents reported that they sometimes left their job early or arrived late due to problems regarding childcare. There were essentially no country differences in this area.

The final question in this set, "Do you ever bring a child to work on occasion due to problems regarding childcare?", elicited much lower agreement. Eighteen per cent overall said that they did this on occasion (15% of men and 22% of women), but there were large country differences. This behaviour was least acceptable in France, with only 9% of parents saying they ever did it, and also infrequent in Italy (12%) and in Ireland (15%). Denmark was unusual in that 36% of parents said that they did bring a child to work on occasion when there were childcare problems. When we look at the Danish sex breakdown we see that 32% of Danish men reported bringing a child to work on occasion and 40% of Danish women did.

Table 9.6. Actual Flexibility: Percentage "Yes" by Country (N=400)

	France %	Italy %	Denmark %	Ireland %	All Countries %		
					Males	Females	Total
Make private calls	89.0	87.0	100.0	91.0	94.0	89.5	91.8
Run private errands	38.0	24.0	55.0	60.0	54.5	34.5	44.5
Leave early/ arrive late due to childcare problems	76.0	69.0	79.0	75.0	73.5	76.4	74.9
Bring a child to work	9.1	12.0	36.0	15.0	14.5	21.6	18.0

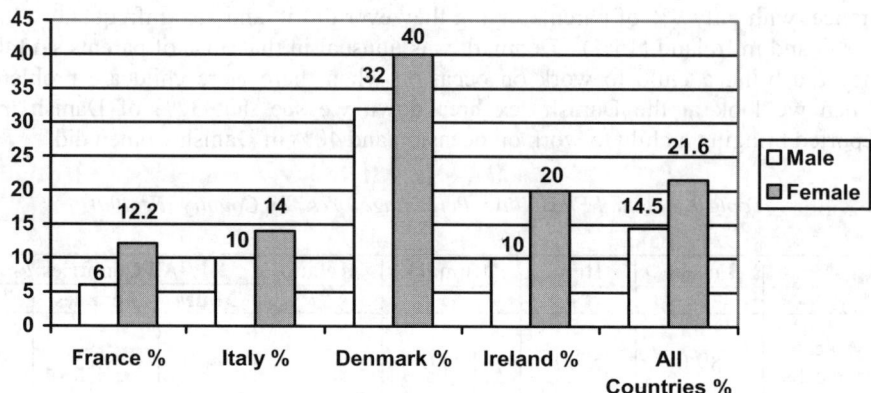

Figure 9.3. Percentage of Parents Who Would Bring a Child to Work due to Childcare Problems: Percentage Distributions By Country and Sex

These results convey a picture of a more relaxed and permissive attitude towards "intrusion" of family-related matters in Danish workplace culture - in comparison with the other countries. The Danish participants experienced both the most potential and the most actual flexibility.

3.3 Potential for Contact between Participants and Children During the Work Day

Participants were asked about how easily they could keep in contact with their children during the working day. Firstly they were asked about how much of the day they were available to their children by phone contact etc., then about how easily they could contact their childminding facility. Lastly they were asked about how easily they could leave work to visit their childminding facility on occasion.

3.3.1.Availability of Participants During the Day
Three-quarters of the sample were available either most of the day or all day for their children via phone messages, etc. However, while this held for Italy, Denmark and Ireland, it was not the case for France. French participants were significantly less likely to be available. The country means are presented below and detailed percentage data is presented in Appendix Table A58. In Denmark and Ireland there appears to be little difference between the public and private sectors on this measure. In France those in the public sector were more available than in the private sector and in the private sector males were less available than females. In Italy the reverse was true: parents working in the private sector were more available to their children

by phone than those working in the public sector; there appeared to be no sex differences here.

Table. 9.7. *How Much of the Workday is the Respondent Available for Their Child/ren Via Phone, Messages, Voicemail, etc.: Mean Scores by Country, Sex and Sector (N=400)*

		France	Italy	Denmark	Ireland
Public Sector	Male	3.4	4.0	4.8	4.6
	Female	3.2	4.1	5.0	4.8
Total Public Sector		**3.3**	**4.1**	**4.9**	**4.7**
Private Sector	Male	2.5	4.8	4.9	4.8
	Female	2.9	4.7	4.8	4.3
Total Private Sector		**2.7**	**4.8**	**4.9**	**4.5**
Total country		**3.0**	**4.4**	**4.9**	**4.6**

(1=not at all, 5 = all day)
Country: $F=92.34$, $df = 3$, $p \leq 0.001$
Country x Sector: $F=9.79$, $df = 3$, $p \leq 0.001$
Country x Sector x Sex $F=2.61$, $df = 3$, $p \leq 0.05$

When looking more closely at the different groupings, all Danish participants were very available to the children during the day: 100% of female public sector participants were available all day (mean = 5 out of 5). In Ireland all groups were very available but female, private sector participants somewhat less so.

3.3.2. Ease of Contacting the Childminding Facility
Parents were also asked how easy or difficult it was for them to keep in contact with the childminder/babysitter, school or facility during the day, by telephone or otherwise. The vast majority of parents (89%) said that they could do this easily, 7.5% said that they could do so with difficulty, and 3% said that they could not do it at all (see Appendix Tables A59 and A60).

French participants were significantly less likely to be able to keep in contact with their childminding facility during the day by telephone or otherwise than were participants from the other countries and this pertained particularly to those in low SES jobs. Those in high SES jobs were significantly more likely to be easily able to keep in contact with the childminding facility.

Table 9.8. Ease of Contact with Youngest Child's Childcare Facility: Mean Scores by Country and SES (N=400)

	France	Italy	Denmark	Ireland	All
Low SES	2.5	2.9	2.9	2.9	2.8
High SES	2.8	2.9	3.0	3.0	2.9
Total	**2.6**	**2.9**	**3.0**	**3.0**	**2.9**

(1=not at all, 3 = easily)
Country: $F=15.63$, $df = 3$, $p \leq 0.001$
SES: $F=7.17$, $df = 1$, $p \leq 0.01$
Country x SES: $F=2.58$, $df = 3$, $p \leq 0.05$

Of those participants who did experience difficulties in contacting their youngest child during the day (10.5%), for a third of them it was lack of access to a telephone that was the difficulty, for 16% it was distance/transport and for 10.5% permission from employer and for 39.5%, "other" (see Appendix Tables A61).

A similar picture is painted for the possibility of participants leaving work on occasion to visit their childminding facility (see Appendix Tables A62 and A63): as before, the French participants found it significantly more difficult to do than the participants of any other country.

Table 9.9. Possibility of Leaving Work to Visit Youngest Child: Mean Scores by Country (N=400)

France	Italy	Denmark	Ireland	All Countries
2.1	2.7	2.7	2.7	2.6

(1=not at all, 3 = easily)
Country: $F=22.01$, $df = 3$, $p \leq 0.001$

For those participants who had difficulties in leaving work to visit their child, almost half reported that it was because they couldn't leave work (Appendix Table A64). The next most common reason was distance/transportation problems, and thirdly that the employer would disapprove of them doing so. In Denmark distance and transportation weren't important but there was more difficulty in them being able to leave work than in the other countries.

4. PERCEPTIONS OF WORKPLACE ATTITUDES

Due to the fact that parents spend so much time at work, the workplace environment - both in terms of policies and attitudes - is a critical factor in coping with issues of work-life balance. The study included several sets of questions to measure the degree of perceived acceptance of workers' family responsibilities. These items were based on the work of Holt (1994) and Hojgaard (1990, 1996b) in Denmark.

4.1 Perceived Attitudes of Colleagues, Supervisors and Employers

Initially, respondents were asked about how understanding their colleagues, supervisors and employers were around their family responsibilities. We collected data on three key areas: how acceptable it was to arrive late or to leave early from work due to problems regarding children, how acceptable it was to bring a child to work on occasion due to childcare problems and how well co-workers took into account the participants' responsibilities for a young child.

4.1.1. Perceived Acceptability of Arriving Late/ Leaving Early

In comparison to the participants from the other countries, the Danish participants were more likely to think it was acceptable amongst their colleagues to leave earlier and/or arrive later due to problems regarding childcare. In Denmark the mean score was 5.1 ("acceptable") out of a possible 6 points, with 6 = "very acceptable." In the other countries the means ranged from 4.6 – 4.8, with 4 = "somewhat acceptable." In all of the four countries, it was more likely to be considered acceptable by co-workers to leave work early and /or arrive late in higher SES occupations than in lower SES ones.

Table 9.10. Perceived Acceptability by Colleagues of Respondent Arriving Late to / Leaving Early from Work due to Childcare Problems: Mean Scores by Country and SES (N=400)

	France	Italy	Denmark	Ireland	Total
Low SES	4.4	4.3	4.9	4.6	4.6
High SES	4.8	4.9	5.3	5.0	5.0
Total	**4.6**	**4.6**	**5.1**	**4.8**	**4.8**

(1 = very unacceptable, 6 = very acceptable)
Country: F =3.21, df = 3; p≤0.05
SES: F =11.24, df = 1; p≤0.001

As in the case of co-workers, respondents in Denmark were more likely than those in other countries to feel that their managers would consider it acceptable for parents to leave work early or to arrive late due to childcare problems. This behaviour was considered least acceptable in Italy. Also, as in the case with co-workers, employees in higher SES jobs were more likely to think their managers would find it acceptable if they left work early or arrived late due to childcare problems.

Table 9.11. Perceived Acceptability by Managers of Respondent Arriving Late to/ Leaving Early from Work due to Childcare Problems: Mean Scores by Country and SES (N=400)

	France	Italy	Denmark	Ireland	Total
Low SES	3.8	3.7	4.4	4.2	**4.2**
High SES	4.3	4.3	5.0	4.6	**4.6**
Total	**4.1**	**3.9**	**4.9**	**4.7**	**4.4**

(1 = very unacceptable, 6 = very acceptable)
Country: $F = 13.27$, $df = 3$; $p \leq 0.001$
SES: $F = 11.00$, $df = 1$; $p \leq 0.001$

4.1.2. Perceived Acceptability of Bringing a Child to Work

It was also perceived as significantly more acceptable by Danish participants to bring a child to work than in the other countries. The Danes were the only ones to feel that amongst their colleagues this would be considered acceptable (i.e., somewhere between "somewhat acceptable" and "acceptable" on average) – parents in the other countries tended to rate it as somewhere between "somewhat unacceptable and somewhat acceptable". There was a moderately significant interaction effect between country, sex and SES – while the Danish participants were all rather similar in their responses, bringing a child to work was considered least acceptable among Italian women working in low SES jobs, and far more acceptable to Italian women in high SES jobs.

Table 9.12. Perceived Acceptability of Respondent Bringing a Child to Work by Colleagues: Mean Scores by Country, Sex and SES (N=400)

		France	Italy	Denmark	Ireland
Male	Low	3.2	3.3	4.5	2.6
	High	3.0	3.5	4.8	3.2
Female	Low	4.0	2.5	4.4	3.5
	High	3.8	4.2	4.4	2.9
Total Country		**3.5**	**3.3**	**4.5**	**3.0**

(1 = very unacceptable, 6 = very acceptable)
Country: $F = 14.84$, $df = 3$; $p \leq 0.001$
Country x Sex x SES: $F = 2.93$, $df = 3$; $p \leq 0.05$

Concerning perceptions of managerial attitudes toward bringing a child to work, there was a highly significant difference between countries. Danish managers were perceived as significantly more accepting of this behaviour than were managers in the other countries. In all of the other countries it was considered unacceptable/somewhat unacceptable to bring a child to work, even if there were childcare problems. However, it was even more unacceptable in lower SES jobs than in higher in all countries.

Table 9.13. Perceived Acceptability of Respondent Bringing a Child to Work by Managers: Mean Scores by Country and SES (N=400)

	France	Italy	Denmark	Ireland	Total
Low SES	2.7	2.4	4.0	2.5	**2.9**
High SES	3.0	3.1	4.5	3.0	**3.4**
Total	**2.9**	**2.8**	**4.2**	**2.8**	**3.2**

(1 = very unacceptable, 6 = very acceptable)
Country: $F = 18.76$, $df = 3$; $p \leq 0.001$
SES: $F = 7.94$, $df = 1$; $p \leq 0.005$

4.1.3. Perceived Attitudes of Colleagues, Supervisor and Employer towards One's Childcare Responsibilities

Respondents were asked, "How well do you think the following people take into account the fact that you have responsibility for a child/ren?" The women in the study were more likely than the men to think that their colleagues were sympathetic to their childcare responsibilities. Surprisingly, this trend was reversed in Italy - male respondents perceived more understanding on the part of their colleagues than did female respondents.

Table 9.14. How Well Colleagues Take into Account Respondents' Childcare Responsibilities Mean Scores By Country and Sex (N=400)

	France	Italy	Denmark	Ireland	Total
Male	3.9	4.1	3.7	3.7	**3.8**
Female	4.1	3.6	4.3	4.0	**4.0**

(1 = not at all well, 5 = very well)
Sex: $F = 3.80$, $df = 1$; $p \leq 0.05$
Country x Sex: $F = 4.82$, $df = 3$; $p \leq 0.005$

Respondents were also asked how well they thought their supervisors took into account their childcare responsibilities. There were slight, but significant differences by country, indicating that most acceptance was perceived by Irish parents and least by French parents. The Italians and the Danes fell in between. In all cases lower SES respondents were less likely to perceive sympathetic attitudes from their supervisors than were higher SES workers; however, this pattern did not hold in Ireland, where there was no difference between high and low SES workers.

Table 9.15. How Well Immediate Supervisor Takes into Account Respondents' Childcare Responsibilities: Mean Scores by Country and SES (N=400)

	France	Italy	Denmark	Ireland	Total
Low SES	3.3	3.5	3.5	3.9	**3.5**
High SES	3.6	3.7	4.0	3.9	**3.8**
Total	**3.4**	**3.6**	**3.7**	**3.9**	**3.7**

(1 = not at all well, 5 = very well)
Country: $F = 2.80$, $df = 3$; $p \leq 0.05$
SES: $F = 5.51$, $df = 1$; $p \leq 0.05$

Co-workers, supervisors and employers are all distinct entities and it cannot be assumed that their attitudes will always coincide. Thus, respondents were also asked about the attitude of their employer toward their childcare responsibilities. There was a moderately significant difference between countries on this measure. As may be seen below, the Italian participants reported their employers took into account their childcare responsibilities the least and Irish participants did the most. Danes and the French fell somewhere in between. There was also a tendency for female workers to perceive more positive employer attitudes than males, particularly in Denmark. However, this pattern was reversed in Italy, in which male workers were more likely to perceive positive employer attitudes than were female workers.

Table 9.16. How Well Employer Takes into Account Respondents' Childcare Responsibilities: Mean Scores by Country and Sex (N=400)

	France	Italy	Denmark	Ireland
Male	3.4	3.4	3.0	3.5
Female	3.5	2.8	3.5	3.7
Total	**3.5**	**3.1**	**3.3**	**3.6**

(1 = not at all well, 5 = very well)
Country: $F = 2.70$, $df = 3$; $p \leq 0.05$
Country x Sex: $F = 3.56$, $df = 1$; $p \leq 0.05$

4.2 Perceived Attitudes towards People Availing of Family Friendly Policies

Participants were asked a series of further questions about the attitudes in their workplace towards people availing of family friendly policies. The reason for the inclusion of these items was to examine whether attitudinal barriers exist in this area and, if so, to what extent. This is important from at least two points of view. One concerns barriers to women's career advancement and the second relates to barriers to men's greater participation in family life.

4.2.1. Perceived Attitudes to Men taking Extended Leave for Childcare Reasons
Respondents were initially asked *"To what extent do you agree that in your workplace:*

> a) "Many employees are resentful when men take extended leaves to care for newborn or adopted children."

Participants generally reported that they disagreed with the statement. We examined whether there were any significant differences based on country, sex, SES or public *vs.* private sector. As may be seen in the Table below, the all country mean was 3.3 out of 7, with 1 = "strongly disagree" and 7 = "strongly agree". A score of 3.3 thus falls between slightly disagree and neutral (4). The mean scores ranged from 1.8 in Italy (moderate disagreement) to 5.7 in France (close to moderate agreement). The mean scores in Denmark (2.8) and Ireland (3.2) were in between, but were closer to the Italian scores, indicating moderate to slight disagreement.

In addition to significant country differences, there was also a significant difference between public and private sector employees. In all of the countries, private sector workers were more likely to think that there was resentment when men took extended leave for childcare reasons in comparison to the public sector (mean scores for private sector were 3.6 and for public sector 2.9).

Table 9.17. Perceived Resentment of Men Taking Extended Leave for Childcare: Mean Scores by Country and Sector (N=400)

	France	Italy	Denmark	Ireland	Total
Public	5.4	1.6	1.5	2.9	2.9
Private	6.0	1.9	2.9	3.6	3.6
Total	5.7	1.8	2.2	3.3	3.3

(1=strongly disagree, 7 = strongly agree)
Country: $F=88.71$, $df=3$, $p \leq 0.001$
Sector: $F=18.24$, $df=1$, $p \leq 0.001$

In general there were not great differences here on the basis of occupational status. There was a slight tendency for higher SES workers in Denmark and Ireland to perceive less resentment when men took leave. In Italy there was no difference based on SES. However, in France there was a very big difference in views of lower and higher SES workers. Here higher SES workers perceived the most resentment if men took leave (mean score = 6.3), whereas lower SES workers perceived less resentment (mean = 5.2). Nevertheless, the French scores were still very different from those in the other countries.

There were no sex differences on this measure. Men and women in all countries had similar attitudes on this issue.

Table 9.18. Perceived Resentment of Men Taking Extended Leave for Childcare: Mean Scores by Country and SES (N=400)

	France	Italy	Denmark	Ireland
Low SES	5.2	1.8	2.4	3.4
High SES	6.3	1.8	2.1	3.1

(1=strongly disagree, 7 = strongly agree)
Country x SES: $F=3.34$, $df = 3$, $p \leq 0.05$

4.2.2. Perceived Attitudes to Women taking Extended Leave for Childcare Reasons
We ordered the questions, males first, since for women to take extended leave is more commonplace. We were interested in spontaneous attitudes toward this relatively new stimulus, and for it not to be influenced by the female statement first.

Perceived attitudes about women taking leave were more permissive, not surprisingly, than were those toward men taking leave. The least resentment towards women taking extended leave was in Italy, followed by Denmark. This may be because of the pro-family attitudes in Italy and the tradition of egalitarian attitudes and family friendly policies in Denmark. The attitudes in Ireland followed, and the French attitudes, as before, were seen as least permissive by the respondents. The French mean was 4.9 as compared with the Italian mean of 1.6, the Danish mean of 1.8 and the Irish mean of 2.8. The socio-economic differences were negligible in Italy and Denmark, as seen below, however in France, as we saw before, there was more perceived resentment towards women taking extended leave in the higher socio-economic group. In Ireland the reverse was true, although the difference was not as great as in France.

Table 9.19. Perceived Resentment of Women Taking Extended Leave for Childcare:
Mean Scores by Country and SES (N=400)

	France	Italy	Denmark	Ireland
Low SES	4.3	1.5	1.6	3.1
High SES	5.4	1.7	1.6	2.5
Total	**4.9**	**1.6**	**1.8**	**2.8**

(1=strongly disagree, 7 = strongly agree)
Country: $F=81.38$, $df = 3$, $p \leq 0.001$
Country x SES: $F=3.89$, $df = 3$, $p \leq 0.01$

In all countries, there was an overall significant effect of sector, whereby more resentment of women taking leave was perceived in the private sector. This was modified by an SES effect, which indicated that in the private sector greater resentment towards women taking leave was felt by lower SES workers, whereas in the public sector, lower SES workers felt there was less resentment than did higher SES workers.

Table 9.20. Perceived Resentment of Women taking Extended Leave for Childcare:
Mean Scores by SES and Sector (N=400)

	Public	Private
Low SES	2.2	3.1
High SES	2.8	2.9
Total	**2.5**	**2.9**

(1=strongly disagree, 7 = strongly agree)
Sector: $F=7.44$, $df = 1$, $p \leq 0.01$
Sector x SES: $F=7.53$, $df = 1$, $p \leq 0.01$

4.2.3. Sex and Country Differences in Perceived Resentment towards Men and Women taking Extended Leave for Childcare

While there were no sex differences concerning men and women taking leave, we were interested in exploring whether there were sex and country differences in attitudes towards men *vs.* women taking leave. Thus, comparisons were carried out comparing male and female attitudes within each country toward men taking leave *vs.* women taking leave. These comparisons are presented below. There were no significant differences between Italian men or women's perceptions of men *vs.* women taking leave. Italian men and women tended not to perceive that there was resentment in either case. The same was true in Ireland, though a somewhat less permissive attitude prevailed than in Italy. On the other hand, both males and females in France and in Denmark felt it was seen as less acceptable for men to take leave than for women. This means that men in France and Denmark would presumably feel less latitude to engage in this behaviour, since it is seen as less acceptable for men to do it than for women. However, more importantly perhaps are the overall mean scores for the countries, indicating that in general there is more perceived resentment if men take extended leave and this is particularly pronounced in France and least in Italy, followed by Denmark.

Table 9.21. *Perceived Resentment of Men Taking Extended Leave for Childcare vs. Women Taking Extended Leave: Mean Scores by Country and Sex (N=400)*

Sample	Means		Statistics		
	Men taking leave	Women taking leave	t	df	Sig.
France	5.7	4.9	5.17	91	$p \leq 0.001$
France – males	5.9	4.8	4.31	46	$p \leq 0.001$
France – females	5.6	4.9	2.98	44	$p \leq 0.005$
Italy	1.8	1.7	1.46	99	n.s.
Italy – males	1.9	1.7	1.12	49	n.s.
Italy – females	1.6	1.7	0.94	49	n.s.
Denmark	2.3	1.6	4.33	98	$p \leq 0.001$
Denmark – males	2.7	1.6	4.01	48	$p \leq 0.001$
Denmark – females	1.9	1.6	1.96	49	$p \leq 0.05$
Ireland	3.3	2.8	1.97	99	$p \leq 0.05$
Ireland – males	3.4	2.9	1.52	49	n.s.
Ireland – females	3.1	2.7	1.25	49	n.s.
All Countries	3.2	2.7	6.21	390	$p \leq 0.001$
All Countries – males	3.4	2.7	5.16	195	$p \leq 0.001$
All Countries - females	3.0	2.7	3.51	194	$p \leq 0.001$

(1=strongly disagree, 7 = strongly agree)

4.2.4. Perceived Attitudes towards Men Working Part-Time or Job-Sharing
One of the ways in which men and women can combine work and family is to work part-time or to job share. This practice is widespread for women in many countries. Indeed, women make up the majority of part-time workers and they are also more likely to avail of job-sharing options than are men. It was one of the aims of the present study to see if there were barriers to men availing of family friendly options such as these. Hence, we asked the question: "To what extent do you agree that in your workplace . . .

"Men who participate in available work-family programmes (e.g., job-sharing, part-time work) are viewed as less serious about their career than those who do not participate in these programmes."

We found that there was a significant difference between countries in response to this statement. French and Irish participants both agreed that men who participate in available work-family programmes (e.g., job-sharing or part-time work) are viewed as less serious about their career than those who do not, whereas both the Italians and Danes disagreed. There was a significant interaction effect between country and SES indicating that in three of the countries - Ireland, France and Denmark, higher SES respondents were more likely to agree with the statement, whereas in Italy there was no effect of class on this. The social class difference was quite pronounced in France and Ireland and to a much lesser extent in Denmark.

Table. 9.22. *Men in Work-Family Programmes Perceived as 'Less Serious' about Career: Mean Scores by Country and SES (N=400)*

	France	**Italy**	**Denmark**	**Ireland**	**Total**
Low SES	4.2	2.1	2.9	4.3	**3.4**
High SES	6.0	2.1	3.5	5.9	**4.5**
Total	**5.1**	**2.1**	**3.2**	**5.1**	**3.9**

(1=strongly disagree, 7 = strongly agree)
Country: $F=56.13$, $df = 3$, $p \leq 0.001$
SES: $F=29.01$, $df = 1$, $p \leq 0.01$
Country x SES: $F=4.35$, $df = 3$, $p \leq 0.005$

Male participants were significantly more likely to think that men who participate in available work-family programmes (e.g. job-sharing, part-time work) are viewed as less serious about their career than those who do not participate in these programmes than were female participants. This is thus likely to create a distinct barrier to men taking up this kind of employment, which could facilitate work-life balance for then.

Table 9.23. Men in Work-Family Programmes Perceived as 'Less Serious' About Career: Mean Scores by Sex and Sector (N=400)

	Male	Female
Public	3.7	3.1
Private	4.7	4.3
Total	**4.2**	**3.7**

(1=strongly disagree, 7 = strongly agree)
Sex: $F=4.50$, $df = 1$, $p \leq 0.05$
Sex x Sector: $F=4.64$, $df = 1$, $p \leq 0.05$

4.2.5. Perceived Attitudes towards Women Working Part-time Work or Job Sharing

The participants from all countries disagreed that women who participate in available work-family programmes (e.g. job-sharing, part-time work) are viewed as less serious about their career than those who do not participate in these programmes, except the Irish who tended to agree slightly. Despite the overall disagreement with the statement, those in low SES jobs were more likely to disagree than those in high SES jobs. When looking more closely at the groups who agreed with the statement, in contrast to the majority who disagreed, the French and Irish high SES participants were the only groups to agree.

Table 9.24. Women in Work-Family Programme Perceived as 'Less Serious' about Career: Mean Scores by SES and Country (N=400)

	France	Italy	Denmark	Ireland	Total
Low SES	3.2	2.0	2.1	3.7	2.7
High SES	4.6	2.0	2.9	5.8	3.8
Total	**3.9**	**2.0**	**2.5**	**4.7**	**3.3**

(1=strongly disagree, 7 = strongly agree)
Country: $F=45.12$, $df = 3$, $p \leq 0.001$
SES: $F=32.02$, $df = 1$, $p \leq 0.001$
Country x SES: $F=5.66$, $df = 3$, $p \leq 0.001$

It is noteworthy that in the case of male participation in work-family programmes there was a sex difference – male participants were more likely to agree that men were viewed as less serious about their careers than women participants. In the case of women in family-work programmes there was no sex difference – both male and female participants generally thought that women were not viewed as being less serious about their careers if they took part in work-family programmes. With respect to women on this issue, the Italians, followed by the Danes, disagreed most strongly that women are viewed as less serious about their careers if in these circumstances. The French tended to be neutral on this, whereas the Irish tended to agree slightly. Participants appear to be more likely to agree that men's, rather than women's, careers are jeopardized, reflecting traditional gender role attitudes.

4.2.6. Sex and Country Differences in Perceptions of Men vs. Women in Work-Family Programmes as 'Less Serious' about Career

When comparing participants' reports of how men and women are compared in the workplace with respect to their participating in work-family programmes, e.g., job sharing and part-time work, the same trends may be seen as in the comparison of men and women taking extended leave for childcare reasons. French and Danish participants, particularly the men, thought there was a difference in how men and women were perceived – men who participated in work family programmes were more likely to be perceived as not taking their careers seriously than women were. The Italians did not see a difference between how men and women were perceived in this regard and neither did Irish males.

Table 9.25. Perceived Attitudes Toward Men vs. Women in Work-Family Programmes: Mean Scores by Country and Sex (N=400)

Sample	Means		Statistics		
	Men in Work-Family Programmes	Women in Work-Family Programmes	t	df	Sig.
France	5.2	3.9	6.09	92	p≤0.001
France – males	5.6	3.9	6.37	46	p≤0.001
France – females	4.7	3.8	2.63	45	p≤0.01
Italy	2.1	2.0	0.92	99	n.s.
Italy – males	2.0	1.8	1.57	49	n.s.
Italy – females	2.2	2.1	0.06	49	n.s.
Denmark	3.2	2.5	4.01	96	p≤0.001
Denmark – males	3.7	2.9	2.96	47	p≤0.005
Denmark – females	2.8	2.1	2.69	48	p≤0.01
Ireland	5.1	4.7	2.40	99	n.s.
Ireland – males	5.2	5.0	0.75	49	n.s.
Ireland – females	5.1	4.4	2.60	49	p≤0.01
All Countries	3.9	3.3	7.08	389	p≤0.001
All Countries – males	4.1	3.4	5.74	194	p≤0.001
All Countries - females	3.7	3.1	4.29	194	p≤0.001

(1=strongly disagree, 7 = strongly agree)

4.3 Perceived Work Pressure

One of the problems in combining work and family life is the problem of work demands. In some jobs employees feel pressure to work over and above the normal hours and to bring work home. In some cases, employees feel that this is necessary in order to get ahead. Thus, not only can employees not contemplate working *fewer* hours to facilitate work-life balance, in many cases they may be expected to work *more* hours. To what extent this was a problem was examined in this part of the study.

Respondents were asked whether they agreed or disagreed with the statement: *"To get ahead employees are expected to work over and above the normal hours, whether at the workplace or at home?"*

Participants in high SES jobs and those working in the private sector were significantly more likely to agree than were those in low SES jobs and those working in the public sector, as illustrated below.

Table 9.26. *Perception that to Get Ahead Employees must Work Over and Above the Normal Hours: Mean Scores by SES and Sector (N=400)*

	Low SES	High SES	Total
Public	3.0	4.5	3.7
Private	4.5	4.9	4.3
Total	**3.4**	**4.7**	**3.3**

(1=strongly disagree, 7 = strongly agree)
Sector: $F=8.61$, $df = 1$, $p \leq 0.005$
SES: $F=37.79$, $df = 1$, $p \leq 0.001$

Participants in France and Ireland tended to agree that to get ahead employees are expected to work over and above the normal hours, whether at the workplace or at home, and those in Italy and Denmark disagreed. When looking more closely at the different groups involved it appears that all the Irish participants agreed with the statement except female participants in low SES jobs. The same situation occurred for the French participants. On the other hand, all Danish participants disagreed with the statement except female high SES participants, who appeared to be most stressed. Female participants in low SES jobs generally disagreed more than the other groups with the above statement, across all countries.

Table 9.27. *Perception that to Get Ahead Employees must Work Over and Above the Normal Hours: Mean Scores by Country, Sex and SES (N=400)*

		France	Italy	Denmark	Ireland
Male	Low SES	4.6	2.1	2.7	5.2
	High SES	5.6	3.3	3.8	6.2
Female	Low SES	3.6	3.3	2.2	3.7
	High SES	5.7	3.0	4.4	5.8
Total country		**4.9**	**2.9**	**3.3**	**5.2**

(1=strongly disagree, 7 = strongly agree)
Country: $F=29.55$, $df = 3$, $p \leq 0.001$
Country x Sex x SES: $F=2.63$, $df = 3$, $p \leq 0.05$

The next related question posed in this series asked respondents to what extent they agreed or disagreed with the statement: *"To be viewed favourably by top management, employees must constantly put their jobs ahead of their families or personal lives."*

French and Irish participants tended to agree that to be viewed favourably by top management, employees must constantly put their jobs ahead of their families or personal lives more than did the Italian or Danish ones, who tended to disagree slightly to moderately. Participants in lower SES jobs tended to disagree with the above statement and those in high SES jobs tended to agree. There was also a significant interaction effect of country, sex, SES and sector. The groups who agreed most strongly with the statement were French male participants in the private sector, working in both high and low SES occupations, French female participants working in high SES jobs in the public sector and Irish male participants working in high SES jobs in the public sector.

Compared to the previous measure, "To get ahead employees are expected to work over and above the normal hours, whether at the workplace or at home," the same effects of country and SES are present, with France and Ireland and high SES participants most likely to agree that "To be viewed favourably by top management, employees must constantly put their jobs ahead of their families or personal lives."

Table 9.28. *To be Viewed Favourably by Top Management Employees must Put Job ahead of Family Life: Mean Scores by Country, Sex, SES and Sector (N=400)*

			France	Italy	Denmark	Ireland	Total SES
Low SES	Male	Public	4.7	1.7	1.9	5.4	
		Private	6.5	1.8	3.3	4.2	3.5
	Female	Public	3.9	2.0	2.8	3.6	
		Private	5.2	3.8	2.2	3.6	
High SES	Male	Public	5.0	2.4	3.9	6.1	
		Private	6.4	2.4	2.5	5.3	4.2
	Female	Public	6.1	2.4	2.3	5.7	
		Private	5.2	2.3	4.5	5.6	
Total Country			5.4	2.3	3.0	4.9	3.9

(1=strongly disagree, 7 = strongly agree)
Country: $F=55.22$, $df = 3$, $p \leq 0.001$
SES: $F=4.35$, $df = 1$, $p \leq 0.001$
Country x Sex x SES x Sector: $F=4.53$, $df = 3$, $p \leq 0.005$

4.4. Summary of Workplace Attitudes

The most striking impression one sees from the data in this section is that the attitudes of the Italians and of the Danes appeared to reflect the most accepting and relaxed workplace cultures, as compared with the French and the Irish. In general the French tended to agree with the statements more than participants of the other countries – that there was resentment when people used work-family measures and that they were expected to put work above family. The Irish also agreed to some extent that there were these pressures in their workplaces. Those in high SES jobs tended to perceive the most pressures of this type, and those in the private sector also. Male participants perceived more pressure about men regarding work-family measures. On many of the statements all participants disagreed except for French participants in high SES jobs who were the group most likely to feel this sort of pressure. The group that appeared to feel the least pressure was female participants in low SES jobs; on the other hand, they have fewer occupational opportunities and therefore may have lower expectations.

French and Danish participants, particularly the men, thought there was a difference in how men and women are perceived – men who participated in work family programmes were more likely to be perceived as not taking their careers seriously than women were. The Italians did not see a difference between how men and women were perceived in this regard and neither did Irish males.

5. WORKPLACE POLICIES

We have described extensively in Chapter 2 – 6 the national policies available to meet the needs of working parents. This was done in relation to individual countries in each of the national literature reviews, and then comparatively in Chapter 6.

In this section, we report on data in which the respondents were asked personally about a variety of potential workplace policies in their place of employment. Participants firstly were asked whether or not each policy was available in their workplace, secondly, whether or not they had used each policy and lastly whether their attitude towards the policy in general was favourable or not.

5.1. National Leave Policies

5.1.1. Paid Maternity Leave
The majority of participants were aware that there was paid maternity leave available in their workplaces, although a quarter of French males and a third of Danish males didn't know whether there was any paid maternity leave available or not in their workplaces.

*Table 9.29. Paid Maternity Leave: Availability, Use and Attitude:
Percentage Distributions by Country and Sex (N=400)*

	France %		Italy %		Denmark %		Ireland %	
	M	F	M	F	M	F	M	F
Availability (% Yes)	50.0	89.8	86.0	94.0	62.7	90.0	81.6	92.0
Availability (% Don't know)	25.0	8.2	10.0	2.0	31.4	6.0	10.2	4.0
Used (% Yes)	0.0	85.4	0.0	82.0	0.0	72.0	0.0	80.4
Do Not Favour	0.0	0.0	0.0	4.0	0.0	0.0	0.0	0.0
Somewhat Favour	26.1	6.4	24.0	4.0	4.0	2.0	8.0	4.0
Strongly Favour	73.9	93.6	76.0	92.0	96.0	98.0	92.0	96.0

Approximately four-fifths of the women interviewed in each country had taken paid maternity leave.

The vast majority of participants were highly favourable towards paid maternity leave. The participants who least enthusiastic about it were a quarter of French males and a quarter of Italian males who only reported that they 'somewhat' favoured it.

5.1.2. Unpaid Maternity Leave

Unpaid maternity leave was most available to Irish participants, followed by the Italians. It was not available to the majority of the Danish participants, and most of the French participants didn't know if it was available or not.

Table 9.30. Unpaid Maternity Leave: Availability, Use and Attitude:
Percentage Distributions by Country and Sex (N= 400)

	France %		Italy %		Denmark %		Ireland %	
	M	F	M	F	M	F	M	F
Availability (% Yes)	33.3	30.9	70.0	77.6	12.2	6.0	90.6	89.8
Availability (% Don't know)	46.7	43.6	20.0	8.2	34.7	8.0	7.5	8.5
Used (% Yes)	0.0	7.3	0.0	36.0	0.0	4.1	0.0	54.2
Do Not Favour	28.6	46.0	16.0	22.0	53.1	84.0	5.8	8.5
Somewhat Favour	47.6	46.0	36.0	28.0	42.9	16.0	25.0	22.0
Strongly Favour	23.8	8.0	48.0	50.0	4.1	0.0	69.2	69.5

The percentages of women using unpaid maternity leave varied greatly by country. Only 4% of Danish women used it, followed by 7% of French women. A third of Italian women had used it and a half of the Irish women had used it. A high proportion of French males and females and Danish males did not know whether or not it was available in their workplace.

Participants were less favourable towards unpaid maternity leave than they were towards paid maternity leave. Danish participants, particularly the women, were not in favour of it as a policy. French participants were divided on the matter, though French females were less favourable than French males. Irish participants were generally favourable. Half of Italian participants strongly favoured it and the rest were divided.

5.1.3. Paid Paternity Leave

Paid paternity leave was available in the workplaces of 83% of the Danish respondents and in approximately two-thirds of those of the Italian participants. Approximately half of Irish men and women said that paid paternity leave was available to them. Among the French, it was available to 43% of the men and 26% of the women. There was a fairly high proportion of 'don't knows', though less so amongst the Danish parents.

Table 9.31. Paid Paternity Leave: Availability, Use and Attitude:
Percentage Distributions by Country and Sex (N=400)

	France %		Italy %		Denmark %		Ireland %	
	M	F	M	F	M	F	M	F
Availability (% Yes)	42.9	26.3	66.0	68.8	82.0	84.0	50.0	47.9
Availability (% Don't know)	26.5	52.6	26.0	14.6	10.0	10.0	14.0	22.9
Used (% Yes)	36.2	0.0	24.0	0.0	66.0	0.0	34.0	0.0
Do Not Favour	2.3	0.0	2.0	6.0	0.0	2.0	0.0	2.1
Somewhat Favour	18.2	28.6	34.0	32.0	2.0	0.0	6.1	2.1
Strongly Favour	79.5	71.4	64.0	62.0	98.0	98.0	93.9	95.8

Fully two-thirds of the Danish fathers in the sample said they had taken paid paternity leave. Approximately one-third of French and Irish fathers reported that they had, as did one quarter of the Italian fathers. The Danish and the Irish participants were overwhelmingly in favour of paid paternity leave. Around three-quarters of the French and two-thirds of the Italian participants strongly favoured it also.

5.1.4. Unpaid Paternity Leave

Unpaid paternity leave was available to 58% of Irish men and in the workplaces of 28% of Irish women. It was also fairly widely available to Italian men, of whom 49% said it was available; similarly 57% of Italian women said it was available at their workplaces. In France and Denmark it was much less available, being reported as available by about a fifth of French parents and 13% of Danish. There was a high degree of 'Don't Know' responses, especially in France, but also in Italy and Ireland.

Table 9.32. *Unpaid Paternity Leave: Availability, Use and Attitude: Percentage Distributions by Country and Sex (N=400)*

	France %		Italy %		Denmark %		Ireland %	
	M	F	M	F	M	F	M	F
Availability (% Yes)	22.4	21.1	49.0	57.4	14.3	12.0	58.3	28.6
Availability (% Don't know)	38.8	52.6	34.7	23.4	14.3	14.0	16.7	36.7
Used (% Yes)	0.0	0.0	8.0	0.0	12.5	0.0	15.7	0.0
Do Not Favour	38.3	33.3	14.0	22.0	63.3	80.0	8.2	12.5
Somewhat Favour	53.2	38.9	42.0	40.0	28.6	14.0	34.7	18.8
Strongly Favour	8.5	27.8	44.0	38.0	8.2	6.0	57.1	68.8

Not a single French male participant had used unpaid paternity leave even though 22% of them reported that it was available in their workplaces. There was very little take-up in any of the other countries either.

Participants were not favourable to unpaid paternity leave as compared to paid paternity leave. The Danish participants stood out as being unfavourable towards it, and the Irish as being in favour. Figure 6 below shows the extent to which paid and unpaid maternity and paternity leave are used. Italy and Ireland have a similar pattern of usage, with paid maternity leave being the most common leave taken, followed by unpaid maternity leave. In France and Denmark paid maternity leave is also the most common, but unpaid maternity leave is little used and is far superseded by paid paternity leave. Danish participants took more paid paternity leave than in any other country – almost as much as maternity leave was taken. It can also be seen that more Irish participants took unpaid maternity and paternity leave than participants from any other country.

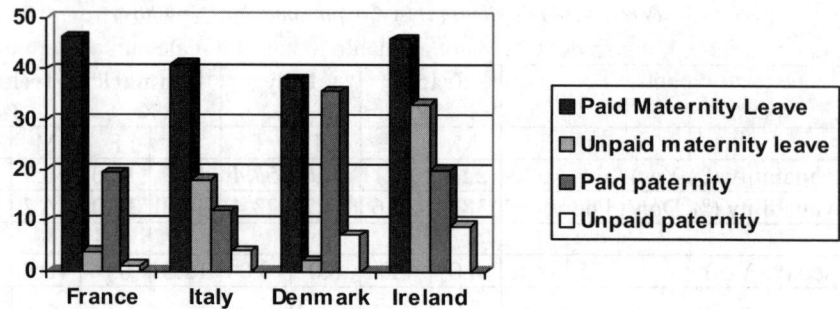

Figure 9.4: Use of Maternity and Paternity Leave by Country: Percentage Distribution by Country

While people in all countries were favourable to paid leave, they were not equally favourable to unpaid leave. Everyone was favourable to paid maternity leave, however, when it came to *unpaid* maternity leave, France and Denmark were much less favourable than Ireland and Italy. The majority of Irish participants were strongly in favour of every one of the policies detailed including the unpaid leave policies that many of the other participants were not in favour of. The Danish participants were the next most favourable overall, due to their favouring very strongly the paid leave and flexible working policies, and not favouring at all the unpaid leave policies. The Italians were the next most favourable overall, followed by the French.

5.1.5. Parental Leave
Parental leave is leave taken for childcare purposes, usually following maternity/ paternity leave or some other time before the child is under three or under five, depending on the country. In Denmark, France and Italy, this leave is paid in varying degrees from 30% in Italy to up-to full salary in Denmark (negotiable with employer) and at a flat rate in France; in Ireland there is only unpaid parental leave. The length of parental leave varies by country and age of child (see Table 6.5, Chapter 6).

5.1.5.1. Availability of Parental Leave
We asked the participants to indicate whether or not they or their partner had paid and/ or unpaid parental leave available to them at their workplace. If they did, they were asked whether or not they had used it, and what their attitude was towards it.

In Italy almost half of the participants had it available to both partners. In France a very high proportion of participants did not know whether or not it was available to them, although it was definitely not available to half the male and a quarter of the female participants. Paid parental leave was not available to 95% of Irish participants.

Table 9.33. Availability of Paid Parental Leave:
Percentage Distributions by Country and Sex (N=400)

	France %		Italy %		Denmark %		Ireland %	
	M	F	M	F	M	F	M	F
My Work only	0.0	25.5	6.0	22.0	8.0	35.3	0.0	0.0
Partners Work only	10.2	0.0	16.0	10.0	14.0	0.0	0.0	0.0
Both	18.4	4.3	46.0	46.0	42.0	21.6	2.0	2.0
Neither	42.9	25.5	10.0	4.0	20.0	35.3	96.0	94.0
Don't know	28.6	44.7	22.0	18.0	16.0	7.8	2.0	4.0
Total	100.0	100.0	100.0	100.0	100.0	100.0	100.0	100.0

Unpaid parental leave was available to both partners in the majority of Irish couples, and to just under half the Italian couples interviewed. The availability was more disparate in Denmark and France.

Table 9.34. Availability of Unpaid Parental Leave:
Percentage Distributions by Country and Sex (N=400)

	France %		Italy %		Denmark %		Ireland %	
	M	F	M	F	M	F	M	F
My Work only	2.0	20.4	4.0	20.0	6.0	6.0	2.0	14.3
Partners Work only	10.2	4.1	14.0	4.0	10.0	24.0	6.0	4.1
Both	46.9	16.3	44.0	42.0	32.0	26.0	78.0	63.3
Neither	6.1	8.2	14.0	8.0	26.0	20.0	6.0	8.2
Don't know	34.7	51.0	24.0	26.0	26.0	24.0	8.0	10.2
Total	100.0	100.0	100.0	100.0	100.0	100.0	100.0	100.0

5.1.5.2. Use of Parental Leave
The groups most likely to have used paid parental leave were Danish, Italian and French females in that order. Paid parental leave is not available in Ireland. Ten per cent of Italian and 8% of Danish men had taken paid parental leave. A fifth of Italian and Irish females had used unpaid parental leave and a quarter of Danish

females had done, but fewer men had: 10% of Irish men, 8% of Danish men, 6% of Italian men and 2% of French men. The statistics on partners' use of parental leave corroborates these findings.

Table 9.35. *Use of Paid and Unpaid Parental Leave by Respondents and their Partners: Percentage of 'Yes' by Country and Sex*

	France %		Italy %		Denmark %		Ireland %	
	M	F	M	F	M	F	M	F
Self – paid leave	0.0	24.5	10.0	44.0	8.0	52.0	0.0	2.0
Self – unpaid leave	2.1	10.4	6.0	20.0	8.0	24.0	10.0	20.0
Partner – paid leave	20.0	2.1	36.0	6.0	48.0	8.0	0.0	2.0
Partner – unpaid leave	12.0	2.1	12.0	6.0	20.8	2.0	28.0	6.0

The low take-up of unpaid parental leave in Ireland may relate to the fact that it cannot be taken very flexibly. The leave must be taken either as a continuous block of 14 weeks or, *by agreement between the employer and the employee*, may be broken up over a period of time. (Parental Leave Act 1998, s. 7(1), in Equality Authority, 1998). Furthermore, an employee must give written notice to the employer of his or her intention to take parental leave, not later than six weeks before the employee proposes to commence the leave (*Ibid.*). The employer may decide to postpone the parental leave if he or she is satisfied that granting the leave would have a substantial adverse effect on the operation of his or her business. Thus it is not surprising that parental leave is not more widely availed of.

5.1.5.3. Attitudes towards Parental Leave
Very few participants were not in favour of paid parental leave. The most favourable were the Danish and the Irish.

*Table 9.36. Attitudes Towards Paid Parental Leave:
Percentage Distributions by Country and Sex (N=400)*

	France %		Italy %		Denmark %		Ireland %	
	M	F	M	F	M	F	M	F
Do Not Favour	0.0	0.0	4.0	0.0	2.0	0.0	6.0	0.0
Somewhat Favour	42.0	28.3	32.0	16.0	12.0	8.0	14.0	14.0
Strongly Favour	58.0	71.7	64.0	84.0	86.0	92.0	80.0	86.0
Total	100.0	100.0	100.0	100.0	100.0	100.0	100.0	100.0

Attitudes were much less favourable to unpaid than to paid parental leave. The Danish and the French were least favourable and the Irish were the most favourable. The positive attitudes towards unpaid parental leave in Ireland relate to the fact that paid parental leave is not yet available and unpaid parental leave has recently been granted and more recently extended in length.

*Table 9.37. Attitudes Towards Unpaid Parental Leave:
Percentage Distributions by Country and Sex (N=400)*

	France %		Italy %		Denmark %		Ireland %	
	M	F	M	F	M	F	M	F
Do Not Favour	48.0	60.0	16.0	34.0	46.0	60.0	14.0	8.0
Somewhat Favour	42.0	33.3	50.0	28.0	38.0	32.0	42.0	40.0
Strongly Favour	10.0	6.7	34.0	38.0	16.0	8.0	44.0	52.0
Total	100.0	100.0	100.0	100.0	100.0	100.0	100.0	100.0

5.1.5.4.Attitudes to Parental Leave if it were Paid More
Every one of the female Danish participants who had not taken paid parental leave would have done so had it been paid more, as compared to only a quarter of the Danish male participants. In France too, twice as many female participants as male would have taken parental leave if it had been paid more. In Italy only 20-30% of participants would have taken it if it had been paid more. As already noted, paid parental leave is not available in Ireland, so this particular question was not applicable to Irish respondents.

Table 9.38. Whether Respondents who did not take Paid Parental Leave Would Have if it were Paid More: Percentage of 'Yes' by Country and Sex

France %		Italy %		Denmark %		Ireland %	
M	F	M	F	M	F	M	F
22.2	56.3	20.0	28.6	25.0	100.0	-	-

Those parents who did not take up *unpaid* parental leave were asked if they would have taken it if it had been paid. Female participants were more likely to say that they would take parental leave if it were paid than male participants. There was strong indication of the potential take-up of paid parental leave among Irish parents (85% of women and 77% of men). There was equally strong support among Danish women (87.5%) and French women (76%). Male interest in paid parental leave was less than that of women, but strong among Irish (77%) and Danish (43%) men and less strong among Italian (21%) and French (30%) men.

Table 9.39. Whether Respondents who did not take Unpaid Parental Leave Would Have if it were Paid: Percentage of 'Yes' by Country and Sex

France %		Italy %		Denmark %		Ireland %	
M	F	M	F	M	F	M	F
30.3	76.2	20.6	53.1	42.9	87.5	76.7	84.6

5.2 Flexible Workplace Policies

5.2.1. Part-time Working

Part-time working was available in the majority of workplaces, the exception being the workplaces of Danish males.

Table 9.40. Part-time Working: Availability, Use and Attitude:
Percentage Distributions by Country and Sex (N=400)

	France %		Italy %		Denmark %		Ireland %	
	M	F	M	F	M	F	M	F
Availability (% Yes)	69.4	73.5	64.0	87.8	29.4	62.0	66.0	83.7
Availability (% Don't know)	6.1	6.1	6.0	0.0	7.8	8.0	2.0	2.0
Used (% Yes)	4.1	43.8	6.0	38.0	6.0	28.0	12.0	42.0
Do Not Favour	25.0	4.3	8.0	6.0	8.0	4.0	6.0	2.0
Somewhat Favour	37.5	17.0	42.0	30.0	40.0	16.0	26.0	6.0
Strongly Favour	37.5	78.7	50.0	64.0	52.0	80.0	68.0	92.0

Around 40% of female participants had worked part-time at some point, except for Danish females of whom only 28% had. Very few males had worked part-time, the highest number being in Ireland (12%).

The majority of women were strongly in favour of part-time working in all countries, including in Denmark, where there was little take-up of it. Male participants were more divided, but the majority either favoured or strongly favoured it except in France where a quarter of French males did not favour it as a policy.

5.2.2. Job-Sharing

There was less certainty about the availability of job-sharing, as compared to part-time working. It was most available in Ireland, where it was available to 60% of men and 54% of women. It was available to approximately a quarter of the French participants, and significantly fewer of the Danish and Italian.

Table 9.41. Job-Sharing: Availability, Use and Attitude:
Percentage Distributions by Country and Sex (N= 400)

	France %		Italy %		Denmark %		Ireland %	
	M	F	M	F	M	F	M	F
Availability (% Yes)	24.5	22.9	8.0	18.4	13.3	13.3	60.0	54.0
Availability (% Don't know)	24.5	29.2	18.0	20.4	23.3	16.7	4.0	10.0
Used (% Yes)	6.3	10.6	2.0	6.0	3.3	3.3	4.0	12.0
Do Not Favour	20.0	23.8	26.0	18.0	22.6	16.7	12.0	6.0
Somewhat Favour	65.0	47.6	48.0	40.0	38.7	36.7	32.0	12.0
Strongly Favour	15.0	28.6	26.0	42.0	38.7	46.7	56.0	82.0

There was very little take-up of job-sharing in any of the countries. In France and Ireland women were more likely to job-share than were men. The Irish participants were generally strongly favourable towards job sharing, especially the women. In the other countries attitudes were more mixed.

5.2.3. Flexible Hours

Participants seemed more certain about whether or not flexible hours were available in their workplace. Flexible hours were available for around half the participants, with the lowest availability being in Italy and the highest in France.

Table 9.42. Flexible Hours: Availability, Use and Attitude:
Percentage Distributions by Country and Sex (N=400)

	France %		Italy %		Denmark %		Ireland %	
	M	F	M	F	M	F	M	F
Availability (% Yes)	62.5	62.5	49.0	36.7	40.0	52.9	48.0	50.0
Availability (% Don't know)	4.2	14.6	4.1	4.1	0.0	2.0	0.0	2.0
Used (% Yes)	51.0	55.6	32.0	24.0	36.0	51.0	36.0	38.0
Do Not Favour	11.4	2.2	6.0	10.0	8.2	10.2	8.2	6.0
Somewhat Favour	36.4	31.1	32.0	28.0	18.4	18.4	18.4	16.0
Strongly Favour	52.3	66.7	62.0	62.0	73.5	71.4	73.5	78.0

There was a comparatively high take-up of flexible hours compared to other workplace policies, with half of French participants of both sexes and half of Danish females having availed of them. Flexible hours had also been availed of by a third of Italian, Danish and Irish males, and a third of Irish females. The lowest take up of this policy was by Italian females, of whom only a quarter had availed of flexible hours.

Male and female participants had very similar attitudes to flexible working: within and across countries: the majority strongly favoured it and only a small minority were not in favour.

5.2.4. Career Breaks

Many participants were not sure whether or not career breaks were available to them. A small majority of Irish, Italian and French participants and three-quarters of the Danish participants reported that career breaks were available in their workplace.

Table 9.43. Career Breaks: Availability, Use and Attitude: Percentage Distributions by Country and Sex (N= 400)

	France %		Italy %		Denmark %		Ireland %	
	M	F	M	F	M	F	M	F
Availability (% Yes)	58.3	61.7	40.0	57.1	70.0	79.6	56.0	52.9
Availability (% Don't know)	25.0	19.1	30.0	16.3	18.0	10.2	10.0	11.8
Used (% Yes)	2.0	14.6	0.0	6.0	22.0	44.9	0.0	8.0
Do Not Favour	28.3	24.4	12.0	14.0	0.0	0.0	10.2	4.0
Somewhat Favour	45.7	35.6	48.0	50.0	12.0	8.2	24.5	24.0
Strongly Favour	26.1	40.0	40.0	36.0	88.0	91.8	65.3	72.0

Only a small proportion of female participants from France, Italy and Ireland had taken career breaks and virtually no male participants. In Denmark, however, a fifth of male participants had used them and almost half of female participants had done so. The Danish and the Irish were the most in favour of career breaks where the French and Italians were more divided.

5.2.5. Term-Time Working

Term-time working is more likely to be available in French and Danish workplaces and less so in Irish and Italian workplaces.

Table 9.44. Term-Time Working: Availability, Use and Attitude:
Percentage Distributions by Country and Sex (N=400)

	France %		Italy %		Denmark %		Ireland %	
	M	F	M	F	M	F	M	F
Availability (% Yes)	31.9	54.3	4.0	10.2	58.1	43.3	24.0	4.0
Availability (% Don't know)	14.9	26.1	34.0	22.4	16.1	23.3	12.0	10.0
Used (% Yes)	8.3	17.0	0.0	0.0	16.1	3.3	10.2	0.0
Do Not Favour	40.5	27.9	22.0	16.0	22.6	16.7	18.8	10.2
Somewhat Favour	45.2	51.2	50.0	34.0	19.4	33.3	22.9	16.3
Strongly Favour	14.3	20.9	28.0	50.0	58.1	50.0	58.3	73.5

The take-up of term-time working was very low. The three groups who were most likely to use it were French females (17%) and Danish (16%) and Irish (10%) males. The most favourable attitudes to term-time working were held by the Irish, followed by the Danes, then the Italians, then the French.

5.2.6. Personalised Working Hours

Personalised working hours were available in 35- 50% of participants' workplaces. This figure appears similar within and between countries.

Table 9.45. Personalised Working Hours: Availability, Use and Attitude:
Percentage Distributions by Country and Sex (N=400).

	France %		Italy %		Denmark %		Ireland %	
	M	F	M	F	M	F	M	F
Availability (% Yes)	40.8	47.8	38.0	34.7	46.0	39.2	44.0	38.0
Availability (% Don't know)	14.3	19.6	8.0	12.2	0.0	3.9	2.0	6.0
Used (% Yes)	29.2	40.9	24.5	22.0	44.0	36.7	34.0	22.0
Do Not Favour	4.4	0.0	12.0	6.0	6.3	8.0	20.0	18.0
Somewhat Favour	31.1	31.0	30.0	28.0	18.8	28.0	22.0	14.0
Strongly Favour	64.4	69.0	58.0	66.0	75.0	64.0	58.0	68.0

At least 22% of participants in all countries had used personalised hours. The highest take-up was by Danish males (44%) and French females (41%) and the lowest take up was by Italians (23%) and Irish females (22%).

The Irish figures for take-up of personalised hours closely mirror those obtained by the CSO in a nationwide study (CSO, 2001). The CSO found that over a fifth of all Irish people in employment planned and scheduled their own working times in the second quarter of 2001, although in Dublin only 17% did so. Men were found to be almost twice as likely to plan their own working time (28%) as women (16%). This sex difference was also apparent in our study in which 34% of Dublin men and only 22% of Dublin women had personalised working hours. The majority of participants were strongly in favour of personalised hours.

5.2.7. Tele-working
Tele-working was not available to the majority of participants. It was most available to Danish males (46%), then to Irish males 35%), and was least available to Italian females (8%).

Table 9.46. Tele-working: Availability, Use and Attitude:
Percentage Distributions by Country and Sex

	France %		Italy %		Denmark %		Ireland %	
	M	F	M	F	M	F	M	F
Availability (% Yes)	19.0	13.6	10.0	8.2	46.0	22.0	34.7	20.0
Availability (% Don't know)	2.4	13.6	2.0	6.1	0.0	2.0	6.1	2.0
Used (% Yes)	17.4	4.5	4.0	6.0	34.0	10.2	10.0	8.2
Do Not Favour	22.2	23.7	16.0	32.0	18.4	20.0	18.4	9.8
Somewhat Favour	38.9	36.8	46.0	28.0	26.5	18.0	26.5	27.5
Strongly Favour	38.9	39.5	38.0	40.0	55.1	62.0	55.1	62.7

The majority of participants had not done tele-working. A third of Danish males had used this policy, however. The majority of Irish and Danish participants were strongly in favour of tele-working, and less than quarter of any group were not in favour.

5.2.8. Summary of Workplace Policies

We constructed an index of 'family-friendliness' of the respondent's workplace by summing the total number of 'yes's in response to each of the questions regarding the availability of workplace policies, e.g. 'Is paid maternity leave available?' Each of the 12 policies to receive a 'yes' was given a score of three; thus the scale ranges from 0 – 36.

There were significant differences found between countries, sectors and SES. The significant country difference indicated that Irish respondents were more likely to have the most family friendly policies available and French respondents the least. There was also a significant difference between participants working in the public *vs.* private sectors, with those in the private sector having somewhat fewer of the policies available to them. Participants in higher SES occupations had a greater availability of the policies than those in lower SES occupations.

Table 9.47. Family-Friendliness of Workplace: Mean Scores by Country, SES and Sector

		France	Italy	Denmark	Ireland	Total SES	Total Sector
Low SES	Public	14.0	19.4	14.6	18.3	Low = 15.9	Pub. = 17.9
	Private	13.0	14.1	15.1	18.5		
High SES	Public	17.5	18.5	15.9	23.7	High = 18.2	Priv. = 16.2
	Private	12.6	17.0	18.1	20.8		
Total Country		14.2	17.2	16.3	20.3	17.0	17.0

(0 = no family friendly policies available,
36 = all family friendly policies available)
Country: $F=14.91$, $df = 3$, $p \leq 0.001$
Sector: $F=7.26$, $df = 1$, $p \leq 0.01$
SES: $F=12.13$, $df = 1$, $p \leq 0.001$

The figure below illustrates these differences in the family friendliness of the workplaces in the different countries.

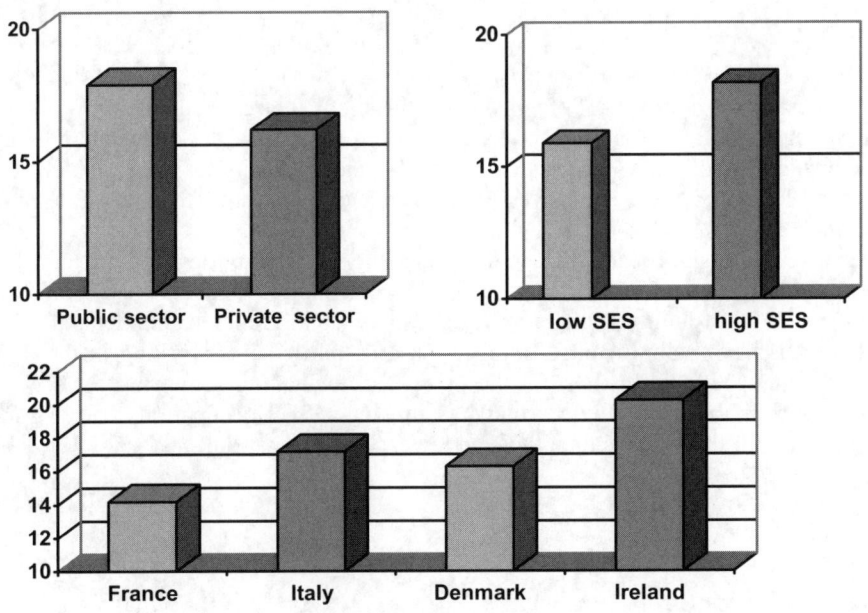

Figure 9.5: Relative Family-Friendliness of Workplace:
Mean Scores by Sector, SES and Country

CHAPTER 10

COMBINING WORK AND FAMILY LIFE

1. RECONCILING WORK AND FAMILY

In the previous two chapters we focused first on children and family life and then on the workplace. In this chapter we bring the two pieces together with the specific aim of finding out how working parents with young children reconcile these two major areas of their lives. Our major focus here is on key dependent measures of well-being. These include the measure of ease *vs.* difficulty of combining work and family life as well as several classic measures which have been widely used in social indicators research, i.e., satisfaction with work, health, partner/spouse, family life and life in general. We also include two measures related to time which cross the boundary of family and work and have major implications for reconciliation – namely 1) the extent to which parents' working schedules create problems with their childcare arrangements; and 2) and parents' ideal working schedule.

Building upon many of the measures presented in the preceding sections, this chapter presents results examining the predictors of successfully (or unsuccessfully) combining work and family life. The most significant predictors are presented for the combined four-country sample and then for males and females separately. Individual country differences are also discussed.

We then examine country differences in well-being, as well as the correlates of the different measures of well-being, drawing upon the key sets of variables presented earlier, including time variables, attitudes in the workplace, extent of help received, etc. Policies in the workplace, such as potential and actual flexibility and overall "family friendliness" of the workplace, are also examined in relation to the various measures of perceived well-being.

1.1. Ease vs. Difficulty in Reconciling Work and Family

Participants were asked how easy or difficult it was for them to combine their work with their family lives. They were asked to respond on a six-point scale, ranging from 1 = "very easy" to 6 = "very difficult." As may be seen below, 56.8% of all parents said it was easy to combine work and family life and 43.2% said it was difficult. Most parents fell into the two categories "somewhat easy" (36.9%) and "somewhat difficult" (30.6%). Of those saying it was difficult, 8.3% said it was "difficult" and 4.3% said it was "very difficult." The full comparative percentage tables by country are presented in Appendix Table A65.

Table 10.1. Ease vs. Difficulty in Combining Work and Family Life: Percentage Distributions for All Countries by Sex

	All Countries %		
	M	F	Total
Very Easy	5.0	3.1	4.0
Easy	15.5	16.3	15.9
Somewhat Easy	40.5	33.2	36.9
Somewhat Difficult	29.0	32.1	30.6
Difficult	7.5	9.2	8.3
Very Difficult	2.5	6.1	4.3
Total	**100.0**	**100.0**	**100.0**

Overall, the Danish parents found it significantly easier to combine their jobs with their family lives than did the parents in the other three countries. The Danes tended to say it was "somewhat easy" (38%) or "easy" (28%), whereas in the other countries the responses tended to fall into the "somewhat easy" to "somewhat difficult" categories. The means for the countries are presented below, confirming the significant effect of country. Two separate analyses of variance were conducted, one with country, sex and SES and the second with country, SES and sector. It was found that there was no significant effect of sex on this measure. In order to further explore possible gender differences, t-tests were conducted on the data comparing male and female scores within each country. These analyses confirmed that there were no significant differences in France, Denmark or Ireland, but that there was a significant gender difference in the Italian data which showed that Italian working mothers found it significantly more difficult (mean = 3.9) than Italian working fathers (mean = 3.3) to combine their work with their family lives (t = -3.34, df = 98; p<0.001).

We therefore present the results for the second ANOVA, involving sector, which did show significant effects. As may be seen below, those parents in lower SES jobs found it significantly easier to combine work and family life. On first glance, this is counter-intuitive, since parents of higher socio-economic status could theoretically afford to purchase more resources (e.g., childcare, domestic help, etc.) to help with reconciliation of work and family. Furthermore, many jobs of lower SES parents very demanding physically, in terms of hours, etc. However, it will be recalled from our results on the workplace that people in higher SES jobs had more pressure at work and this may help to explain their greater difficulty combining work and family life. There was a moderately significant interaction effect of SES and sector indicating that there was virtually no difference within the public sector; however, within the private sector those in higher SES jobs found it much more difficult that those in lower SES jobs

Table 10.2. Ease vs. Difficulty in Combining Work and Family Life: Mean Scores by Country and SES

	France	Italy	Denmark	Ireland	Total
Low SES	3.4	3.5	2.7	3.2	3.2
High SES	3.7	3.7	3.2	3.7	3.5
Total	**3.5**	**3.6**	**2.9**	**3.4**	**3.4**

(1 = very easy, 6 = very difficult)
Country: $F = 7.54$, $df = 3$; $p \leq 0.001$
SES: $F = 10.25$, $df = 1$; $p \leq 0.001$

Table 10.3. Ease vs. Difficulty in Combining Work and Family Life: Mean Scores by Sector and SES

	Public	Private
Low SES	3.4	3.0
High SES	3.5	3.6

(1 = very easy, 6 = very difficult)
SES-Sector: $F = 4.42$, $df = 1$; $p \leq 0.05$

1.2. Issues of Time

In most countries the schedules of workplaces and childcare centres and schools are not synchronised. Moreover, because most people work similar schedules, traffic is generated at peak times which means it is even more difficult to quickly get from work to the childcare facility and *vice versa*. This situation frequently necessitates parents needing to arrange complex childcare arrangements, often involving several modes and sources of care, ranging from childcare centres to childminders to grandparents.

We were interested in finding out the extent to which the hours one worked created problems with one's childcare arrangements. Over all countries it was found that 34% of parents said "not at all," 35% said "not very much," 25% said "yes, to some extent," and 6% said "yes, a great deal." The full percentage data by country is contained in Appendix Table A66.

Analysis of variance revealed that there was a significant difference on this question among the four countries. French participants were most likely to report that the hours they worked caused problems with their childcare arrangements and Irish and Danish participants reported the least problems.

Table 10.4. The Extent to which Working Hours Create Problems with Childcare Arrangements: Mean Scores by Country

France	Italy	Denmark	Ireland
2.4	2.1	1.9	1.8

(1 = not at all, 4 = yes, a great deal)
$F = 8.64$, $df = 3$; $p \leq 0.001$

We also asked participants what their "ideal working schedule" would be (with no change in salary). The most common response was that they would like to work shorter days (27.5%). The next most common response was that participants were happy with their current schedules (23%). This was followed by 18% preferring to be able to work flexible hours and 17% opting for more holiday time. Approximately 16% said they would prefer longer days, but fewer days. French participants, particularly the women (40%), preferred to keep their schedule the way it was. Among Danish females there was a tendency to favour shorter days (43%). However, generally speaking, approximately 20% or so in every country favoured one of the options. This clearly indicates that there is no one solution to meeting people's needs in this area, but rather a need for a variety of flexible options.

Chi-square tests were carried out to compare male and female responses. No significant differences were found, indicating that male and female parents in all of the countries are basically similar in imagining a wide variety of optimal working patterns.

Table 10.5. Respondents' Ideal Working Schedule:
Percentage Distributions by Country and Sex

	France %		Italy %		Denmark %		Ireland %		All Countries %		
	M	F	M	F	M	F	M	F	M	F	Total
Longer day/ Fewer days	4.0	6.0	19.9	12.0	6.3	16.0	35.1	27.1	16.3	15.3	15.8
Shorter days	25.5	19.8	16.3	28.0	27.8	42.7	30.8	29.4	25.1	30.0	27.5
Flexible hours	18.3	19.7	23.9	20.0	19.8	12.2	12.2	16.7	18.5	17.1	17.8
More holiday time	22.5	24.5	8.2	10.2	22.4	17.4	17.2	14.1	17.6	16.5	17.1
Stay the same	31.1	40.4	27.7	27.9	21.8	7.8	10.0	18.0	22.7	23.5	23.1
Other	6.2	5.4	4.0	3.7	1.9	10.3	2.4	9.9	3.6	7.3	5.5

Note: As respondents could give more than one answer, totals do not add up to 100%

Our results may be compared with a 1999 study conducted in the European Union member states and Norway by the European Foundation for the Improvement of Living and Working Conditions in Dublin (Latta & O'Conghaile, 2000) which found that there was a desire to reduce the length of the working week by both male and female individuals interviewed. The length of the current working week was 39 hours, and the ideal length was 34 hours. This compares with an actual average of 38 hours worked per week in our sample (42 hours for men and 32 hours for women).

The women interviewed in the Latta and O'Conghaile (2000) study, while also wishing to reduce their working week, preferred to work long part-time (21-30 hours) rather than short part time (<20 hours). Over a quarter of the women interviewed (27%) expressed the wish to work long part-time while only 14% were actually doing so. On examining the reasons for wanting a shorter working week, the most common reason for women aged 30-39 was to have 'more time for children' (77%), followed by 'more time for yourself and own activities' (66%), and thirdly, 'to reduce the strains resulting from full-time job' (55%)(*Ibid*).

Of the men interviewed across Europe, 13% reported that they would like to work part-time, while less than 4% were actually doing so. The reasons of men in the 30-39 age group for wanting to reduce the length of their working week, were primarily to have 'more time for yourself and own activities' (80% of the men reported this as a reason). Over half the men interviewed reported that they would like 'more time for children' (58%) and under half 'to reduce the strains resulting from full time job' (44%) (*Ibid*).

Research carried out by Bielenski & Kappuninen in Europe (1999) on working time found that ten times as many couples would prefer both partners to be working part-time than did so at the time of the study (see figure below).

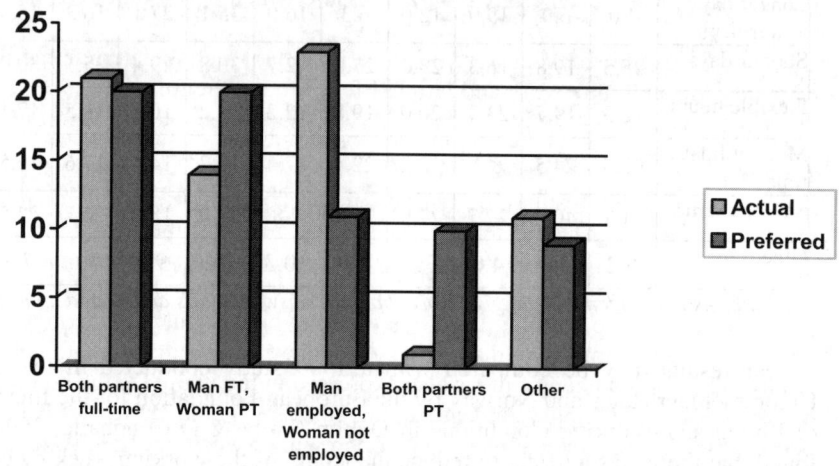

Figure 10.1. Actual and Preferred Working Patterns of European Couples (Adapted from Bielenski & Kauppinen, 1999, p. 6)

Most couples where both partners were in employment were happy with their choice, with a tendency towards preferring part-time work for the woman where both are in full-time work, and part-time work for both partners where the woman is already in part-time employment. This latter trend was particularly noteworthy amongst Scandinavian men, of whom 26% would prefer for both partners to be in part-time work, as compared to 10% of the men in the Mediterranean countries. The differences between the actual situations of couples in the Mediterranean and Scandinavian countries were much larger than the differences between the preferred work-sharing options (*Ibid*).

The happiest couples of all were those in which both partners were working the same number of hours – either both full-time or both part-time, and conversely, the traditional model of working whereby the man works full-time and the women does not working at all has very low popularity. These results therefore, make a strong case for the availability of part-time work (*Ibid*).

1.3 Predictors of Ease vs. Difficulty in Combining Work and Family Life

As was seen earlier, there were significant differences between the four countries in terms of the ease or difficulty parents experienced in combining work and family life. This was found to be much easier in Denmark than in the other three countries and it was also more difficult for those in higher occupational status jobs, which may be related to the generally greater pressure which was found to exist for people in these jobs.

When we examined what were the most important factors determining the ease or difficulty in combining work and family life we found the following:

1.3.1. All Countries – Males and Females

When looking at the results of a multiple regression analysis for the total sample of all four countries, male and female, we see that many of the things we might have expected to be significant are not - like age, education or number of children (See Table 10.6). Amongst the most important factors was found to be time. The length of one's partner's commuting time was found to be particularly important ($p \leq .001$). The longer the commuting time, the less time they will be available to help with the family. The importance of time is also expressed in the item "Do the hours you work create problems in your childcare arrangements?" The more this was true for people, the more difficulty they had in combining work and family life ($p \leq .001$). Not surprisingly, the more hours a person worked per week the more difficulty they had combining work and family ($p \leq 0.01$).

Another very significant predictor was the amount of help a person got with domestic and childcare responsibilities. The more help one got, the easier it was to combine work and family ($p \leq 0.001$). Attitudes in the workplace were also very important. Most important was a feeling that in a pinch one could bring one's child to work for a little while if childcare arrangements broke down. If working parents felt that this was accepted by colleagues in particular, but also by their managers, they were more likely to say that combining work and family was easier. Such behaviour was more likely to be considered unacceptable in Ireland, France and Italy, as opposed to Denmark. As this question was tapping such a sensitive issue, it is interesting that it is a good predictor, as it clearly is tapping into the relative acceptance of childcare responsibilities in the workplace culture.

Table 10.6. Predictors of Ease vs. Difficulty in Combining Work and Family Life: Multiple Regression for All Countries – Total Sample Males and Females (N =400)

	Predictor Variables	Beta	Sig.
1.	Age	0.03	-
2.	Level of education	-0.01	-
3.	Partner's education	0.02	-
4.	Occupational Status	0.14	-
5.	Partner's Occupational Status	0.06	-
6.	Own Commuting Time	0.10	-
7.	Partner's Commuting Time	0.16	***
8.	Length of Work Week	0.16	**
9.	Length of Partner's Work Week	-0.05	-
10.	Number of children	-0.02	-
11.	HELPINDEX Index of Help with Domestic Responsibilities	-0.25	***
12.	Acceptability of arriving late/leaving early		
12a.	among your colleagues	0.09	-
12b.	your managers	-0.10	-
13.	Acceptability of bringing child to work		-
13a.	among your colleagues	-0.31	***
13b.	your managers	0.20	-
14.	How well the following people take into account your responsibility for a child:		
14a.	your colleagues	-0.02	-
14b.	your immediate supervisor	-0.10	-
14c.	your employer	0.07	-
15.	Extent to which the hours you work create problems with childcare arrangements	0.29	***

$R = 0.54$, $R^2 = 0.292$, Adj $R^2 = 0.252$, Standard Error = 0.96

Table 10.6a. ANOVA for Total Equation

	Sum of Squares	df	Mean Square	F	Sig.
Regression	928.99	19	6.79	7.41	***
Residual	313.45	342	0.91		
Total	442.44	361			

$* \leq .05$ $\quad\quad ** \leq .01 \quad *** \leq .001$

1.3.2. All Countries – Males Only

Looking at the data for males only in the four countries, it was found again that if the hours one works create problems in one's childcare arrangements, the more likely one is to have difficulty combining work and family life. Not surprisingly, the longer the working week, the greater the difficulty. Also important was colleagues' acceptance of one's childcare responsibilities, as manifested in the item concerning acceptability of bringing a child to work say for an hour if one had difficulty in childcare arrangements (Table 10.7).

1.3.3. All Countries – Females Only

What were the key predictors of successfully combining work and family for women? Again time was a crucial factor. One's own commuting time was significant, as was one's partner's. The shorter the commuting time, the easier it was to combine work and family. Women whose hours created problems with their childcare arrangements also had more difficulty reconciling work and family life. The amount of help women received was also significantly related to successfully combining work and family. The less help they received from their partner, the more difficulty they experienced combining work and family life – the more help they received the easier it was. Finally, colleagues' attitudes were also important, as were those of the woman's immediate supervisor. The more accepting the attitudes concerning the woman's childcare responsibilities, the easier she found it to combine work and family (Table 10.7).

Table 10.7. Predictors of Ease vs. Difficulty in Combining Work and Family Life: Multiple Regression for All Countries – Males and Females (Males, N = 200 and Females, N = 200)

		Males		Females	
	Predictor Variables	Beta	Sig.	Beta	Sig.
1.	Age	0.00	-	0.06	-
2.	Level of education	-0.13	-	0.15	-
3.	Partner's education	0.01	-	-0.02	-
4.	Occupational Status	0.11	-	0.08	-
5.	Partner's Occupational Status	0.22	*	0.00	-
6.	Own Commuting Time	0.03	-	0.15	*
7.	Partner's Commuting Time	0.17	*	0.18	**
8.	Length of Work Week	0.22	***	0.13	-
9.	Length of Partner's Work Week	-0.06	-	-0.08	-
10.	Number of children	-0.00	-	-0.00	-
11.	HELPINDEX Index of Help with Domestic Responsibilities	-0.05	-	-0.16	*
12.	Acceptability of arriving late/leaving early		-		-
12a.	among your colleagues		-	0.07	-
12b.	your managers	-0.13	-	0.02	-
13.	Acceptability of bringing child to work				
13a.	among your colleagues	-0.37	**	-0.28	*
13b.	your managers	0.25	-	0.18	-
14.	How well the following people take into account your responsibility for a child:				
14a.	your colleagues	0.02	-	-0.12	-
14b.	your immediate supervisor	0.04	-	-0.25	**
14c.	your employer	0.08	-	0.07	-
15.	Extent to which the hours you work create problems with childcare arrangements	0.36	0.000	0.20	**

Males: $R = .583$, $R^2 = .34$, Adj $R^2 = .259$, Standard Error = .92
Females: $R = .59$, $R^2 = .35$, Adj $R^2 = .275$, Standard Error = .97

Table 10.7a. ANOVA for Total Equation

		Sum of Squares	df	Mean Square	F	Sig.
Male	Regression	67.62	19	3.56	4.20	***
	Residual	131.32	155	0.85		
	Total	198.94	174			
Female	Regression	83.87	19	4.17	4.72	***
	Residual	156.29	167	0.94		
	Total	240.16	186			

$* \leq .05 \quad ** \leq .01 \quad *** \leq .001$

1.3.4. Results for Individual Countries: Ireland
The factors that were significant in the all country data were also significant for Ireland, and in most cases even more significant. The most significant factors for Irish parents were:
- Partner's Commuting Time
- The Number Hours Worked per week
- The Amount of Help received with Domestic Chores and Childcare at Home
- The Extent to which one's Hours create problems with Childcare Arrangements

The multiple regression for Ireland explained a greater degree of variance in the dependent measure than did the multiple regressions for the all country data (See Table 10.8). In the Irish data set, 39% of the variance in the dependent measure was explained, based on the adjusted R^2. Again the total equation was highly significant.

1.3.5. Results for Italy
The results for Italy have some similarities with the previous sets of results and some differences. In Italy one's occupational status was related to difficulty in combining work and family. Those of higher occupational status had more difficulty, presumably because of the greater pressure found in this group. The longer the commuting time, the greater the difficulty participants had in combining work and family. As in the case in Ireland, the Italian multiple regression explained more variance in the dependent measure (35%, based on the adjusted R^2) than did the all country data.

1.3.6. French and Danish Results
The full data for France and Denmark are not presented because the overall equations did not reach significance, as did the Italian and Irish data. However, the Danish and French data did show that similar variables were predictive to those that were significant in the all country data.

Table 10.8. Predictors of Ease vs. Difficulty in Combining Work and Family Life:
Multiple Regression for Ireland Only (N = 100)

		Predictor Variables	Beta	Sig.
1.		Age	0.06	-
2.		Level of education	0.07	-
3.		Partner's education	0.02	-
4.		Occupational Status	0.09	-
5.		Partner's Occupational Status	-0.02	-
6.		Own Commuting time	-0.06	-
7.		Partner's Commuting time	0.31	***
8.		Length of Work Week	0.31	***
9.		Length of Partner's Work Week	-0.07	-
10.		Number of children	-0.06	-
11.		HELPINDEX Index of Help with Domestic Responsibilities	-0.46	***
12.		Acceptability of arriving late/leaving early		
12a.		among you and colleagues	0.21	-
12b.		by managers	-0.14	-
13.		Acceptability of bringing child to work		
13a.		among you and colleagues	-0.35	*
13b.		by managers	0.29	-
14.		How well the following people take into account your responsibility for a child:		
14a.		Colleagues	0.02	-
14b.		Immediate Supervisor	-0.18	-
14c.		Employer	0.24	-
15.		Extent to which the hours you work create problems with childcare arrangements	0.48	***

$R = .71$, $R^2 = .50$, Adj $R^2 = .39$, Standard Error = 1.03

Table 10.8a. ANOVA for Total Equation

	Sum of Squares	Df	Mean Square	F	Sig.
Regression	91.82	19	4.83	4.57	***
Residual	93.03	88	1.06		
Total	184.85	107			

* ≤ .05   ** ≤ .01   *** ≤ .001

Table 10.9. *Predictors of Ease vs. Difficulty in Combining Work and Family Life: Multiple Regression for Italy Only (N= 100)*

		Predictor Variables	Beta	Sig.
1.		Age	0.07	-
2.		Level of education	-0.23	-
3.		Partner's education	0.02	-
4.		Occupational Status	0.38	*
5.		Partner's Occupational Status	-0.12	-
6.		Own Commuting Time	0.23	*
7.		Partner's Commuting Time	-0.14	-
8.		Length of Work Week	0.10	-
9.		Length of Partner's Work Week	0.05	-
10.		Number of children	-0.14	-
11.		HELPINDEX Index of Help with Domestic Responsibilities	-0.10	-
12.		Acceptability of arriving late/leaving early		
	12a.	among your colleagues	0.03	-
	12b.	your managers	-0.31	P<0.06
13.		Acceptability of bringing child to work		
	13a.	among your colleagues	-0.17	-
	13b.	your managers	0.08	-
14.		How well the following people take into account your responsibility for a child:		
	14a.	among your colleagues	0.09	-
	14b.	your immediate supervisor	-0.20	-
	14c.	your employer	-0.16	-
15.		Extent to which the hours you work create problems with childcare arrangements	0.21	-

$R = .73$, $R^2 = .53$, Adj $R^2 = .35$, Standard Error = .77

Table 10.9a. *ANOVA for Total Equation*

	Sum of Squares	df	Mean Square	F	Sig.
Regression	33.77	19	1.78	3.02	***
Residual	29.98	51	0.59		
Total	63.72	70			

* ≤ 0.05 ** ≤ 0.01 *** ≤ 0.001

2. WELL-BEING

In this section we examine several global measures of satisfaction which have been widely used, particularly in social indicator research. Participants were asked to record their satisfaction on five measures of well-being: their health, their work, their family life, the relationship with their partner and their life in general.

2.1. Health

Most participants appeared satisfied with their health with most saying they were either satisfied or very satisfied. Percentage distributions showed that 87% were on the satisfied side of the continuum and 13% on the dissatisfied side. Of those who were satisfied with their health, 21.6% were "somewhat satisfied", 41.6% were "satisfied" and 23.6% were "very satisfied" (Appendix Table A67). There was a significant difference between countries with Danish participants reporting the highest level of satisfaction with their health, and Italy and France the least.

Table 10.10: Satisfaction with Present State of Health:
Mean Scores by Country and Sex

	France	Italy	Denmark	Ireland	Total
Male	4.6	4.6	5.0	4.5	**4.7**
Female	4.4	4.5	5.1	4.9	**4.8**
Total	**4.5**	**4.5**	**5.1**	**4.7**	**4.7**

(1= very dissatisfied, 6 = very satisfied)
Country: F=5.25, df = 3, p≤0.001

2.2. Work

The results for satisfaction with work are very similar to those for satisfaction with health: most participants reported being satisfied with a few being very and a few being somewhat satisfied (Appendix Table A68). There was a significant difference between countries showing the same trends: The Danish are the most satisfied followed by the Irish.

Table 10.11. Satisfaction with Present Work: Mean Scores by Country and Sex

	France	Italy	Denmark	Ireland	Total
Male	4.4	4.4	5.0	4.4	**4.5**
Female	4.3	4.5	4.8	4.8	**4.6**
Total	**4.3**	**4.4**	**4.9**	**4.6**	**4.6**

(1= very dissatisfied, 6 = very satisfied)
Country: $F=4.96$, $df = 3$, $p \leq 0.005$

In the case of work satisfaction, there was also a significant interaction effect of sex and SES. Male participants in lower SES jobs were the group least satisfied with their work, and male participants in higher SES jobs were the most satisfied. Conversely, women in lower SES jobs were more satisfied than their higher SES counterparts, which is surprising, given the nature of the work available in low and high SES occupations. However, as we have noted earlier, women in higher SES occupations reported significantly more pressure than did women in lower SES jobs, which may be a contributing factor. Nevertheless, the means still range from 4.3 to 4.8 out of a possible 6, indicating relatively high levels of work satisfaction.

Table 10.12. Satisfaction with Present Work: Mean Scores by Sex and SES

	Male	Female
Low SES	4.3	4.7
High SES	4.8	4.5

(1= very dissatisfied, 6= very satisfied)
Sex x SES: $F=8.97$, $df = 1$, $p \leq 0.005$

2.3. Family Life

The majority of participants reported being either satisfied or very satisfied with their family lives (Appendix Table A69). There were no significant differences of sex, SES or country.

Table 10.13. Satisfaction with Family Life: Mean Scores by Country and Sex

	France	Italy	Denmark	Ireland	Total
Male	4.9	5.2	5.2	5.2	**5.2**
Female	4.9	5.1	5.2	5.2	**5.1**
Total	**4.9**	**5.1**	**5.2**	**5.2**	**5.1**

(1= very dissatisfied, 6 = very satisfied)

2.4. Relationship with Partner

Participants' satisfaction with their relationships with their partners shows the same trends as for their satisfaction with their health and their work: most are satisfied, with the Danes being the most satisfied, followed by the Irish (Appendix Table A70).

Table 10.14. Satisfaction with Partner: Mean Scores by Country and Sex

	France	Italy	Denmark	Ireland	Total
Male	5.1	5.2	5.3	5.3	**5.2**
Female	4.9	4.8	5.3	5.4	**5.1**
Total	**5.0**	**5.0**	**5.3**	**5.4**	**5.2**

(1= very dissatisfied, 6 = very satisfied)
Country: $F=4.53$, $df = 3$, $p \leq 0.005$

2.5. Life in General

The same trends can be seen for satisfaction with life in general: the majority of participants were satisfied. The Danish participants were the most satisfied, followed by the Irish, then the Italians and lastly the French (Appendix Table A71). There was also a moderately significant sex difference on this measure with female participants reporting higher levels of satisfaction with their life in general than male participants.

Table 10.15. Satisfaction with Life in General: Mean Scores by Country and Sex

	France	Italy	Denmark	Ireland	Total
Male	4.6	4.8	5.3	4.9	**4.9**
Female	4.6	5.0	5.5	5.2	**5.1**
Total	**4.6**	**4.9**	**5.4**	**5.1**	**5.0**

(1= very dissatisfied, 6 = very satisfied)
Country: $F=14.48$, $df = 3$, $p \leq 0.001$
Sex: $F=4.51$, $df = 1$, $p \leq 0.05$

2.6. Summary of Satisfaction Measures

In looking at the results for the satisfaction measures, it is apparent that Denmark stands out as having the highest levels of satisfaction on three of the five measures (health, work and life in general) and shares the highest satisfaction scores with Ireland concerning relationship with partner. Ireland had the second highest mean satisfaction scores on health, work and life in general. There were no significant country differences on satisfaction with family life. The greater satisfaction which is apparent in the Danish data may reflect three things: 1) the relatively even distribution of working hours between the sexes (backed up by a more equal distribution of household labour between women and men); 2) a high level of relatively affordable public day-care provision and a high degree of paid maternity and parental leave; and 3) a workplace culture with a relatively relaxed and permissive attitude towards reconciling work and family life.

It is thus clear that the nature of the Danish workplace, the greater public provision of childcare facilities and the greater sharing of roles in the home are reflected in higher levels of well-being in several spheres on the part of the Danish respondents (Højgaard, 2002).

Table 10.16. Summary Table of Satisfaction Levels:
Mean Scores by Country

Satisfaction with:	France	Italy	Denmark	Ireland	Sig.
Health	4.5	4.5	**5.1**	4.7	$p<0.001$
Work	4.3	4.4	**4.9**	4.6	$p<0.005$
Family Life	4.9	5.1	5.2	5.2	N.S.
Partner	5.0	5.0	**5.3**	5.4	$p<0.005$
Life in General	4.6	4.9	**5.4**	5.1	$p<0.001$

(1= very dissatisfied, 6 = very satisfied)

However, while this interpretation is no doubt true, it should be noted that country differences have been systematically observed in social indicator studies of well-being, in the direction of larger countries, such as France and Italy, tending to express lower levels of satisfaction, whereas smaller countries, such as Denmark, Ireland, and the Netherlands tending to express higher levels. This tendency was observed by Davis *et al.* (1982) in a study of determinants of perceived well being in eight European countries, and by Davis and Fine-Davis (1991) in a comparative study of social indicators of living conditions in the same eight European countries. Inglehart and Rabier (1985) in noting this phenomenon suggest "that the cross-national differences have an important cultural component . . . they probably . . . reflect different cultural norms. Quite possibly these cultures differ in the extent to which it is permissible to express unhappiness and dissatisfaction with one's life (*Ibid*, p. 12)."

3. CORRELATES OF WELL-BEING

In this section we examine the relationships between a wide range of respondent characteristics and measures of their well-being. These include time-related variables, variables related to domestic and childcare help, attitudes in the workplace, and the degree of family friendliness of the workplace in terms of policies available to facilitate reconciliation of work and family life.

The dependent measures of well-being consist of measures of satisfaction in several life domains:
- health
- work
- family life
- relationship with spouse/partner
- life in general

3.1   Relationships between Time-related Variables and Measures of Well-Being

3.1.1. All Countries – Males and Females
As was noted earlier in the section which examined predictors of Ease *vs.* Difficulty in Combining Work and Family Life, time is of critical importance. In this section we examine the relationships between various measures of time and the dependent measures of satisfaction in various life spheres in order to see to what extent time is related not only to combining work and family, but also to more general measures of well-being.

The following table presents data for the entire male and female sample of working parents from all of the four countries (N=400). The first two variables concerning time (in the left-hand column of the table) concern length of commuting time – the first, the commuting time of the respondent and the second, the commuting time of the respondent's partner. It may be seen that there is a low, but significant relationship between the length of commuting time and satisfaction with family life ($p \leq 0.05$). Both the respondent's own commuting time and that of his/her partner is significantly related to satisfaction with family life in the direction of shorter commuting time being associated with greater satisfaction and longer time with greater dissatisfaction. There were also low, but still significant relationships between the length of partner's commuting time and both satisfaction with one's health and with one's work. The shorter the partner's commuting time the greater one's satisfaction with one's health and with one's work.

While the length of one's own working week (as measured in hours) was not significantly related to well-being, the length of one's *partner's* working week was. The fewer hours per week that one's partner worked, the greater the respondent's own satisfaction both with family life and with their relationship with their spouse/partner ($p \leq 0.05$).

Table 10.17. Relationships between Time-related Variables and Measures of Well-being: Correlations for All Countries, Males and Females (N = 400)

Time-related Variables	Measures of Well-being: Satisfaction with:				
	Health	Work	Family life	Relationship with Spouse/Partner	Life
Length of commuting time	-0.03	-0.06	-0.12*	-0.00	-0.05
Length of partner's commuting time	-0.10*	-0.10*	-0.12*	-0.01	-0.07
Length of work week	-0.07	0.01	-0.09	-0.03	-0.08
Length of partner's work week	0.08	0.06	-0.10*	-0.11*	0.04
Amount of time would like to spend with family (1 = much less, 5 = much more)	-0.15**	-0.08	-0.10*	-0.02	-0.04
Amount of personal time would like to have (1 = much less, 5 = much more)	-0.23***	-0.15**	-0.27***	-0.24***	-0.26***

* $p \leq .05$ ** $p \leq .01$ *** $p \leq .001$

The final two time-related variables examined concerned the amount of time one would like to spend with the family (i.e., much more, more, the same amount, less, or much less) and the amount of personal time one would like to have. It may be seen that the less a respondent expressed a need to spend more time with the family, the more satisfied they were with their health. Conversely, the more they expressed a need or wish to spend time with the family, the less satisfied they were with their health ($p \leq .01$). This suggests that spending enough time with family is related to greater health satisfaction, whereas not spending enough time with one's family is related to poorer health satisfaction. Given that satisfaction with health has been found in other studies to be related to actual health, this is noteworthy.

In the same vein, the more personal time a respondent wanted, the less satisfied they tended to be on the five measures of well-being. The more personal time wanted, the less satisfaction was expressed with one's health, one's work, one's family life, one's relationship with one's partner and with one's life in general. Four out of five of these relationships were significant at the $p \leq .001$ level. This suggests that if one does not get sufficient personal time, this unmet need is felt in other key domains of one's life. Conversely, if one has a sufficient amount of personal time, one is more likely to manifest well-being in all of the key domains of health, work, family life, relationship with partner, and life in general.

3.1.2. Male-Female Differences

An examination of these correlational relationships for males and females separately are presented in the following tables. It may be seen that the table for female participants has a far greater number of significant relationships (Table 10.19). Thus, most of the relationships between time and well-being hold more strongly for women than for men. In particular, it can be seen that for women the length of their commuting time is significantly related to their work satisfaction ($p \leq 0.01$) and their satisfaction with family life ($p \leq 0.01$). The shorter the commuting time, the greater their satisfaction with work and family life. The longer their commute, the greater their dissatisfaction.

The more the mothers in the sample expressed a desire to spend more time with their families the less likely they were to say they were satisfied with their health, work, family life and life in general. For them, greater well-being was related to not needing to see more of their family. In the male sample, the results were quite different. None of the relationships were significant and in some cases, the correlation was in the opposite direction to that of the women.

In the case of needs for personal time, men and women were the same in terms of directionality, but for women the relationships were stronger in most cases. This was particularly true in the case of health and life satisfaction. The more a woman craved more personal time, the less satisfied she was with her health and with her life in general ($r = -0.32$ and $r = -0.34$ respectively, $p \leq 0.001$ in both cases). The relationships were also very strong in the cases of work satisfaction, satisfaction with family life and satisfaction with spouse/partner ($p \leq 0.001$ in all cases). The converse of these relationships is that working mothers who have enough personal time are more likely to express satisfaction in all of the five life domains examined here. For men, the relationships were strongest for satisfaction with family life, relationship with partner and life in general (p≤0.001).

Table 10.18. Relationships between Time-related Variables and Measures of Well-being: Correlations for All countries, Males only (N =200)

Time-related Variables	Measures of Well-being: Satisfaction with:				
	Health	Work	Family life	Relationship with Spouse/ Partner	Life
Length of partner's commuting time	0.02	-0.06	-0.09	-0.06	-0.01
Length of work week	-0.10	-0.01	-0.10	-0.07	-0.02
Length of partner's work week	0.13	0.02	-0.08	-0.05	0.03
Amount of time would like to spend with family (1 = much less, 5 = much more)	-0.12	0.10	0.02	0.13	0.13
Amount of personal time would like to have (1 = much less, 5 = much more)	-0.16*	-0.07	-0.28***	-0.23***	-0.21**

* $p \leq 0.05$ ** $p \leq 0.01$ *** $p \leq 0.001$

Table 10.19. Relationships between Time-related Variables and Measures of Well-being: All countries, Females only (N = 200)

Time-related Variables	Measures of Well-being: Satisfaction with:				
	Health	Work	Family life	Relationship with Spouse/Partner	Life
Length of commuting time	-0.06	-0.17**	-0.17**	-0.05	-0.18**
Length of partner's commuting time	-0.21**	-0.14*	-0.13*	0.04	-0.14*
Length of work week	-0.02	0.03	-0.13*	-0.08	-0.08
Length of partner's work week	0.02	0.10	-0.10	-0.11	-0.01
Amount of time would like to spend with family (1 = much less, 5 = much more)	-0.17**	-0.23***	-0.19**	-0.12	-0.17**
Amount of personal time would like to have (1 = much less, 5 = much more)	-0.32***	-0.23***	-0.26***	-0.24***	-0.34***

* $p \leq 0.05$ ** $p \leq 0.01$ *** $p \leq 0.001$

3.2 Relationships between Variables related to Domestic Help and Childcare and Measures of Well-Being

In earlier sections of the Report, we presented extensive data on who does what in the household. It will be recalled that respondents were asked who carried out each of twelve household and childcare activities: "Me", "My Partner", "Both of Us" or "Other". In the following analysis we explored whether or not there was a relationship between who carries out domestic and childcare chores and measures of well-being. Specifically, we looked at the "Both of Us" measure and the Total Amount of Domestic/Childcare Help (HELPINDEX). The first measure ("Both of Us") is the summation of the number of tasks in which respondents said both carried them out. The HELPINDEX is a summary index reflecting amount of help received, i.e., if respondent generally carried out the task, a score of 1 was given, if both did it a score of 2 was given, if partner or "other "did it, a score of 3 was given. Thus, the fewer "Me's" and the greater the number of "Both of Us" and/or "Partner" or "Other", the more the help was received.

It may be seen that the more both partners carried out domestic and childcare tasks the greater their satisfaction with family life, relationship with partner ($p \leq 0.001$ in both cases) and with life in general ($p \leq 0.05$). The greater the total amount of help received, the greater the satisfaction with spouse/partner ($p \leq 0.05$).

Table 10.20. *Relationships between Variables related to Domestic Help/Childcare and Measures of Well-being: Correlations for All Countries, Males and Females (N = 400)*

Variables related to domestic help/childcare	Measures of Well-being: Satisfaction with:				
	Health	Work	Family life	Relationship with Spouse/Partner	Life
Number of domestic/childcare tasks carried out by "both of us"	0.05	-0.01	0.18***	0.22***	0.10*
HELP INDEX Total amount of domestic/childcare help	-0.04	0.03	0.06	0.11*	-0.04
Satisfaction with childcare arrangements	0.14**	0.13**	0.28***	0.25***	0.23***

* $p \leq 0.05$ ** $p \leq 0.01$ *** $p \leq 0.001$

However, when we examine the male and female data separately, we see a somewhat different picture. It may be seen that receiving help with domestic tasks and childcare is more significantly related to women's well-being than it is to men's. For example, the HELPINDEX (i.e. amount of help received) is significantly correlated with women's satisfaction with their spouse/partner ($p \leq 0.01$), whereas it is not significantly related at all for men. It can also be seen that the more *both* partners carry out domestic tasks and childcare, the more likely women are to report feeling satisfied with their family life ($p \leq 0.01$), with their spouse/partner ($p \leq 0.001$) and with their life in general ($p \leq 0.05$). For men, there are also significant positive correlations with satisfaction with partner and family life, but these relationships are not as strong as they are for women ($p \leq 0.05$) and there is no relationship with overall life satisfaction for men, as there is for women.

Table 10.21. *Relationships between Variables related to Domestic Help/Childcare and Measures of Well-being: Correlations for All Countries, Females Only (N = 200)*

Variables related to domestic help/childcare	Measures of Well-being: Satisfaction with:				
	Health	Work	Family life	Relationship with Spouse/ Partner	Life
Number of domestic/childcare tasks carried out by "both of us"	0.01	-0.00	0.17**	0.23***	0.14*
HELP INDEX Total amount of domestic/childcare help	0.01	0.07	0.12	0.17**	0.10
Satisfaction with childcare arrangements	0.26***	0.19**	0.25***	0.24***	0.25***

* $p \leq 0.05$ ** $p \leq 0.01$ *** $p \leq 0.001$

Table 10.22. Relationships between Variables related to Domestic Help/Childcare and Measures of Well-being: Correlations for All Countries, Males Only (N = 200)

Variables related to domestic help/childcare	Measures of Well-being: Satisfaction with:				
	Health	Work	Family life	Relationship with Spouse/ Partner	Life
Number of domestic/childcare tasks carried out by "both of us"	0.11	-0.02	0.16*	0.16*	0.08
HELP INDEX Total amount of domestic/childcare help	-0.08	0.06	-0.04	-0.05	-0.05
Satisfaction with childcare arrangements	0.01	0.06	0.33***	0.27***	0.20**

$* \quad p \leq 0.05 \qquad ** \quad p \leq 0.01 \qquad *** \quad p \leq 0.001$

The global measure of Satisfaction with Childcare Arrangements was also examined in relation to the five measures of well-being. When we look at the total sample data, including both males and females, we see that there is a pattern of significant positive correlations between being satisfied with one's childcare arrangements and each of the five measures of well-being. All relationships are significant at the p≤0.01 or p≤0.001 level. Particularly strong are relationships between satisfaction with childcare arrangements and satisfaction with family life, partner and life in general (Table 10.20).

When we examine the correlations separately for men and women, we see some similarities and some differences. In the case of women, satisfaction with childcare arrangements is significantly correlated with all five measures of well-being – not only with family, partner and life in general, but also with satisfaction with health and work. For men, it is only correlated with satisfaction with family, partner and life in general. It does not impinge on health or work satisfaction. This suggests that to get childcare right is absolutely critical to women's well-being in all spheres. If this isn't right, all areas of a woman's life suffers, whereas for men, it would appear that they can compartmentalise at least health and work. However, it is interesting to note that the relationship for men between satisfaction with childcare arrangements and satisfaction with family life is even stronger than that for women (r = 0.33 for men; r = 0.25 for women, both p≤0.001). It is also ever so slightly more strongly related to satisfaction with partner for men (r = 0.27 *vs.* r = 0.24 for women, p≤0.001 in both cases). This indicates the centrality of successful childcare arrangements to men's satisfaction in the personal sphere. However, for women it is central to all areas of their well-being (Table 10.21 and Table 10.22).

3.3. Relationships between Perceived Attitudes in the Workplace and Working Parents' Well-being

Three sets of items tapping attitudes in the workplace were included in the study to help us to understand the attitudinal milieu in which working parents operate. In particular, we wanted to see if we could gain a better understanding of how attitudes in the workplace mitigate against men playing a larger role in family life. These attitudinal variables have already been discussed in terms of country differences, gender differences and differences related to socio-economic status and public *vs.* private sector. In this section we examine the relationships between these workplace attitudes and the five measures of well-being.

The first question posed was: "Is it acceptable that one may leave earlier and/or arrive later due to problems regarding children?" First, people were asked whether or not this was acceptable among themselves and their colleagues and then by their managers. The response continuum ranged from "very unacceptable" (1) to "very acceptable" (6). It may be seen in the following three tables, that the more acceptable it was to leave earlier or arrive later due to childcare problems, the more likely the respondents were to express satisfaction with work and with life in general. These significant relationships held for the whole sample and for males and females separately. Interestingly, the relationships were stronger for males than for females. In the case of both variables, the correlations for males were very high (r = 0.33 re colleagues and r = re managers, p≤0.001 in both cases).

Table 10.23. Relationships between Perceived Attitudes in the Workplace and Measures of Well-being: Correlations for All Countries, Males and Females (N=400)

Attitudes in the workplace	Measures of Well-being: Satisfaction with:				
	Health	Work	Family life	Relationship w/ spouse/ partner	Life
Acceptability of leaving earlier/arriving later (colleagues)	0.09	0.25 ***	0.01	0.09	0.19 ***
Acceptability of leaving earlier/arriving later (managers)	0.08	0.29 ***	0.03	0.09	0.20 ***
Acceptability of bringing child to work (colleagues)	0.02	0.19 ***	0.06	0.08	0.19 ***
Acceptability of bringing child to work (managers)	0.01	0.18 ***	0.05	0.07	0.19 ***
How well colleagues take account of childcare responsibilities	0.12 *	0.21 ***	0.13 **	0.12 *	0.21 ***
How well supervisor takes account of childcare responsibilities	0.11 *	0.35 ***	0.12 *	0.14 **	0.25 ***
How well employer takes account of childcare responsibilities	0.06	0.28 ***	0.06	0.12 *	0.13 **
Perceived resentment when men take extended leave for childcare	-0.10 *	-0.13 **	-0.16 ***	-0.10 *	-0.23 ***
Perceived resentment when women take extended leave for childcare	-0.05	-0.16 ***	-0.11 *	-0.08	-0.22 ***
Perception that men in PT/job share viewed as less serious about career	-0.02	-0.01	-0.16 ***	-0.11 *	-0.16 ***
Perception that women in PT/job share viewed as less serious about career	-0.04	-0.04	-0.12 *	-0.09	-0.17 ***
Perception that employees expected to work over and above normal hours	-0.07	-0.00	-0.13 **	-0.10 *	-0.14 **
Perception that to be viewed favourably by management, must put job ahead of family/personal life	-0.05	-0.12 *	-0.15 **	-0.12 *	-0.19 ***

*p ≤ 0.05   ** p ≤ 0.01   *** p ≤ 0.001

Table 10.24. Relationships between Perceived Attitudes in the Workplace and Measures of Well-being: Correlations for All Countries, Males Only (N=200)

Attitudes in the workplace	Measures of Well-being: Satisfaction with:				
	Health	Work	Family life	Relationship w/ Spouse/ Partner	Life
Acceptability of leaving earlier/arriving later (colleagues)	0.09	0.33 ***	-0.00	0.08	0.20 **
Acceptability of leaving earlier/arriving later (managers)	0.05	0.37 ***	0.00	0.07	0.23 ***
Acceptability of bringing child to work (colleagues)	0.08	0.28 ***	0.08	0.09	0.26 ***
Acceptability of bringing child to work (managers)	0.01	0.22 **	0.02	0.08	0.21 **
How well colleagues take account of childcare responsibilities	0.07	0.18 *	0.08	0.06	0.10
How well supervisor takes account of childcare responsibilities	0.03	0.28 ***	0.04	0.09	0.13
How well employer takes account of childcare responsibilities	0.01	0.19 **	-0.01	0.02	0.03
Perceived resentment when men take extended leave for childcare	-0.07	-0.11	-0.19 **	-0.10	-0.24 ***
Perceived resentment when women take extended leave for childcare	-0.05	-0.22 **	-0.11	-0.09	-0.27 ***
Perception that men in PT/job share viewed as less serious about career	0.00	0.02	-0.21 **	-0.15 *	-0.14
Perception that women in PT/job share viewed as less serious about career	-0.01	0.04	-0.10	-0.16 *	-0.10
Perception that employees expected to work over and above normal hours	-0.05	0.12	-0.16 *	-0.11	-0.12
Perception that to be viewed favourably by management, must put job ahead of family/personal life	-0.01	-0.05	-0.13	0.08	-0.17 *

*p ≤ 0.05   ** p ≤ 0.01   *** p ≤ 0.001

Table 10.25. Relationships between Perceived Attitudes in the Workplace and Measures of Well-being: Correlations for All Countries, Females Only (N=200)

Attitudes in the workplace	Measures of Well-being: Satisfaction with:				
	Health	Work	Family life	Relationship w/ spouse/ partner	Life
Acceptability of leaving earlier/arriving later (colleagues)	0.09	0.18 **	0.04	0.10	0.18 **
Acceptability of leaving earlier/arriving later (managers)	0.11	0.22 ***	0.05	0.10	0.17 *
Acceptability of bringing child to work (colleagues)	-0.04	0.12	0.05	0.08	0.12
Acceptability of bringing child to work (managers)	0.01	0.16 *	0.07	0.07	0.17 *
How well colleagues take account of childcare responsibilities	0.16 *	0.24 ***	0.18 **	0.18 **	0.30 ***
How well supervisor takes account of childcare responsibilities	0.19 **	0.40 ***	0.20 **	0.19 **	0.34 ***
How well employer takes account of childcare responsibilities	0.10	0.36 ***	0.13	0.21 **	0.22 **
Perceived resentment when men take extended leave for childcare	-0.13	-0.15 *	-0.13	-0.11	-0.21 **
Perceived resentment when women take extended leave for childcare	-0.05	-0.12	-0.11	-0.07	-0.19 **
Perception that men in PT/job share viewed as less serious about career	-0.03	-0.04	-0.13	-0.09	-0.17 *
Perception that women in PT/job share viewed as less serious about career	-0.07	-0.12	-0.13	-0.04	-0.22 ***
Perception that employees expected to work over and above normal hours	-0.09	-0.11	-0.11	-0.10	-0.15 *
Perception that to be viewed favourably by management, must put job ahead of family/personal life	-0.07	-0.19 **	-0.17 *	-0.15 *	-0.20 **

$*p \leq 0.05$ $**p \leq 0.01$ $***p \leq 0.001$

Two questions were included concerning bringing a child to work (say for an hour) if one had problems regarding childcare. It will be recalled that this was more acceptable in Denmark than in the other countries and was particularly unacceptable in Ireland and in France. Given the controversial nature of this behaviour, it is interesting that it is significantly related to two measures of working parents' well-being – work satisfaction and life satisfaction. The feeling that it would be considered acceptable by one's colleagues to bring a child to work was highly significantly correlated with work satisfaction on the part of men, as well as to their overall life satisfaction ($p \leq 0.001$ in both cases). For women, colleagues' acceptance was not significantly related; however, managers' attitudes were important for women; their acceptance was significantly related to women's work satisfaction and overall life satisfaction ($p \leq 0.05$ in both cases). Whereas for men, managers' attitudes, while very significant (greater acceptance on the part of managers being related to greater work satisfaction and life satisfaction on the part of fathers) ($p \leq 0.01$), were not as important as colleague's attitudes.

How well one's colleagues, immediate supervisor and employer took account of one's childcare responsibilities was also strongly related to working parents' well-being. This was true for men in the case of work satisfaction. The better one's colleagues, supervisor and employer were perceived as taking into account one's childcare responsibilities the greater the work satisfaction of men. In the case of women this was also true, but it also extended into all of the other areas of their well-being as well – their satisfaction with their health, their family life, their relationship with their partner and with their life in general. For women, the attitude of their immediate supervisor appeared to be the most important. Thus, the attitude of colleagues and managers to working parents' childcare responsibilities is of critical importance to their work satisfaction and, in the case of women, to their overall well-being.

Three further types of question were also posed to the respondents concerning workplace attitudes. The first was designed to see if people felt that there was resentment in the workplace if parents took extended leave to look after newborn (or adopted) children. Respondents were asked whether they thought such resentment existed in their workplace, first in the case of men taking extended leave and then in the case of women. These results have been presented earlier and, as will be recalled, such feelings were fairly common. In the present analysis, we looked at whether the presence of such attitudes in the workplace were related to the respondent's sense of well-being. As may be seen in the previous three tables, the less working parents, both men and women, perceive that such resentment exists when parents take extended leave for childcare, the greater their sense of well-being on a number of measures (particularly, work satisfaction, life satisfaction and satisfaction with family life). Interestingly enough the effects were stronger for males than for females, particularly in relation to work satisfaction and life satisfaction.

One of the ways that women frequently combine work and family is to work part-time or to job share. This kind of working is less prevalent among men, although it is increasingly being discussed as a way for men also to reconcile work and family life. Respondents were asked whether they agreed or disagreed with the following statement:

> "Men who participate in available work-family programmes (e.g., job-sharing, part-time work) are viewed as less serious about their career than those who do not participate in these programmes."

They were also presented with the same statement but the word "men" was replaced with "women." As in the case of the previous two questions, where critical attitudes were perceived, employees expressed lesser well-being on a range of measures. However, when there was acceptance of job-sharers and those working part-time and they were not seen as less serious, respondents expressed higher levels of well-being. This applied to men and to women. It was manifested in higher levels of satisfaction on the part of men in the areas of family life and relationship with spouse. For women it manifested itself in higher levels of life satisfaction. Conversely, one could argue that those with higher levels of satisfaction are less likely to perceive negative attitudes in the workplace.

Finally, respondents were asked 1) whether they felt that in order to get ahead employees were expected to work over and above the normal hours, and 2) whether they felt that to be viewed favourably by top management, employees must constantly put their jobs ahead of their families or personal lives. Their agreement or disagreement with these statements was inter-correlated with their measures of well-being. It was found that for both men and women, if they felt a sense of pressure that they needed to work over and above the normal working hours and to put their jobs ahead of their families, that this resulted in lower well-being, on almost all of the measures, particularly life satisfaction, satisfaction with family life and to some extent, work satisfaction, particularly in the case of women.

3.4. Relationships between the Family Friendliness of the Workplace and Respondents' Well-Being

We have described in an earlier section the summary measure of a number of family friendly policies in the workplace. We have referred to this measure as "family friendliness of the workplace." In the earlier section we examined the effects of country, sex, socio-economic status and public *vs.* private sector on this measure. In this section we shall examine family friendliness of the workplace in relation to a wider number of variables. We have also referred earlier to Potential Flexibility and Actual Flexibility in the Workplace. Potential Flexibility referred to whether employees were able to do certain things in the workplace, such as make personal calls, do errands, etc. Actual Flexibility referred to the extent to which they actually did things like this at work.

In the next analysis, we examine the Flexibility and Family Friendliness of the Workplace in relation to respondents' well-being; as before, data are presented for the total sample, followed by males only and then females only.

Firstly, it may be seen that Potential Flexibility in the Workplace is significantly related to satisfaction with health for the total sample ($p \leq 0.01$), for males ($p \leq 0.01$) and for females ($p \leq 0.05$). In contrast Actual Flexibility is not significant for males or for the total sample, but it is for females, though not at a high level of significance ($p \leq 0.05$). What this suggests is that the freedom to have flexibility has a salutary effect on health, even though one may not need to use that freedom.

Table 10.26. Relationships between Measures of Family Friendliness of the Workplace, Combining Work and Family and Measures of Well-being: Correlations for All Countries, Males and Females (N=400)

Attitudes in the workplace	Measures of Well-being: Satisfaction with:				
	Health	Work	Family life	Relationship w/ Spouse/ Partner	Life
Potential Flexibility at Work	0.18 ***	0.21 ***	0.05	0.11 *	0.18 ***
Actual Flexibility at Work	0.09	0.10 *	-0.08	-0.06	0.03
Total Number of Family Friendly Policies in Workplace	-0.03	0.17 ***	-0.03	0.05	0.08
Combining Work and Family	Health	Work	Family life	Relationship w/ Spouse/ Partner	Life
Hours worked create problems with childcare arrangements	-0.16 ***	-0.23 ***	-0.25 ***	-0.17 ***	-0.27 ***
Ease/difficulty combining work and family life	-0.25 ***	-0.23 ***	-0.38 ***	-0.22 ***	-0.33 ***

$*p \leq 0.05$ $** p \leq 0.01$ $*** p \leq 0.001$

Table 10.27. *Relationships between Measures of Family Friendliness of the Workplace, Combining Work and Family and Measures of Well-being: Correlations for All Countries, Males Only (N=200)*

Attitudes in the workplace	Measures of Well-being: Satisfaction with:				
	Health	Work	Family life	Relationship w/ spouse/ partner	Life
Potential Flexibility at Work	0.22 **	0.29 ***	0.13	0.16 *	0.24 ***
Actual Flexibility at Work	0.04	0.19 **	-0.11	-0.10	0.08
Total Number of Family Friendly Policies in Workplace	-0.03	0.20 **	0.02	0.08	0.07
Combining Work and Family	Health	Work	Family life	Relationship w/ spouse/ partner	Life
Hours worked create problems with childcare arrangements	-0.19 **	-0.21 **	-0.33 ***	-0.14 *	-0.27 ***
Ease/difficulty combining work and family life	-0.14 *	-0.15 *	-0.33 ***	-0.21 **	-0.25 ***

*p ≤ 0.05   ** p ≤ 0.01   *** p ≤ 0.001

Potential and Actual Flexibility were also significantly correlated with work satisfaction for men, and to a lesser extent Potential Flexibility was related to work satisfaction for women. Potential Flexibility was also significantly correlated with Life Satisfaction for both men and women, but more strongly for men (p≤0.001 for men, p≤0.05 for women). For men only, Potential Flexibility was correlated with Satisfaction with Relationship with Partner (p≤0.05), suggesting that when men perceive a flexible workplace, they are happier at home.

The level of Family Friendliness of the Workplace, as measured in terms of number of family friendly policies available in the workplace, was significantly correlated with work satisfaction of men and women, but more strongly for men.

Table 10.28. Relationships between Measures of Family Friendliness of the Workplace, Combining Work and Family and Measures of Well-being: Correlations for All Countries, Females Only (N=200)

Attitudes in the workplace	Measures of Well-being: Satisfaction with:				
	Health	Work	Family life	Relationship w/ spouse/ partner	Life
Potential Flexibility at Work	0.15 *	0.14 *	-0.01	0.07	0.14 *
Actual Flexibility at Work	0.14 *	0.04	-0.07	-0.05	0.01
Total Number of Family Friendly Policies in Workplace	-0.03	0.14 *	0.04	0.04	0.09
Combining Work and Family	**Health**	**Work**	**Family life**	**Relationship w/ spouse/ partner**	**Life**
Hours worked create problems with childcare arrangements	-0.13	-0.25 ***	-0.19 **	-0.21 **	-0.26 ***
Ease/difficulty combining work and family life	-0.36 ***	-0.30 ***	-0.41 ***	0.21 **	-0.42 ***

*p ≤ 0.05   ** p ≤ 0.01   *** p ≤ 0.001

The last two measures in these tables specifically concern combining work and family. The first question asked: *"Do the hours you work create problems in your childcare arrangements?"* The second question was, *"How easy/difficult is it for you to combine your job and family life?"* The responses to these questions were also correlated with the five measures of well-being. These two questions were highly significantly correlated with all five measures at the p≤0.001 level, in all cases in the same direction. The less one's working hours created problems with childcare arrangements, the greater one's well-being. The easier it was to combine work and family life, the greater one's well-being. These results held strongly for men and for women. The only case in which a relationship was significant for men and not for women was in the case of satisfaction with health. For men, if the hours they worked created problems with childcare arrangements, they were less likely to be satisfied with their health (p≤0.001). For women, this did not reach significance. This is likely to be because women worked on average fewer hours than men. While virtually all of the relationships were strong, the strongest for men related to satisfaction with family life. If their hours created problems with childcare arrangements and if they had difficulty combining work and family, the less satisfied they were with their family life (r =0.33, p≤0.001 in both cases). For women, ease *vs.* difficulty in combing work and family life was very strongly related to satisfaction with family life (r = -0.41) to life satisfaction (r =0.42), to satisfaction with health (p≤0.001 in all cases). It was also related to work satisfaction (r = -0.30, p≤0.001) and to satisfaction with relationship with partner (r = -0.21; p≤0.01).

3.5. Relationships between Measures of Well-Being

We have been examining five dependent measures of well-being in relation to other variables, such as workplace attitudes, time-related variables, etc. We now shall examine these five measures on their own to see to what extent the various measures of well-being are related to each other. An examination of the next table with the data for men and women together from all four countries shows that every measure of well-being is significantly related to every other variable. Thus, if one is satisfied with one's work, one is more likely to feel overall life satisfaction. If one is satisfied with one's partner, one is more likely to be satisfied with family life and life in general, etc. The greatest contributors to overall life satisfaction are satisfaction with partner (r=0.62; p≤.001) and satisfaction with family life (r = 0.59; p≤0.001). Satisfaction with work comes next (r=0.48; p≤0.001), followed by satisfaction with health (r = 0.40; p≤0.001). The levels of correlation are very similar for men and for women, as may be seen in the separate male and female tables, which follow. One interesting difference, however, is that for men satisfaction with their work is unrelated to their satisfaction with family life (r = 0.08; N.S.) whereas for women, it is highly correlated (r = 0.37; p≤0.001), suggesting that men may be able to compartmentalise to some extent, whereas it would appear from this, as well as some of the previous data presented, that for women their work and family lives are inextricably interrelated.

Table 10.29. Relationships between Measures of Well-Being:
Correlations for All Countries, Males and Females (N=400)

Measures of Well-Being	Measures of Well-being: Satisfaction with:				
	Health	Work	Family life	Relationship w/ spouse/ partner	Life
Satisfaction with health	-	0.31 ***	0.30 ***	0.29 ***	0.40 ***
Satisfaction with work		-	0.24 ***	0.20 ***	0.48 ***
Satisfaction with family life			-	0.65 ***	0.59 ***
Satisfaction with relationship with spouse/ partner				-	0.62 ***
Life satisfaction					-

*p ≤ 0.05   ** p ≤ 0.01   *** p ≤ 0.001

*Table 10.30. Relationships between Measures of Well-Being:
Correlations for All Countries, Males Only (N=200)*

Measures of Well-Being	Measures of Well-being: Satisfaction with:				
	Health	Work	Family life	Relationship w/ Spouse/ Partner	Life
Satisfaction with health	-	0.27 ***	0.29 ***	0.31 ***	0.39 ***
Satisfaction with work		-	0.08	0.18 *	0.41 ***
Satisfaction with family life			-	0.67 ***	0.59 ***
Satisfaction with relationship with spouse/ partner				-	0.63 ***
Life satisfaction					-

$*p \leq .05$ $**p \leq .01$ $***p \leq .001$

Table 10.31. Relationships between Measures of Well-Being: Correlations for All Countries, Females Only (N=200)

Measures of Well-Being	Measures of Well-being: Satisfaction with:				
	Health	Work	Family life	Relationship w/ spouse/ partner	Life
Satisfaction with health	-	0.35 ***	0.31 ***	0.30 ***	0.41 ***
Satisfaction with work		-	0.37 ***	0.23 ***	0.54 ***
Satisfaction with family life			-	0.63 ***	0.60 ***
Satisfaction with relationship with spouse/ partner				-	0.63 ***
Life satisfaction					-

*p ≤ .05   ** p ≤ .01   *** p ≤ .001

CHAPTER 11

SUMMARY AND DISCUSSION

1. BACKGROUND

Demographic and social changes throughout Europe have led to a changing social situation requiring new policies. The increasing labour force participation of women, particularly those in the childbearing years, has been accompanied by increasing needs for childcare, flexible working arrangements and greater demands for equality in the workplace. The challenge which still faces even the most advanced of the EU member states is how to facilitate more egalitarian sharing of roles, that is - how to relieve women of the double burden of employment and domestic duties, while encouraging men to take an active part in family and domestic life.

The present study brought together an interdisciplinary team of social scientists who had been working in different countries with different experiences. Denmark is an example of a Scandinavian country with a female participation rate among the highest in the world. In 1998 it was 73.2 %, where the male participation rate was 81.6 % (Ligestillingsradet & Danmarks Statistik 1999). The female participation rate is characterised by a so-called "plateau-model", that is, working without interruption. Generally women keep their connection with the labour market while they have babies/small children. In spite of this and the fact that it has strong public provision of childcare, it too is still struggling with the question of how to involve men in greater sharing of roles. France also has a long tradition of provision of public childcare, though it has experimented with different forms of childcare policy than Denmark (Fagnani, 2002b). Both Denmark and France also have generous leave policies for working parents. It is noteworthy that they are also demonstrating a new pattern of high female labour force participation in the childbearing age group together with high total fertility rates, which is in contrast to the previous pattern in which high fertility was associated with decreasing participation. This new trend reflects the success of family friendly policies in maintaining both the birth rate and the participation of women in employment.

Italy has traditionally had lower rates of female participation and its current rate of 39% is the lowest in the European Community, yet this has been changing, particularly in Northern Italy. Where it formerly had low rates of female participation and high birth rates, its birth rate is now among the lowest in Europe. This is explained in terms of the fact that the roles of wife and mother are no longer seen by women as the only possible life courses as they were in the past; now such roles may be the result of conscious choices between different possible alternatives (Bimbi, 1993a). This is, of course, also true of women in all of the countries. However, the timing of the trends observed in each country is different and relates to relative rates of social change, including the availability of the social policies and provisions referred to above in relation to Denmark and France which help support childbirth as well as female employment.

While its public child care provision is far less extensive than that in Denmark and France, leave provisions for parents in Italy are quite liberal. Like Italy, Ireland has also had a relatively traditional pattern, though in the last 30 years the labour force participation of married women has dramatically increased from 7.5% in 1971 to 46.4% in 2001, with an even higher percentage in the childbearing age group 25-34 (64.7%). The economy has recently experienced a boom and there has been an even greater demand for female labour. While the provisions for leave are improving, there is still no paid parental leave, as there is in the other three countries studied here. In addition there is no public provision of child care before the age of four, except for disadvantaged children and children at risk. The childcare issue has only relatively recently come on to the political agenda and the optimal solution to this issue is still a matter of public debate (Fine-Davis, 2001, 2003).

In spite of the different labour force participation rates in these countries of women in general, it is noteworthy that the participation rates for women with children under six are similar for Italy (42%) and Ireland (41%) and higher for France (51%) (OECD, 2001) and Denmark, though precisely comparable figures are not available. Those figures that are available suggest that it is likely that it is in the range of 80 - 90% (Danmarks Statistik, 2002, Table 3.2.1, p. 66). Thus, it is clear that while there are some differences, there are also a lot of commonalities between these countries. All are currently grappling with similar issues, due to the convergence of economic and social conditions in the Community and their Welfare states are undergoing quite significant changes (Pierson, 2001). We are thus in a state of social transition in gender roles and have not sufficiently adapted to the transition we are experiencing. While policies are gradually being developed to accommodate the needs of dual breadwinner couples, it is clear that attitudes have not kept pace with the social changes which constitute the reality of people's lives. This is true of employers, it is true of fathers and, to some extent, it is also true of women themselves. Individual countries are responding with varying levels of social support. Employers are also responding with partial, but not sufficient workplace flexibility.

There is clearly a need for more information in all of these areas so as to gain greater understanding of the processes operating as well as to help inform developing social policy, both at the workplace and at governmental level. It is our hope through this collective research to contribute to a better understanding of the realities of life of young working parents in their attempt to exercise the roles of parent and worker. We also hope to highlight the critically important role played by public, social and family policies in facilitating equal opportunities and quality of life for this group of workers. Finally and most importantly, we hope to shed light on those factors which are associated with work-life balance and well-being, so that workplace policies as well as social policies at the more macro level may be further developed in order to enhance opportunities for women and men to optimally combine their multiple roles of worker, parent and individual.

2. THE STUDY

The main purpose of the present study was to explore the attitudes and experiences of European working parents with young children, with a view to understanding the barriers to greater reconciliation of work and family life. A second major purpose was to develop new social indicators to measure issues of work life balance which may be utilised in studies with larger more representative samples.

A comparative study was carried out on samples of 100 men and women in each of four countries (France, Italy, Denmark and Ireland), for a total of 400 respondents, all of whom were 1) employed; 2) living in a couple with a partner/spouse who was also employed; and 3) had at least one child under six. The sample was stratified by sex, socio-economic status and employment in the public *vs.* the private sector. These sampling parameters held for all of the four countries participating in the study and hence the samples are comparable. All of the respondents were from major cities in each of the respective countries; all of the French respondents were from Paris, the Danish from Copenhagen, the Irish from Dublin and the Italian from Bologna.

Prior to collecting the data a review of the literature was carried out in each of the four countries on national policies, the current availability of family friendly policies and attitudinal studies related to them; as well as attitudinal studies concerning gender roles, child care and work life balance, to the extent that these were available. This also entailed identifying instruments and items from previous research, which had been used to measure the topics of the current research. A new instrument was then constructed which reflected the best of the items located in previous research conducted primarily in Denmark, Italy, France and Ireland.

The questionnaire was translated from English into the languages of the other three participating countries – French, Danish and Italian, and the interviews were conducted in the native language of respondents by native speakers. Interviews were carried out by interviewers on a one-to-one basis, each interview lasting approximately 45 minutes. Interviews were generally carried out in the respondent's workplace, although some were carried out in the respondents' homes and a few were carried out in the workplace of the interviewer, i.e., at the university. All interviewing took place between October 2001 and January 2002.

Below we present the key findings of the study with interpretation from both a social psychological and social policy perspective. Wherever possible we have compared our findings with related findings from other studies in the four countries, as well as throughout the world. In addition, we have compared them with national and international statistics where these were available. It is important to bear in mind that a main goal of the study was to develop measures – new social indicators – in the area of work-life balance. This study particularly focused on the work-life balance issues of working parents with young children. It is to be hoped that the measures we have developed will be used by other researchers on larger, more representative, national and cross-national samples.

We shall summarise and discuss below the key findings under the major headings of the study.

3. CHILDREN AND FAMILY LIFE

The sample consisted of half males and half females, all of whom were working parents living with their partner and with at least one child under six. Most respondents were in their mid-thirties, with a mean age of 35 years for all countries. Approximately three-quarters of the respondents were married (73%), and one-quarter co-habiting (27%). The highest percentage of co-habiting couples was in the French sample (42%), the next highest in the Danish (32%), followed by the Irish (22%), and then the Italian (11%). These figures are consistent with Eurostat (2001) data for 1999 indicating that the proportion of births outside of marriage is highest in Denmark and France (45 % and 41% respectively), followed by Ireland (31%) and lowest in Italy (9%) . Socio-economic status (SES) was one of the stratification variables in the sampling design. Thus 50% of the sample were categorised as "lower SES" and 50% as "higher SES", based on their occupational status. Sector of employment was also one of the key independent variables in the stratification design. We systematically sampled respondents so as to have half who were public sector employees and half employed in the private sector.

Most of the respondents had either one or two children. The average age of the youngest child was 2 ½ and the average age of the next youngest child was six.

3.1. Effects of the Birth of the Youngest Child

Following the birth of their youngest child, 50% of women and 27% of the men in the sample modified their working time. Danish women were least likely do do so (34%), compared with Irish, Italian and French women (54-56% of whom did). French men were least likely to do so (8%), compared with men from Italy, Ireland and Denmark (24-36%). The majority of those who modified their working time tended to decrease it. Almost one-fifth of Irish and Danish fathers did so.

While Danish mothers were less likely to modify their working time following the birth, Danish parents, both mothers and fathers, were more likely than any other group to temporarily interrupt their working activity over and above paid maternity leave, following the birth of their youngest child, utilising the provision of paid paternity leave and paid parental leave. This was true of 62.5% of Danish men and 92% of Danish women, whereas it only applied to 21% of French women, 38% of Italian women and 46% of Irish women. Men in the other three countries were even less likely to interrupt their work on the birth of the youngest child: 16% of Irish men, 8% of Italian men and no French men. In addition to standing out as being the most likely to take time off work following the birth of the youngest child, Danish parents also reported experiencing the fewest effects on their lives as a result of the birth in terms of life habits, free time etc.

Previous Italian research has observed that fathers rarely reduce their paid working time after the birth of their children and there is even a tendency to increase it in order to face additional economic needs (Bimbi and Castellano, 1990; Sabbadini and Palomba, 1994; Ventimiglia, 1996; Pattaro, 2000). Only a minority of fathers, moreover, opt to use parental leave, even though this is perceived by both fathers and mothers to be an optimal solution for promoting good paternal involvement in childcare and for achieving good family-work reconciliation more easily (Zanatta, 1999). It is also noteworthy that the attitudes differ from behavioural practices. Italian research suggests that there are several reasons for this and they are linked to the presence of objective constraints, relating to the dominant structures and patterns at the workplace (Saitta, 1996; Irer, 1998). Paid work - even though it is no longer regarded, as in the past, as an exclusive sphere for the definition and self-realization of the male figure, continues to be the priority on a day-to-day level.

3.2 Time with the Family, Partner's Time with the Family and Time for Oneself

It was found that the majority of respondents from all countries wanted to spend more time with their families: 52% wanted to spend "more time" and 23% said they wanted to spend "much more time." There was also a wish for one's partner to spend more time with the family. In the all-country sample, 50% said they would like their partner to spend more time with the family and 18.5% said they would like them to spend "much more time"; female respondents were significantly more likely to express this desire. The parents in our sample also expressed a wish for more personal time; 59% would like "more time" and 16.5% would like "much more time." French parents expressed the greatest wish for more personal time and the Danes the least. These results may be compared with a recent European-wide survey in which, the 25-39 age group (which includes most parents with young children) reported a greater desire for more free time (personal time) than any other age group at 12% (Eurostat, 2001).

3.3. Domestic and Childcare Arrangements

One of the main areas of the study was an examination of domestic and child care activities and a comparison of mothers and fathers in terms of who did what and the reciprocal perceptions of who carried out which activities.

The study found that mothers carried out significantly more of the domestic and child-care tasks in the home than fathers did in all of the four countries. There were large discrepancies between male and female perceptions of who did what. Fathers were more likely to think *both* of the partners carried out tasks than mothers did. Mothers were more likely to report that *they* carried out the tasks. Where fathers excelled was in relation to taking care of the children. This was true in the case of feeding, bathing, taking to school/crèche, and changing nappies/dressing children. But most of all, it was true in the case of playing with the children.

Our data show that, in all countries there exists a wide gap between what both partners express and perceive about the various activities they carry out in their daily lives. The results of the present study confirm what previous research has shown in Italy (Bimbi & Castellano, 1990; Ventimiglia, 1994; Giovannini *et al*, in press) regarding the fact that fathers are more likely to overestimate their contribution in the home and their participation in child-care, as compared with mothers. Bimbi (1990) suggests that fathers are aware of the "asymmetry" that is present in their family. However, they do not participate more and, in many cases, do not even show a willingness to change, except where child-care is concerned.

Qualitative research in France has also emphasised the fact that many young fathers say they would like to play a bigger part in their children's lives (Castelain-Meunier, 1998, Neyrand, 1999). This mirrors the attitude change which has been occurring from generation to generation over the last few decades in France. However, as demonstrated by the data in our survey, French men have difficulties in steering clear of most obstacles to changes at the workplace: cultural norms, professional constraints and reluctance from employers to accept the idea that men can also claim their right to devote more time to their children. Our data have also shown in this regard that men are less likely than women to work in "family-friendly" environments. Moreover, when mothers reduce their working time or work less than their partner, they feel less justified in being demanding regarding their partner's help (Fagnani, 2000).

The fact that fathers in our study tended to be more involved in activities with children, rather than in domestic work, and particularly in play activities is consistent with earlier Italian research. Studies carried out in the Emilia-Romagna region by Bimbi and Castellano (1990) and by Giovannini and Ventimiglia (1994) emphasised the considerable emotional involvement of fathers in the life of their children. The majority of the fathers interviewed expressed the desire to have more free time to spend with their own children. Moreover, the return home from work was perceived by individuals as the most important and rewarding moment of the day. Fathers interviewed by Giovannini and Ventimiglia (1994) also underlined the sense of reward they feel in playing with them, in being together, in being physically affectionate with them. The emotional proximity to the child and the participation in her/his growth are considered fundamental elements not only for the development and the growth of the child, but also for themselves (Badolato, 1993; Ventimiglia, 1994). Fathers seem to perceive them as moments for personal growth, enrichment and as a primary source of satisfaction and reward.

However, Bimbi & Castellano (1990) have suggested that we face a situation in which even those fathers who would like to spend more time with their family and with their children are nevertheless satisfied with the level of their contribution to the various household activities, and do not feel that they should be more involved in a domain that they do not perceive as pertaining to them.

Concerning the Italian context, the roots of such attitudes can be found in the comparison with an ideal model: some fathers who are in reality not very "collaborative" in the family domain may compare themselves favourably with their even more "housework and childcare-distant father", and will perceive themselves as much more "present" and, therefore, overestimate their contribution to the family. A further explanation for such male overestimation may be found in the relatively lesser experience of fathers with respect to household activities, which may lead them to think of their contribution as appropriate, when in fact it is quite limited, because they do not realise the totality of things it would be necessary for them to do. As much previous research in Italy has found (e.g., Balbo *et al.*, 1990; Bimbi and Castellano, 1990; Balbo, 1991; Bernardi and Mancini, 1994; Palomba and Sabbadini, 1994; Ventimiglia, 1996 and 1999), men and women have very different strategies for coping with the demands of their lives. A typically female strategy emphasises time-crossing (*trasversalità*) and the co-management of different spaces, through a constant commuting - of a psychological nature – between family needs, children, and professional work tasks. This strategy differs from the 'single-tasked' man (*monotematicità maschile*), who tends to divide his different life areas and to run the different spheres within "exclusive" and separated moments: working time, family time, time for oneself, time with children, and free time.

3.4 Childcare Arrangements

As childcare is of key importance in the reconciliation of work and family life of working parents with young children, it was a main focus of the study. It was found that the youngest child (aged under six) was most commonly cared for in a childcare center/crèche/nursery or école maternelle. These children were in the care of someone other than their parents for an average of 33 hours per week, with a high of 37 hours per week in France and a low of 30 hours per week in Ireland. The majority of parents also used their partners or another relative to supplement their main arrangement. The second youngest child (aged under 12) was usually cared for in school, child care center or créche during the day, and again, partners and other relatives usually supplemented this care.

In Denmark child-care is considered a public task and is the responsibility of the municipalities. The vast majority (88%) of the Danish children were being looked after in public day care. Couples in France also more frequently used public facilities than their counterparts in Ireland or in Italy, both countries where public provision for children is less developed and where the family network (in particular, grandparents) plays a major role in childcare. In Italy and in Ireland, mothers work more often on a part-time basis, which accounts for the fact that respectively 22% and 23.5% of the fathers answered that their youngest child is cared for by their partner. Moreover, relying on a registered childminder is more common in France than anywhere else: there is an extensive network of childminders, in particular in the outskirts of Paris, and parents who rely on them are provided with AFEAMA, an allowance which considerably reduces the cost of childcare.

The mean cost of parents' childcare arrangements was €76 per week. Irish parents spent the most on childcare and Italian parents the least. In France and Ireland the socio-economic status (SES) of the parents was significantly related to the amount they spent on child care. French parents of lower SES spent on average €40 per week; high SES parents spent €130 (before tax rebates). In Ireland, those of lower SES spent on average €57 and those of higher SES €116.

The majority of respondents reported that they were satisfied with their childcare arrangements. There was a significant difference between countries, with Italian parents reporting the least and Irish the most satisfaction.

In this context it is interesting to note that other cross-national research carried out in nine European countries (Nebenfuhr, 1998) asked parents which would most facilitate work-life balance: better care facilities for children under three or for children between three years and school age. Whilst both alternatives were seen to be helpful in promoting work-life balance, the vast majority of all the groups studied reported that better care facilities for children under three years old would promote the combination of work and family life. This would clearly have implications for Ireland, which as the lowest public provision for the under threes of all of the countries studied here.

3.5 Alternative Childcare Arrangements

Even in the case of good childcare arrangements, emergencies can occur, breakdowns in arrangements can occur, etc. and alternative arrangements need to be found. Respondents were asked about their back-up arrangements when their usual child care arrangements were not available, such as during holidays, when the crèche was closed, grandparents unavailable, or the child was sick. It was found that the most common option in this situation was to rely on a relative. Over 80% of Danish, French and Italians resorted to this solution to some extent, but only half the Irish parents did. This is consistent with results of a recent study on child-care arrangements of working parents (Fagnani and Letablier, 2003b) which showed that grandparents, in particular the grandmother, often looks after the child when it is necessary.

Approximately 42% of the parents in our sample in all of the countries used their own annual leave "sometimes," "often" or "always" in this situation. Irish parents were the most likely to do so and Danish parents least likely. There was also a significant sex effect illustrating that mothers were more likely to take annual leave in this situation than working fathers. The results for Ireland replicate findings obtained in a previous study, using a nationwide representative sample of employed Irish mothers, which found that mothers commonly had to use their own annual leave, sick leave or unpaid leave in the case of a child's illness (Fine-Davis, 1983b).

Only a third of respondents in the present study used flexi-time when their usual childcare arrangement became unavailable – most of these being Danish and, to a lesser extent, French parents. In addition to this highly significant country difference, there was also a significant effect of socio-economic status: respondents in higher SES jobs were also significantly more likely to use flexi-time than respondents in lower SES jobs when their usual childcare arrangements became unavailable, indicating the availability of a greater degree of flexibility to employees in higher SES occupations. It was observed that this effect was particularly true in the private sector.

It is important to note that in Denmark, Italy and France there are specific leave provisions for working parents in the case of a child being sick (see Chapter 6). While there is a limited amount of *force majeur* leave available in Ireland, it is for emergencies of all kinds and not targeted specifically at children's normal illnesses. Were parental leave able to be taken more flexibly in Ireland this could theoretically be used for this purpose; however, at present its use needs to be signalled and planned in advance with the employer, so that it is not amenable to being used flexibly for child's illness; moreover the fact that it is unpaid discourages some parents from using it and indeed many parents cannot afford to take it at all.

It is clear that parents have to resort to a wide variety of *ad hoc* arrangements when their usual childcare arrangements break down. Not only is this likely to lead to stress for parents, but in many cases it deprives them of their own entitlement to sick leave and annual leave, which is clearly not in the interest of the well-being of the parents. The fact that social class differences were detected in relation to informal arrangements, indicates that there are unequal conditions accruing to parents in different social circumstances.

4. THE WORKPLACE

The first part of the study focused on the family part of the work-life balance. In this chapter we focus on the other half of the equation – namely the workplace.

We began with such issues as commuting to work, hours worked, and the effect the birth of the youngest child on the working arrangements of the parents. We then examined the nature of the workplace in terms of its potential and actual flexibility for working parents, as well as attitudes in the workplace. These included attitudes of colleagues, supervisor and employer concerning one's childcare responsibilities. We were particularly interested in the extent to which these attitudes were perceived as supportive and flexible or non-supportive and inflexible.

A key set of questions in this section concerned attitudes in the workplace toward people who avail of "family friendly" policies, such as extended leave for childcare, part-time working, job sharing, etc. Our purpose here was to see 1) if such individuals were perceived in a less favourable light, e.g., as "less serious" about their career; 2) whether respondents felt such attitudes differed depending on the sex of the employee concerned; and 3) whether there were differences between men and women in their perceptions of such attitudes. Attitudes towards the "long-hours culture" were also explored as potential barriers to work-life balance. Finally, we examined the availability of a range of family friendly policies, the extent to which respondents availed of these and their attitudes towards each of the policies.

4.1 Commuting

The average commuting time for all countries was just about a half hour (32 minutes). Commuting times were longest for Irish respondents (39 minutes on average) and for French respondents (38 minutes). Italian respondents had significantly shorter commuting times (24 minutes), as did Danes (26 minutes).

In all countries, the car was the most common form of transport to work (58% in all countries). This figure was the highest for Ireland – 70%, and lowest for France, at 47%. The French were even more likely to use the Metro (train) to get to work. Approximately 50% used this form of transport. The great reliance on the car in Ireland relative to the other countries may be partly responsible for the longer commuting times due to traffic congestion. The Irish results in the present study largely corroborate results of a nationwide Irish study which found that over half of Irish people in employment drove a car to work in the first quarter of 2000 (CSO, 2000). Two thirds of these car journeys were of less than 10 miles duration. This implies that many people are using the car for short journeys which could potentially be done using other forms of transport such as bus, train or bike.

Those countries that relied more on trains and cycling and less on cars had shorter commuting times. As commuting time was found to be a key predictor in successfully combining work and family, changes in transport modes may assist in this area.

Due to the long commuting time for the French parents interviewed, all of whom lived in the metropolitan Parisian area where commuting time is more time consuming than anywhere else in France, working parents are obliged to spend a lot of time outside of the home. This is particularly true if they have a full-time job and have to navigate both spatial and time constraints. These working conditions have a strong impact on the daily life of their children who spend a lot of time either outside of the home or at home with a childminder. It is not surprising that 59% of working parents having at least one child aged under six declare that they don't see enough their child(ren), according to a recent survey (2001) conducted among 500 parents who were part of a representative national sample of the French population (Fagnani, 2002a).

4.2 Working Hours

The average working time for fathers was 42 hours, for mothers 34 hours, with an overall average of 38 hours for parents of both sexes. This compares with Eurostat figures for the 15 member countries in 1998 of an average working week of 40 hours (Eurostat, 2001). Among the men in the present study, Danish men had the shortest working week (40 hours) and Irish men the longest (45 hours). Among the women, the Irish had the shortest working week (32 hours) and the French and Danish women the longest working week (35 hours).

The women in the four participating countries of this study thus work roughly similar hours, with only three hours difference between the lowest and the highest, whereas the difference in working time among the men is much larger - five hours. The least divergence was between Danish men and women (only five hours) and the greatest divergence was between Irish men and women (13 hours). The relatively small gap between Danish men and women is not due to the fact that Danish women work more than the other women but rather to the fact that Danish men work less. So the Danish men get a lot of help from the women in the economic support of the family – or put in another way - there is greater equality between the sexes with respect to labour market participation.

4.3. Perceived Acceptance of Working Parents' Childcare Responsibilities

Due to the fact that parents spend so much time at work, the workplace environment, both in terms of policies and attitudes is a critical factor in coping with issues of work-life balance. The study included several sets of questions to measure the degree of perceived acceptance of workers' family responsibilities. Initially, respondents were asked about how understanding their colleagues, supervisors and employers were around their family responsibilities. We collected data on three key areas: how acceptable it was to arrive late or to leave early from work due to problems regarding children, how acceptable it was to bring a child to work on occasion due to childcare problems and how well co-workers took into account the participants' responsibilities for a young child.

It was found that Danish workplace attitudes were the most positive regarding parents' family commitments, followed by Irish attitudes. French parents experienced the most pressure in their workplaces around work-life balance, especially those in higher SES jobs. The attitudes of the Italians and the Danes appeared to reflect more accepting and relaxed workplace cultures, as compared with those of the French and the Irish, who experienced more stress in the workplace in relation to combining work and family life.

Parents working in higher SES jobs experienced more understanding in their workplaces around work-family issues than did those in lower SES jobs. Where there were sex differences, women generally tended to report more positive attitudes in the workplace than did male workers; however, in Italy women were *less* likely to report positive attitudes than were their male counterparts. Those working in the private sector also tended to experience less tolerant attitudes.

4.4. Potential and Actual Flexibility in the Workplace

Participants were asked first about what was possible or acceptable in their workplace regarding flexible working, and then they were asked about what kinds of flexibility they actually experienced. They were also asked about the existence of various family friendly policies in their workplace.

The Danish parents reported both the most *potential* and the most *actual* flexibility. This can be seen most clearly in the measure 'bringing a child to work' in the case of a childcare problem, where the Danes were the only ones to really be able to do so at all, and it was only considered acceptable by them, whereas it was not in the other countries.

The vast majority of respondents were able to make private calls at work; however, there was more variability in the possibility of running private errands. This was more acceptable in Denmark and in Ireland than in Italy or France. There were virtually no sex differences on any of these measures except for running private errands, where it was found that men were more likely to be able to do so than women (54% *vs.* 37%). Given that women were found to have greater responsibility for domestic and child care, their lesser ability to run private errands during working time must add to their pressure in balancing work and family life.

4.5 Family Friendly Workplace Policies

In each of the national literature reviews contained in Chapters 2 – 5 the national policies available to meet the needs of working parents were discussed; these were then compared in Chapter 6.

In the study itself respondents were asked about a 14 different potential workplace policies in their place of employment. These included paid and unpaid maternity leave, paid and unpaid paternity leave, paid and unpaid parental leave, flexible hours, part-time working, job-sharing, term time working, personalised (flexible) working hours, teleworking, career breaks, and emergency/ special leave Respondents were first asked whether or not each policy was available to them in their workplace, secondly, whether or not they had used each policy and lastly whether their attitude towards the policy in general was favourable or not.

We constructed an index of 'family-friendliness' of the respondent's workplace by summing the total number of 'yes's in response to each of the questions regarding the availability of workplace policies. There were significant differences found between countries, sectors and SES. The significant country difference indicated that Irish respondents had, on average, the greatest number of family friendly policies available to them (with the exception of certain key paid leave policies such as paid paternity leave and paid parental leave) and French respondents had the fewest. There was also a significant difference between participants working in the public *vs.* private sectors, with those in the private sector having somewhat fewer policies available to them. Participants in higher SES occupations were found to have a greater availability of the policies than those in lower SES occupations. It was notable that many parents *did not know* whether many of the workplace policies were available to them or not. In some of the interviews with Irish respondents it was felt that employers did not always want employees to be aware of all of their entitlements, as they then might be more likely to take advantage of them, which might not suit the employer.

In relation to the some of the specific policies for flexible working - more Irish males said that they would have taken parental leave had it been paid than in any other country – around three-quarters. In Ireland, mothers have only recently been given a longer period of paid leave and also more unpaid leave and would appear to be grateful for it, since they did not have it before. There was more support for unpaid policies in Ireland for this reason, as opposed to attitudes in the other countries, where unpaid policies were not favoured. All of the Irish mothers in the sample expressed support for paid parental leave, as did 94% of the Irish fathers. This policy is currently being discussed at policy level and clearly would find favour among Irish working parents.

Part-time working was available in the majority of workplaces, the exception being the workplaces of Danish males. Approximately 40% of female participants had worked part-time at some point, except for Danish females of whom only 28% had. Very few males had worked part-time, the highest number being in Ireland (12%). The majority of women were strongly in favour of part-time working in all countries, including in Denmark, where there was little take-up of it. Male participants were more divided, but the majority either favoured or strongly favoured it except in France where a quarter of French males did not favour it as a policy.

Several European studies have found support for part-time employment. A study in nine European countries found that of all work combinations, part-time working was given a high preference in all income brackets (Nebenfuhr, 1998). It was also the most common preference for all three groups of mothers – those working full-time, part-time and those having taken a permanent career break.

A preference for part-time work has been observed for more than two decades. In a study conducted in 1978 with nationwide representative samples in eight EU countries, between 10 and 24% of housewives under 40 expressed a desire to work full-time and over 50% a desire to work part-time. Thus, between two-thirds and four-fifths (depnding on their age) of housewives aged 18-40 desiring to work, expressed a preference for part-time employment, yet the lack of existing part-time job opportunities was one of the main reasons such women gave for not being currently employed. Another important reason was the lack of alternative childcare arrangements (Fine-Davis, 1985).

In this context, it is interesting to note that in Ireland, the numbers in part-time employment increased in the first quarter of 2002 and most of this was accounted for by women, who already account for over three-quarters of those in part-time employment (CSO, 2002), suggesting that this form of employment is favoured by a significant proportion of Irish women. It was observed in Chapter 6 that part-time employment of women living with a partner and with children under six increased in France, Italy and Ireland over the period 1984 to 1999. In Denmark the trend was different – part-time employment decreased. However, in all of the countries full-time employment on the part of this group was far more prevalent than part-time.

4.6 Perceived Attitudes towards People Availing of Family Friendly Policies

Participants were asked a series of questions about the attitudes in their workplace towards people availing of family friendly policies. These items were included in order to examine whether attitudinal barriers exist in this area and, if so, to what extent. This is important from at least two points of view. One concerns barriers to women's career advancement and the second relates to barriers to men's greater participation in family life. The perceived attitudes towards men and women who avail of family friendly policies are discussed individually below.

4.6.1 Perceived Attitudes towards Working Parents taking Extended Leave for Childcare Reasons

It was found that perceived attitudes toward women taking leave for childcare reasons were more permissive than were those toward men taking leave. The least resentment towards women taking extended leave was in Italy, followed by Denmark. This may be because of the pro-family attitudes in Italy and the tradition of egalitarian attitudes and family friendly policies in Denmark. The attitudes in Ireland followed, and the French attitudes were seen as the least permissive by the respondents.

French and Danish parents, particularly the fathers, thought there was a difference in how fathers and mothers are perceived – fathers were thought more likely to be resented and taken less seriously if they utilised work-life balance policies in the workplace. The Italians and Irish did not perceive a difference between how fathers and mothers were perceived in this regard.

There were no significant differences between Italian men or women's perceptions of men *vs.* women taking leave. Italian men and women tended not to perceive that there was resentment in either case. The same was true in Ireland, though a somewhat less permissive attitude prevailed than in Italy. On the other hand, both males and females in France and in Denmark felt it was seen as less acceptable for men to take leave than for women. This means that men in France and Denmark would presumably feel less latitude to engage in this behaviour, since it is seen as less acceptable for men than for women.

4.6.2 Perceived Attitudes toward Working Parents Working Part-time or Job-Sharing

One of the ways in which men and women can combine work and family is to work part-time or to job share. This practice is widespread for women in many countries.

Indeed, women make up the majority of part-time workers and they are also more likely to avail of job-sharing options than are men. It was one of the aims of the present study to see if there were barriers to men availing of family friendly options such as these.

We found that there was a significant difference between countries in response to this issue. French and Irish respondents both agreed that men who participate in family friendly programmes (e.g. job-sharing, part-time work) are viewed as less serious about their career than those who do not, whereas both the Italians and Danes disagreed.

Male respondents were significantly more likely than females to think that men who participate in available work-family programmes are viewed as less serious about their career than those who do not.

In light of these results it is interesting to note that in a European-wide survey conducted in 1998 it was men rather than women, particularly in the 20-39 age group, who felt that working part-time would damage their career prospects, and that part-time workers were generally worse-off (Latta & O'Conghaile, 2000).

> "Men's higher wages and traditional expectations combine to make it unusual for fathers to take time off work to care for young children. *It seems reasonable to presume, even without evidence*, that taking time off would incur penalties in terms of their seniority, promotion, lifetime earnings and future pension" (Dex & Joshi, 1999, p. 651)(our italics)

It is noteworthy than even as recently as 1999 it was assumed that men would be penalised if they took time off work to care for young children; such attitudes undoubtedly reinforce the widely held assumption that the childcare role on the part of employed people is reserved for women. These attitudes are likely to create a distinct barrier to men taking up the kinds of working arrangements which could facilitate work-life balance for them and their partners.

4.6.3 Perceived Work Pressure
One of the key problems in combining work and family life is the issue of work demands. In some jobs employees feel pressure to work over and above the normal hours and to bring work home. In some cases, employees feel that this is necessary in order to get ahead and is expected by management. Thus, not only can employees not contemplate working *fewer* hours to facilitate work-life balance, in many cases they may be expected to work *more* hours. To what extent this was a problem was examined in the study.

It was found that respondents working in higher SES jobs were significantly more likely to perceive this kind of pressure at work. Working parents in France and Ireland tended to agree that to get ahead employees are expected to work over and above the normal hours, whether at the workplace or at home, whereas those in Italy and Denmark were more likely to disagree that this was the case.

4.7. Summary of Workplace Attitudes

The most striking impression to emerge from the data in this part of the study was that the attitudes of the Italians and of the Danes consistently reflected the most accepting and relaxed workplace cultures, compared with those of the French and the Irish. The Danish workplace culture appears - all in all – to be more relaxed with respect to the daily work-family flexibility routines and more permissive, together with Italy, on questions of leave and career demands. This helps to explain other aspects of the study in which the Danish parents expressed significantly different views to those of parents in the other participating countries on combining job and family life and in relation to satisfaction in various life domains.

In general the French tended to agree with the statements more than participants of the other countries – that there was resentment when people used work-family measures and that they were expected to put work above family. The Irish also agreed to some extent that there were these pressures in their workplaces. Those in higher SES jobs tended to perceive the most pressure of this type, as did those working in the private sector. Male participants perceived that there was less acceptance for men to partake of family friendly programmes in the workplace.

Due to the fact that parents spend so much time at work, the workplace is a critical factor in dealing with the dilemmas of balancing work and family life. The results of the study convey a picture of a more relaxed and permissive attitude towards child care responsibilities in Danish workplace culture - in comparison with the other countries. Hence, the results point towards a greater latitude for fathers in the work-place culture in Denmark. This may indicate an acceptance and encouragement of fathers and fathering but it may also be related to the relatively high gender segregation of the Danish labour market. A survey Csonka (2000) carried out among almost 3000 public and private companies found that three quarters of the companies were gender segregated, where segregation was defined as a gender majority of 60% or above - thus men tend to work with men and women tend to work with women. This means that work / family issues are more likely to impinge on female workplaces because mothers traditionally have been carrying most of the childcare responsibility – whereas this area is new in primarily male working environments and fewer fathers take advantage of the possibilities – perhaps making it easier to express an accepting attitude.

The results showed that the greater latitude for fathers with respect to daily work-life interferences did not hold when it came to taking leave and participation in work family programmes – a traditional perception of gender roles surfaces here – even in

Denmark where the labour market participation and the working hours are the most gender-equal.

In this climate, it will be more difficult to promote family friendly working arrangements and a greater sharing of gender roles unless there is attitude change.

5. COMBINING WORK AND FAMILY LIFE

In the initial parts of the study we focussed on the family and on the workplace. In the final part we examined the two pieces together with the specific aim of finding out how working parents with young children reconcile these two major areas of their lives and what were the effects on their well-being. Our major focus here was on key dependent measures of well-being. These included the measure of ease *vs.* difficulty of combining work and family life as well as several classic measures which have been widely used in social indicators research, i.e., satisfaction with work, health, partner/spouse, family life and life in general. We also included two measures related to time which cross the boundary of family and work and have major implications for reconciliation – namely 1) the extent to which parents' working schedules create problems with their childcare arrangements; and 2) and parents' ideal working schedule.

5.1 Predictors of Ease vs. Difficulty in Combining Work and Family Life

Overall, the Danish parents found it significantly easier to combine their jobs with their family lives than did the parents in the other three countries. This undoubtedly relates to the generous public provision of child care and leave related to child care both for men and for women. It also reflects the more permissive workplace culture in relation to work-life balance issues. When socio-economic status was examined, it was found in all countries that it was significantly more difficult for those in higher occupational status jobs to combine work and family, which may be related to the generally greater pressure which was found to exist for people in these jobs.

In an analysis of the potential predictors of successfully combining work and family, the following factors emerged as significant:

Amongst the most important factors was found to be time. The length of one's *partner's* commuting time was found to be particularly important. The longer the commuting time, the less time they would be available to help with the family. The importance of time is also expressed in the item "Do the hours you work create problems in your childcare arrangements?" The more this was true for people, the more difficulty they had in combining work and family life. Not surprisingly, the more hours a person worked per week the more difficulty they had combining work and family. Another very significant predictor was the amount of help a person got with domestic and childcare responsibilities. The more help one got, the easier it was to combine work and family; this effect was particularly true for women. Attitudes in the workplace were also very important. Most important was a feeling that in a pinch one could bring one's child to work for a little while if childcare arrangements broke down. If working parents felt that this was accepted by colleagues in particular, but also by their managers, they were more likely to say that combining work and family was easier.

5.2. Well Being

An analysis of the results on well-being indicated that most parents reported being satisfied with their health, their work, their family lives, their relationships with their partners and their life in general. Danish parents were the most satisfied followed by the Irish, then the Italians, and lastly the French.

On the basis of the data obtained in the present study, as well as on the Danish situation, as outlined in the literature review for Denmark, the following four factors may be seen as contributing to Danish parents' sense of well-being: 1) the relatively even distribution of working hours between the sexes (backed up by a more equal distribution of household chores between mothers and fathers); 2) a high level of relatively cheap public day-care provision, widely acknowledged and appreciated; 3) a generous provision of paid maternity and parental leave; and 4) a workplace culture exhibiting a relatively relaxed and permissive attitude towards the problems of reconciling work and family life. It would thus appear that the nature of the Danish workplace, the greater public provision of childcare facilities, and the greater sharing of domestic and childcare responsibilities in the home are contributing to the higher levels of well-being expressed in several areas by the Danish respondents (Hojgaard, 2002).

5.3 Correlates of Well-being

In this section we examine the relationships between a wide range of respondent characteristics and measures of their well-being. These include time-related variables, variables related to domestic and childcare help, attitudes in the workplace, and the degree of family friendliness of the workplace in terms of policies available to facilitate reconciliation of work and family life.

The dependent measures of well-being consist of measures of satisfaction in several life domains:

- health
- work
- family life
- relationship with spouse/partner
- life in general

5.3.1 Relationships between Time-related Variables and Well-being
While the length of one's own working week (as measured in hours) was not significantly related to well-being, the length of one's *partner's* working week was. The fewer hours per week that one's partner worked, the greater the respondent's own satisfaction both with family life and with their relationship with their spouse/partner.

Both the respondent's own commuting time and that of his/her partner was significantly related to satisfaction with family life in the direction of shorter commuting time being associated with greater satisfaction and longer time with greater dissatisfaction. There were also low, but still significant relationships between the length of partner's commuting time and both satisfaction with one's health and with one's work. The shorter the partner's commuting time the greater one's satisfaction with one's health and with one's work.

The study found that the less one's working hours created problems with childcare arrangements, the greater one's well-being. Conversely, when the hours fathers worked created problems with child-care arrangements and if they had difficulty combining work and family, the less satisfied they were with their family life

Other findings suggested that if one did not get sufficient personal time, this unmet need was felt in other key domains of one's life. Conversely, if one had a sufficient amount of personal time, one was more likely to manifest well-being in all of the key domains of health, work, family life, relationship with partner, and life in general. While these relationships were found to be true for men and women, in most cases they were stronger for women. This was particularly true in the case of health and life satisfaction. The more a woman craved more personal time, the less satisfied she was with her health and with her life in general.

All of these results point to the fact that if too much time is spent at work and in commuting it has deleterious effects in many spheres of a person's life.

SUMMARY AND DISCUSSION

5.3.2 Relationships between Variables related to Domestic Help and Childcare and Measures of Well-Being

It was found that the greater the total amount of help received with domestic and child care tasks, the greater the satisfaction with spouse/partner. However, when the male and female data were examined separately, it was found that receiving help with domestic tasks and childcare was more significantly related to women's well-being than it was to men's. It was also found that the more both partners carried out domestic tasks and childcare, the more likely women were to report feeling satisfied with their family life, with their spouse/partner, and with their life in general . For men, there were also significant positive correlations with satisfaction with partner and family life, but these relationships were not as strong as they were for women and there was no relationship with overall life satisfaction for men, as there was for women.

Satisfaction with Childcare Arrangements was also examined in relation to the five measures of well-being. When we examined the correlations separately for men and women, we saw some similarities and some differences. In the case of women, satisfaction with childcare arrangements was significantly correlated with all five measures of well-being. For men, it was correlated with satisfaction with family, partner and life in general, indicating the centrality of successful childcare arrangements to men's satisfaction in the personal sphere. However, it did not impinge on their health or work satisfaction. This suggests that to get childcare right is absolutely critical to women's well-being in all spheres. If this isn't right, all areas of a woman's life suffers.

These findings corroborate research carried out in the U.S. by Shinn *et al.* (1987) which showed that the frequency of mothers arriving late to work or leaving early due to a breakdown in their childcare arrangements was associated with lower scores on measures of well-being and mental health in both the mothers and the fathers.

5.3.3 Relationships between Workplace Flexibility and Well-Being
Potential and actual flexibility in the workplace were examined in relationship to working parents' well-being. Several significant relationships were found:
Potential Flexibility in the Workplace was significantly related to satisfaction with health: the greater the degree of flexibility, the greater the respondent's satisfaction with their health. While *Potential* Flexibility was significantly related to measures of well-being, *Actual* Flexibility was not. This suggests that the freedom to have flexibility has a salutary effect on health, even though one may not need to use that freedom.

The level of Family Friendliness of the Workplace, as measured in terms of number of family friendly policies available to the respondent in their workplace, was significantly correlated with work satisfaction of fathers and mothers, but more strongly for fathers.

These results are corroborated by two American studies which have shown that good work-family policies may enhance the well-being of working mothers (Pleck, 1998). Christenson and Staines (1990) showed that flexi-time was associated with lower levels of perceived conflict between work and family roles. Other studies have found that family-friendly workplace policies were positively associated with a decision to return to work following childbirth, rather than interrupting one's labour force participation (Glass and Riley, 1998). Supervisor and co-worker support were also important determinants of the decision to stay in work. Supportive family-friendly policies and a positive workplace culture, therefore, encourage women to stay in work following childbirth and hence decrease turnover and its associated costs.

Some studies investigating how parents' adoption of flexi-time changes the time that is spent with the children have shown that more time is spent with the children by both mothers and fathers when that parent adopts a flexible schedule (Winett and Neale, 1980). A study conducted in 1990 (Staines) found that the more common kind of flexibility whereby workers have a core set of hours around which they can be flexible did not have much impact on perceived work-life balance, as compared with those workers who had greater flexibility in the form of *personalised hours*. Working mothers who adopted this latter kind of flexibility reported higher levels of job satisfaction, parenting-satisfaction and lower levels of work-life balance conflict (Pleck, 1998).

5.3.4. Relationships between Attitudes in the Workplace and Subjective Well-Being
An analysis of the correlations between attitudes in the workplace and the subjective well-being of respondents also revealed several significant relationships. It was found that the more acceptable it was to leave earlier or arrive later due to childcare problems, the more likely the respondents were to express satisfaction with work and with life in general. The relationships were stronger for males than for females.

The feeling that it would be considered acceptable by one's colleagues to bring a child to work was highly significantly correlated with work satisfaction on the part of fathers, as well as to their overall life satisfaction. For mothers, managers' attitudes were more important than those of colleagues; their acceptance was significantly related to mothers' work satisfaction and overall life satisfaction. The better one's colleagues, supervisor and employer were perceived as taking into account one's child-care responsibilities the greater the work satisfaction of fathers. For mothers this was true also, but it also extended into all of the other areas of their well-being as well – their satisfaction with their health, their family life, their relationship with their partner and with their life in general.

Other research (e.g., Aryee *et al.*,1998) has also found that a family-friendly attitude of the supervisor had a significant, positive effect on organisational commitment and turnover intentions, which backs up the theory that a positive workplace culture is essential if family-friendly policies are to have the intended outcomes (Bowen, 1998; Galinsky & Stein, 1990; Thompson, Thomas & Maier, 1992).

The less working parents perceived resentment towards parents who take extended leave for child-care, the greater their sense of well-being. Equally, the more acceptance there was in the workplace of job-sharers and those working part-time, the greater the likelihood that respondents expressed higher levels of well-being, even if they themselves were not working part-time or job sharing. Obviously the perceived acceptance made them feel comfortable also that this was a safe atmosphere for working parents to be working in.

It was found that for both fathers and mothers, if they felt a sense of pressure that they needed to work over and above the normal working hours and to put their jobs ahead of their families, this resulted in lower well-being on almost all of the measures, particularly life satisfaction, satisfaction with family life and to some extent, work satisfaction, particularly in the case of mothers.

Measures of well-being (satisfaction with health, work, family, relationship with partner, life) were all positively correlated in all cases, except that for fathers, satisfaction with their work was unrelated to their satisfaction with family life whereas for mothers, it was highly correlated, suggesting that fathers may be able to compartmentalise to some extent, whereas it would appear from this, as well as some of the previous data presented, that for mothers their work and family lives are inextricably interrelated.

This reflects the enduring asymmetry between the sexes in family involvement and the persistence of the normative imperative to maintain separate roles for males and females. As women are still assumed to bear the main burden of family life, these two pieces of their lives constitute more major components than they do for men. Thus, for them an imbalance in one sphere is more likely to impinge on the other sphere. This is why we see such strong relationships in the well-being domains.

5.3.5. Relationships between Combining Work and Family and Well-Being
Overall, the easier parents found it to combine work and family life, the greater their well-being; conversely, greater difficulty in combining work and family life, the poorer their well-being.

For mothers, ease *vs.* difficulty in combing work and family life was very strongly related to satisfaction with family life, health, work satisfaction and to satisfaction with their relationship with their partner.

5.4. Advantages of Family Friendly Working Policies

Various advantages for employers have been identified of utilising flexible working policies in their organisations. These include :

- The ability to match work provisions more closely with customer/ product demand (Emmott and Hutchinson, 1998);
- Reduced fixed costs, e.g. by use of teleworking (*Ibid.*);
- Enhanced company image (*Ibid.*);
- Improved staff motivation (*Ibid.*);
- Improved attraction and retention of employees and a wider pool of potential employees. It has been shown in the U.S. that good work-family policies are specifically associated with better retention of female employees (NCJW Center for the Child, 1988);
- Potentially increased productivity and efficiency through reduced operating costs. A study carried out in the pharmaceutical industry (Shepard, Clifton & Kruse, 1996) gave evidence of a 10% increase in productivity when flexible schedules were implemented;
- Reduced stress, sick leave and absenteeism

(Humphreys, *et al.*, 2000).

Similar benefits have been found concerning the effects of workplace childcare. Various studies carried out in the UK, Germany, the U.S. and Ireland have shown that childcare in the workplace is directly responsible for reducing absenteeism, increasing productivity and reducing turnover, while at the same time increasing staff morale and job satisfaction and contributing to the retention of qualified staff who are then available for promotion (Fine-Davis, 1989b).

Flexible working policies may provide greater equality of opportunity for women by allowing certain groups of women better access to the labour market. However it can also be argued that flexible working practices may lead to a two-tier system of working whereby women adopt more flexible working practices than men, thus reinforcing the horizontal and vertical segregation of women in the workforce, whilst continuing to do the majority of work in the home (Emmott and Hutchinson, 1998).

Crowley (2002) argues that in the absence of an equality perspective, there is a risk that the imbalance in the take-up of family-friendly working arrangements between men and women may degenerate into a strategy for women to manage increased stress and the dual roles of caring and working. Drew and colleagues (2002) echo this concern, noting that their research showed that the take up of work life balance policies was "highly gendered". The options that implied no loss of pay, such as flexitime and tele-working tended to be more favoured by men, whereas women were more likely to opt for reduced hours, e.g. part-time work and job sharing. These authors assert that "a major challenge will be to avoid a twin track in which men are in the *fast lane* involving continuous and often excessive hours in full-time employment . . . and women in the *"slow lane"* working or seeking reduced hours and or opting for career breaks" (*Ibid p. 138*). Crowley (*op. cit.*) further argues that strategies to achieve a family friendly workplace need to be integral to human resource management strategies and therefore integral to employment equality strategies.

It is well documented by Lewis and Cooper (1995) that workplaces which do not take into account work-life balance pay the price in terms of absenteeism (Goff *et al.*, 1992); presenteeism (being present but psychologically unavailable) (Cooper and Williams, 1994; Hall and Parker, 1993); turnover (Grover and Crooker, 1995); accidents and the loss of productivity (Ganster and Schaubroeck, 1991); and wasted human potential (Wagner and Neal, 1994). For example, in the UK in 1993, £513 per employee on average was lost due to absenteeism, making a total of £11 billion for the UK economy (CBI, 1994). Cost-benefit analyses have generally shown that the costs of family-friendly policies are outweighed by the benefits (Hillage & Simkin, 1992).

On the other hand, studies of changing labour markets suggest that, by introducing and extending flexible working practices (especially against the background of the 35-hour work law in France) (Pélisse, 2002; Lurol and Pélisse, 2001), employers are seeking to increase the productivity of labour, efficiency and performance, and are not paying sufficient attention to the impact of imposed flexibility on families.

6. CONCLUSIONS AND SOCIAL POLICY IMPLICATIONS

It is clear that parents are under pressure, both time-wise and in terms of work pressures and are finding it difficult to combine work and family life. There were differences between countries, with Danes on the positive side of the continuum in terms of supportive workplace attitudes and policies and the French on the more negative side of the continuum in terms of workplace attitudes and time pressures. Although, it must be said that the French child care policies, both facilities and subsidies, are very advanced and help considerably in enabling parents to combine work and family life. The French attitudes need to be seen in the French institutional and legislative context: French employers have to deal with a very large number of legislative and mandatory family-friendly measures: generous maternity and paternity leave, parental leave, sick leave for children, time-off related to the 35-hour law, etc., which entail a lot of bureaucratic procedures. As a result, many simply comply with the legislation and are often reluctant to provide other flexible arrangements. The issue related to the rights of fathers to be more involved in family life is also not as high on the political agenda in France as it is in Denmark. These factors may help to explain the observed disparities in the attitudes of respondents in these two countries.

The issues of time which were present in the data in various ways, from working hours to commuting time, to difficulty with the hours of child care, were significant predictors of ease *vs.* difficulty in combining work and family life. This points to the need for better transportation systems, notably in Ireland, where the commuting time was the longest and where the use of the car for commuting was the highest. It also points to the need for greater availability of flexible working arrangements, and greater public policy thought given to the synchronsiation of schedules between workplaces, schools and child care facilities. Some research in this area is already taking place. For example there are now time-studies which include investigations on the "time of towns" (Belloni, 1984; Le Nove, 1990; Balbo, 1991; Bimbi, 1991b), examining the structure of urban space-time relations, in relation to the issue of the reconciliation between different life spheres. Innovative work in this area is also being carried out in the Netherlands concerning optimal arrangements of community facilities so as to facilitate work-life balance and quality of life for parents and children (Dutch Ministry of Social Affairs and Employment, 2002). The town of Oeiras in Portugal is also experimenting with optimal synchonisation of transportation with working schedules of the population and similar measures to facilitate reconciliation of work and family life (de Brito, 2003).

Another key area for social change concerns the attitudes in the workplace. People generally were more likely to see barriers to men's taking extended leave for child care reasons and to their working part-time or job sharing than they were in the case of women. Often these attitudes were held by men and not by women, suggesting that men's attitudes need to become more relaxed in this area, so that they can allow themselves and each other the kinds of flexibility that will enable them to more optimally balance their family and work lives, which it is clear they would like to do.

In this context it is important to emphasise that the attitudes of others in the workplace were found to be critically important. These included colleagues, supervisors and employers. Where these were found to be positive, the well-being of the employees ensued – often in many spheres of life, not only work satisfaction, but satisfaction with health, family life and life in general. In view of this, efforts need to focus on sensitising employers and in particular supervisors about the importance of positive *attitudes*, as well as supportive policies in the workplace. It is significant that research has shown that it is often not the most senior managers who tend to resist such changes, but rather lower level managers who tend to focus on more short-term interests (Emmott and Hutchinson, 1998). Thus efforts should focus initially on senior managers who are in a position to give out the signal to middle managment that new behaviours are acceptable. As research on the benefits of flexible working have clearly shown - these not only have social benefits, but economic benefits as well. As a result, this should not be an overly difficult message to convey.

Relatively little research on fathering has been carried out in the context of the plethora of studies in other related areas. Italy stands out as one of the very few countries where innovative studies have been conducted. Some of this research has indicated that new fathers show a great emotional/ relational involvement with their children and that contact with their children greatly contributes to their own sense of well-being and quality of life; however, this involvement mainly revolves around play and does not extend to care-giving (Bimbi and Castellano, 1990; Giovannini and Ventimiglia, 1994; Badolato, 1993; Giovannini 1998). McKeown et al.(1998) add that fathers' interaction with their children is also extremely positive for the children. Their main conclusion was that:

> "There appears to be virtual unanimity among researchers that the more extensive a father's involvement with his children the more beneficial it is for them in terms of cognitive competence and performance at school as well as for empathy, self-esteem, self-control, life-skills and social competence; these children also have less sex-stereotyped beliefs and a more internal locus of control " (*Ibid.*, p. 423).

However, McKeown *et al.* also noted that while the international evidence on fathers' involvement suggests that there has been some increase in participation in childcare and domestic activities, fathers' behaviour has not kept pace with changing attitudes and cultural expectations in this area (*Ibid.*). The results of our study also illustrate that men do not contribute as much time to the household activities and child care as do women. This is not news. But what is interesting is that men perceive that they are giving more than women think the men are giving. If men had more flexibility at work, they could perhaps give more to their families. It is apparent that they want to, as a large majority expressed the wish to spend more time with their families. The more that men contributed to domestic and child care tasks, the more women expressed well-being. However, it was not obvious that men wanted to contribute more to *domestic tasks*. Their primary input in the home was in the area of child care and primarily playing with children. Given that women's well-being was related to how much help they receive with domestic tasks *and* child care, it is clear that men need to begin to contribute in more ways than simply child care, important though this is. As McKeown *et al.* have argued:

> "public policy should seek to create family-friendly measures, especially in the workplace, which maximise the choices men and women have to negotiate roles and responsibilities and will allow fathers as well as mothers the time and space for childcare" (*Ibid.*, p. 427).

Reconciling work and family is now on the social and political agenda. It is to be hoped that EU and national policies encourage measures to promote work-life balance, for, as we see from these cross-national results, people's well-being very much depends on it.

APPENDIX A

TABLES

CHAPTER 7: 2.CHARACTERISTICS OF THE SAMPLE

Table A1.
Age by Country: Mean Scores (N=400)

France	Italy	Denmark	Ireland	All Countries
33	36	34	37	35

Table A2. Marital/ Cohabitation Status: Percentage Distributions by Country (N=400)

	France %	Italy %	Denmark %	Ireland %	All Countries %
Married	58.0	89.0	68.0	77.8	73.2
Co-habiting	42.0	11.0	32.0	22.2	26.8
Total	**100.0**	**100.0**	**100.0**	**100.0**	**100.0**

Table A3.

Socio-Economic Status:
Percentage Distributions by Country (N=400)

	France %	Italy %	Denmark %	Ireland %	All Countries %
1. Manual Routine	3.0	4.0	17.2	10.0	**8.5**
2. Semi-Skilled	17.0	16.8	13.1	12.0	**14.8**
3. Skilled-Manual	11.0	26.7	14.1	10.0	**15.5**
4. Clerical White-Collar	19.0	2.0	6.1	18.0	**11.3**
5. Supervisory (Lower Grade)	10.0	13.9	7.1	12.0	**10.8**
6. Supervisory (Higher Grade)	15.0	7.9	18.2	21.0	**15.5**
7. Managerial and Executive	21.0	16.8	12.1	11.0	**15.3**
8. Professionally Qualified/ High Admin.	4.0	11.9	12.1	6.0	**8.5**
	100.0	**100.0**	**100.0**	**100.0**	**100.0**

Table A4.
Level of Education: Percentage Distributions by Country (N=400)

	France %		Italy %		Denmark %		Ireland %		All Countries %	
	M	F	M	F	M	F	M	F	M	F
Primary	6.1	2.0	0.0	0.0	12.2	4.0	2.0	4.0	5.0	2.5
Secondary (inter cert)	14.3	16.0	31.4	26.5	22.4	40.0	18.0	18.0	21.1	25.1
Secondary (leaving cert)	24.5	16.0	35.3	44.9	20.4	10.0	42.0	46.0	30.7	29.1
Cert/diploma	0.0	0.0	0.0	0.0	0.0	0.0	6.0	6.0	1.5	1.5
University degree	16.3	30.0	27.5	22.4	22.4	28.0	18.0	20.0	21.6	25.1
Postgraduate degree	38.8	36.0	5.9	6.1	22.4	18.0	14.0	6.0	20.1	16.6
Total	100.0	100.0	100.0	100.0	100.0	100.0	100.0	100.0	100.0	100.0

Table A5. Sector Respondent Works in: Percentage Distributions by Country (N=400)

	France %	Italy %	Denmark %	Ireland %	All Countries %
Public	48.0	48.0	48.0	48.0	48.0
Private	52.0	52.0	52.0	52.0	52.0
Total	100.0	100.0	100.0	100.0	100.0

Table A6. Number of Children in Respondents Family:
Percentage Distributions and Mean Scores by Country (N=400)

	France %	Italy %	Denmark %	Ireland %	All Countries %
1	57.0	48.0	37.0	40.4	45.5
2	35.0	43.0	51.0	32.3	40.5
3	6.0	5.0	10.0	21.2	10.5
4	1.0	4.0	2.0	5.1	3.0
5	1.0	0.0	0.0	1.0	0.5
Total	100.0	100.0	100.0	100.0	100.0
Mean	1.5	1.7	1.8	2.0	1.7

Table A7. Age of Youngest and Next-Youngest Child:
Mean Ages by Country (years) (N=400)

	France	Italy	Denmark	Ireland	All Countries
Youngest Child	2.7	2.3	2.7	2.4	2.6
Next Youngest Child	6.6	5.9	6.4	6.4	6.3

CHAPTER 8: 1. THE EFFECT OF THE BIRTH OF THE YOUNGEST CHILD ON WORK AND FAMILY LIFE

Table A8.

Changes in the Way Respondents Organised their Day:
Percentage Distributions by Country (N=400)

	France %	Italy %	Denmark %	Ireland %	All Countries %
None	5.9	6.0	7.0	11.0	7.5
A little	28.7	15.0	23.0	18.0	21.2
A fair amount	21.8	43.0	30.0	30.0	31.2
Very much	43.6	36.0	40.0	41.0	40.1
Total	100.0	100.0	100.0	100.0	100.0

Table A9.

Changes in the Life Habits of Respondents:
Percentage Distributions by Country (N=400)

	France %	Italy %	Denmark %	Ireland %	All Countries %
None	6.0	6.0	10.0	11.0	8.3
A little	31.0	24.0	35.0	16.0	26.5
A fair amount	30.0	38.0	33.0	39.0	35.0
Very much	33.0	32.0	22.0	34.0	30.3
Total	100.0	100.0	100.0	100.0	100.0

Table A10.
Changes in the Professional Tasks of Respondents:
Percentage Distributions by Country (N=400)

	France %	Italy %	Denmark %	Ireland %	All Countries %
None	62.0	26.0	51.0	37.4	43.9
A little	17.0	32.0	25.0	21.2	23.9
A fair amount	12.0	25.0	12.0	23.2	18.0
Very much	9.0	17.0	12.0	18.2	14.2
Total	**100.0**	**100.0**	**100.0**	**100.0**	**100.0**

Table A11.
Changes in the Amount of Domestic Chores of Respondents:
Percentage Distributions by Country (N=400)

	France %	Italy %	Denmark %	Ireland %	All Countries %
None	4.0	1.0	18.0	9.0	8.0
A little	30.3	27.0	33.0	21.0	28.0
A fair amount	37.4	43.0	33.0	36.0	37.3
Very much	28.3	29.0	16.0	34.0	26.8
Total	**100.0**	**100.0**	**100.0**	**100.0**	**100.0**

Table A12.

Changes in the Friendships of Respondents:
Percentage Distributions by Country (N=400)

	France %	Italy %	Denmark %	Ireland %	All Countries %
None	34.0	25.0	23.0	44.4	31.8
A little	46.0	37.0	41.0	24.2	37.1
A fair amount	14.0	26.0	30.0	23.2	23.1
Very much	6.0	12.0	6.0	8.1	8.0
Total	**100.0**	**100.0**	**100.0**	**100.0**	**100.0**

Table A13.

Changes in the Free Time of Respondents:
Percentage Distributions by Country (N=400)

	France %	Italy %	Denmark %	Ireland %	All Countries %
None	4.0	5.0	13.0	5.0	7.0
A little	15.0	18.0	32.0	16.0	20.1
A fair amount	30.0	38.0	36.0	37.0	35.1
Very much	51.0	39.0	19.0	42.0	37.8
Total	**100.0**	**100.0**	**100.0**	**100.0**	**100.0**

Table A14.

Changes in the Respondents' Relationship with their Partner:
Percentage Distributions by Country (N=400)

	France %	Italy %	Denmark %	Ireland %	All Countries %
None	32.0	14.0	23.0	31.0	25.1
A little	41.0	26.0	39.0	29.0	33.7
A fair amount	21.0	47.0	26.0	23.0	29.1
Very much	6.0	13.0	12.0	17.0	12.1
Total	**100.0**	**100.0**	**100.0**	**100.0**	**100.0**

Table A15.

How the Respondents' Relationship with their Partner Changed:
Percentage Distributions by Country

	France %	Italy %	Denmark %	Ireland %	All Countries %
Very negatively	0.0	0.0	0.0	2.9	0.7
Negatively	1.5	3.5	0.0	2.9	2.2
Somewhat negatively	33.8	15.3	17.6	26.5	23.3
Somewhat positively	21.5	42.4	7.8	26.5	26.7
Positively	32.3	30.6	49.0	26.5	33.3
Very positively	10.8	8.2	25.5	14.7	13.7
Total	**100.0**	**100.0**	**100.0**	**100.0**	**100.0**

CHAPTER 8: 3. CHILDCARE

Table A16.

Childcare Arrangement for Youngest Child when Parent is at Work (Next Most Often): Percentage Distributions by Country (N=400)

	France %	Italy %	Denmark %	Ireland %	All Countries %
Self	2.0	0.0	0.0	0.0	0.5
Partner	37.0	29.3	35.0	25.7	31.8
Grandparent	15.0	30.3	31.0	27.7	26.0
Other relative	5.0	2.0	5.0	4.0	4.0
Work crèche/ childcare ctr/nursery	0.0	2.0	0.0	0.0	0.5
Other crèche/ childcare ctr/nursery	2.0	10.1	1.0	4.0	4.3
School/ école maternelle	2.0	0.0	1.0	5.0	2.0
Child minder (registered)	6.0	0.0	1.0	1.0	2.0
Childminder(unreg)/ babysitter/neighbour	20.0	8.1	2.0	2.0	8.0
Other	2.0	0.0	3.0	2.0	1.5
N/A	9.0	18.2	21.0	28.7	19.5
Total	**100.0**	**100.0**	**100.0**	**100.0**	**100.0**

Table A17.

Childcare Arrangement for Youngest Child when Parent is at Work (Third Most Often): Percentage Distributions by Country (N=400)

	France %	Italy %	Denmark %	Ireland %	All Countries %
Self	1.0	1.0	4.0	0.0	1.5
Partner	21.2	17.8	11.0	6.1	13.9
Grandparent	14.1	16.8	21.0	14.3	16.6
Other relative	7.1	5.9	10.0	6.1	7.6
Other crèche/ childcare ctr/nursery	0.0	2.0	2.0	2.0	1.5
School/ école maternelle	1.0	0.0	0.0	0.0	0.3
Childminder(unreg)/ babysitter/neighbour	10.1	4.0	3.0	7.1	5.8
Other	0.0	4.0	1.0	1.0	1.5
N/A	45.5	48.5	48.0	63.3	51.4
Total	**100.0**	**100.0**	**100.0**	**100.0**	**100.0**

Table A18.
Mean Number of Hours Youngest Child is in Care per Day and per Week:
Mean Scores by Country (N=400)

	France	Italy	Denmark	Ireland	All countries
Hours per day	7.8	6.4	7.1	6.7	7.3
Hours per week	36.6	32.4	34.6	30.2	33.4

Per day: $F = 6.61$, $df = 3$; $p \leq 0.001$
Per week: $F = 5.73$, $df = 3$; $p \leq 0.001$

Table A19.
The Second Youngest Child's Childcare Arrangements when Parent is at Work (Most Often): Percentage Distributions by Country (N=400)

	France %	Italy %	Denmark %	Ireland %	All Countries %
Self	2.5	0.0	0.0	0.0	0.5
Partner	0.0	4.2	1.7	3.4	2.5
Grandparent	2.5	2.1	1.7	1.7	2.0
Work crèche/childcare ctr/ nursery	0.0	0.0	1.7	5.2	2.0
Other crèche/childcare ctr/ nursery	0.0	58.3	50.8	15.5	32.8
School/ école maternelle	80.0	35.4	44.1	72.4	56.9
Childminder (registered)	7.5	0.0	0.0	0.0	1.5
Childminder(unreg)/ babysitter/neighbour	5.0	0.0	0.0	1.7	1.5
Other	2.5	0.0	0.0	0.0	0.5
Total	**100.0**	**100.0**	**100.0**	**100.0**	**100.0**

Table A20.

The Second Youngest Child's Childcare Arrangements when Parent is at Work (Next Most Often): Percentage Distributions by Country (N=400)

	France %	Italy %	Denmark %	Ireland %	All Countries %
Self	2.5	0.0	0.0	0.0	0.5
Partner	22.5	31.9	28.3	33.9	29.3
Grandparent	15.0	48.9	35.0	16.1	29.3
Other relative	5.0	0.0	1.7	1.8	2.0
Work crèche/ childcare ctr/ nursery	0.0	0.0	1.7	1.8	1.5
Other childcare/ childcare ctr/ nursery	0.0	2.1	8.3	10.7	5.9
School	10.0	2.1	0.0	5.4	3.9
Childminder (registered)	7.5	0.0	1.7	1.8	2.4
Childminder(unreg)/ babysitter/neighbour	22.5	8.5	1.7	8.9	9.8
Other	10.0	0.0	13.3	0.0	5.9
N/A	5.0	6.4	8.3	19.6	9.8
Total	**100.0**	**100.0**	**100.0**	**100.0**	**100.0**

Table A21.
The Second Youngest Child's Childcare Arrangements when Parent is at Work (Third Most Often): Percentage Distributions by Country (N=400)

	France %	Italy %	Denmark %	Ireland %	All Countries %
Self	5.1	0.0	3.4	0.0	2.0
Partner	25.6	23.4	16.9	8.8	17.6
Grandparent	5.1	19.1	18.6	21.1	17.2
Other relative	5.1	6.4	8.5	3.5	5.9
School	0.0	2.1	3.4	0.0	1.5
Childminder(unreg)/ babysitter/neighbour	5.1	4.3	1.7	12.3	5.9
Other	0.0	2.1	1.7	3.5	2.0
N/A	53.8	42.6	45.8	50.9	48.0
Total	**100.0**	**100.0**	**100.0**	**100.0**	**100.0**

Table A22.
Reasons for Having Chosen a Childcare Centre / Crèche:
Percentage Distributions by Country (N=400)

	France %	Italy %	Denmark %	Ireland %	All Countries %
Both parents work	13.6	56.8	78.8	31.2	45.4
Relieve grandparents	1.8	12.2	4.0	3.4	5.4
Stimulate child	21.0	56.0	73.0	28.5	44.9
Professional skills	9.0	7.9	20.8	9.2	11.7
Other	0.0	1.0	13.1	20.7	8.8
N/A	77.9	21.9	10.9	52.6	40.5
Total	**24.5**	**25.3**	**25.3**	**25.0**	**100.0**

Note: Respondents could select more than one answer and so the figures add up to more than 100%.

Table A23.

Reasons for Not Having Chosen a Childcare Centre / Crèche
Percentage Distributions by Country (N=400)

	France %	Italy %	Denmark %	Ireland %	All Countries %
High cost of crèche	6.7	4.0	0.9	11.5	5.8
Unfavourable to crèche	2.6	2.0	3.8	3.1	2.9
Relative better	5.8	4.1	0.9	15.5	6.6
Child has problems in adapting to crèche	0.0	0.9	0.9	0.0	0.5
Shortage of places	25.1	3.1	6.3	2.9	9.4
Child too young	0.7	15.5	4.9	7.1	7.0
Schedule doesn't suit	14.0	0.0	0.0	1.7	3.9
Favorable only to crèche on part-time basis	4.7	4.1	4.0	23.3	9.0
Other	59.2	72.2	55.2	55.2	68.6
Total	**25.0**	**24.9**	**24.9**	**24.9**	**100.0**

Note: Respondents could select more than one answer and so the figures add up to more than 100%

Table A24.

Reasons for Dissatisfaction with Childcare Arrangements: Percentage Distributions by Country and Sex (N=400)

	France %		Italy %		Denmark %		Ireland %		All Countries %	
	M	F	M	F	M	F	M	F	M	F
Too expensive	0.0	71.7	0.0	0.0	15.0	0.0	0.0	0.0	9.7	17.1
Not easily accessible	0.0	0.0	0.0	0.0	0.0	15.0	0.0	0.0	9.7	0.0
Not enough confidence in personnel	0.0	0.0	100	0.0	57.2	0.0	39.6	34.7	56.3	15.4
Don't feel comfortable about it	0.0	28.3	0.0	0.0	0.0	0.0	0.0	34.7	0.0	22.1
Hours are too rigid	0.0	28.3	0.0	0.0	0.0	32.4	0.0	0.0	0.0	17.1
Several modes of childcare /too complicated	0.0	0.0	0.0	0.0	0.0	0.0	26.8	0.0	7.1	0.0
Would prefer another mode of care	0.0	0.0	100	0.0	16.3	0.0	39.6	45.3	29.9	20.1
Other	0.0	0.0	0.0	0.0	44.1	67.6	73.2	65.3	47.9	50.5

Note: Respondents could select more than one answer and so the figures add up to more than 100%

Table A25.
Use of Respondent's Own Sick Leave as an Alternative Childcare Arrangement:
Percentage Distributions by Country (N=400)

	France %	Italy %	Denmark %	Ireland %	All Countries %
Never	73.7	77.8	67.7	69.3	72.1
Rarely	8.1	5.1	12.1	20.8	11.6
Sometimes	15.2	11.1	18.2	5.0	12.3
Often	2.0	6.1	1.0	4.0	3.3
Always	1.0	0.0	1.0	1.0	0.8
Total	**100.0**	**100.0**	**100.0**	**100.0**	**100.0**

Table A26.
Use of Respondent's Own Sick Leave as an Alternative Childcare Arrangement:
Mean Scores by Sex and SES (N=400)

	Male	Female	Total
Low SES	1.4	1.8	1.6
High SES	1.3	1.5	1.4
Total	1.4	1.6	1.5

(1 = never, 5 = always)
Sex: $F = 9.86$, $df = 1$; $p \leq 0.01$
SES: $F = 5.68$, $df = 1$; $p \leq 0.05$

Table A27.
Use of Partners' Sick Leave as an Alternative Childcare Arrangement:
Percentage Distributions by Country (N=400)

	France %	Italy %	Denmark %	Ireland %	All Countries %
Never	69.4	82.7	66.7	74.0	73.2
Rarely	8.2	7.1	11.1	13.0	10.1
Sometimes	17.3	7.1	18.2	9.0	12.9
Often	4.1	3.1	3.0	2.0	2.8
Always	1.0	0.0	1.0	2.0	1.0
Total	100.0	100.0	100.0	100.0	100.0

Table A28.
Use of Partners' Sick Leave as an Alternative Childcare Arrangement:
Mean Scores by Country and Sex (N=400)

	France	Italy	Denmark	Ireland	Total
Male	2.0	1.3	1.7	1.4	**1.6**
Female	1.3	1.3	1.6	1.5	**1.4**

(1 = never, 5 = always)
Sex: $F = 7.07$, $df = 1$; $p \leq 0.01$
Country x Sex: $F = 2.71$, $df = 3$; $p \leq 0.05$

Table A29.
Use of Respondent's Own Annual Leave as an Alternative Childcare Arrangement:
Percentage Distributions by Country (N=400)

	France %	Italy %	Denmark %	Ireland %	All Countries %
Never	48.0	43.0	41.4	28.0	39.8
Rarely	12.2	8.0	27.3	23.0	17.8
Sometimes	22.4	24.0	26.3	25.0	24.3
Often	12.2	20.0	2.0	15.0	12.5
Always	5.1	5.0	3.0	9.0	5.5
Total	100.0	100.0	100.0	100.0	100.0

Table A30.
Use of Respondent's Own Annual Leave as an Alternative Childcare Arrangement:
Mean Scores by Country and Sex (N=400)

	France	Italy	Denmark	Ireland	Total
Male	1.9	2.0	2.1	2.4	2.1
Female	2.4	2.7	1.8	2.7	2.4
Total	**2.2**	**2.4**	**2.0**	**2.5**	**2.3**

(1 = never, 5 = always)
Country: $F = 4.40$, $df = 3$; $p \leq 0.005$
Sex: $F = 7.11$, $df = 1$; $p \leq 0.01$

Table A31.
Use of Partners' Annual Leave as an Alternative Childcare Arrangement:
Percentage Distributions by Country (N=400)

	France %	Italy %	Denmark %	Ireland %	All Countries %
Never	52.5	46.5	57.6	42.0	49.6
Rarely	13.1	13.1	20.2	17.0	15.9
Sometimes	16.2	19.2	16.2	25.0	19.1
Often	12.1	12.1	4.0	8.0	8.8
Always	6.1	9.1	2.0	8.0	6.5
Total	**100.0**	**100.0**	**100.0**	**100.0**	**100.0**

Table A32.
Use of Partners' Annual Leave as an Alternative Childcare Arrangement:
Mean Scores by Country, Sex and Sector (N=400)

		France	Italy	Denmark	Ireland
Public	Male	1.9	2.0	1.4	3.2
	Female	2.0	2.5	1.6	2.1
Public Total		**2.0**	2.3	1.5	**2.6**
Private	Male	2.4	2.2	1.7	1.7
	Female	1.9	2.2	1.7	2.1
Private Total		**2.1**	**2.2**	**1.7**	**1.9**
Total		**2.0**	**2.2**	**1.6**	**2.2**

(1 = never, 5 = always)
Country: $F = 5.19$, df = 3; $p \leq 0.005$
Country x Sector: $F = 3.14$, df = 3; $p \leq 0.05$
Country x Sector x Sex: $F = 3.82$, df = 3; $p \leq 0.01$

Table A33.
Use of Respondents' Flexi-time as an Alternative Childcare Arrangement:
Percentage Distributions by Country (N=400)

	France %	Italy %	Denmark %	Ireland %	All Countries %
Never	56.7	75.8	50.5	77.8	64.9
Rarely	8.2	4.0	10.1	9.1	8.1
Sometimes	23.7	11.1	27.3	5.1	16.9
Often	8.2	6.1	5.1	7.1	6.6
Always	3.1	3.0	7.1	1.0	3.5
Total	**100.0**	**100.0**	**100.0**	**100.0**	**100.0**

Table A34.
Use of Respondents' Flexi-time as an Alternative Childcare Arrangement:
Mean Scores by Country and SES (N=400)

	France	Italy	Denmark	Ireland	Total
Low SES	1.8	1.4	1.8	1.3	1.6
High SES	2.0	1.8	2.3	1.6	1.9
Total	**1.9**	**1.6**	**2.0**	**1.5**	**1.8**

(1 = never, 5 = always)
Country: $F = 6.26$, $df = 3$; $p \leq 0.001$
SES: $F = 8.81$, $df = 1$; $p \leq 0.005$

Table A35.
Use of Respondents' Flexi-time as an Alternative Childcare Arrangement:
Mean Scores by Sex, Sector and SES (N=400)

		Male	Female
Low SES	Public	1.5	1.6
	Private	1.8	1.5
High SES	Public	2.2	2.0
	Private	1.5	2.0

SES x Sector x Sex: $F = 6.36$, $df = 1$; $p \leq 0.01$

Table A36.
Use of Respondents' Flexi-time as an Alternative Childcare Arrangement:
Mean Scores by Country, SES, Sex and Sector (N=400)

			France	Italy	Denmark	Ireland
Low SES	Public	M	2.1	1.0	1.6	1.2
		F	1.6	1.6	1.9	1.1
	Private	M	1.8	1.4	2.1	1.8
		F	1.8	1.5	1.5	1.2
High SES	Public	M	2.0	2.2	2.6	2.0
		F	2.8	1.5	2.3	1.3
	Private	M	1.6	1.3	1.6	1.5
		F	1.8	2.2	2.7	1.5

Country x SES x Sector x Sex: $F = 3.08$, $df = 3$; $p \leq 0.05$

Table A37.
Use of Partners' Flexi-time as an Alternative Childcare Arrangement:
Percentage Distributions by Country (N=400)

	France %	Italy %	Denmark %	Ireland %	All Countries %
Never	60.2	86.7	58.6	80.0	71.2
Rarely	11.2	1.0	13.1	5.0	7.6
Sometimes	21.4	8.2	17.2	9.0	13.9
Often	5.1	1.0	4.0	4.0	3.8
Always	2.0	3.1	7.1	2.0	3.5
Total	**100.0**	**100.0**	**100.0**	**100.0**	**100.0**

Table A38.
Use of Partners' Flexi-time as an Alternative Childcare Arrangement:
Mean Scores by Country and SES (N=400)

	France	Italy	Denmark	Ireland	Total
Low SES	1.7	1.2	1.8	1.2	**1.4**
High SES	1.9	1.5	2.1	1.7	**1.8**
Total	**1.8**	**1.3**	**1.9**	**1.4**	**1.6**

(1 = never, 5 = always)
Country: $F = 6.62$, $df = 3$; $p \leq 0.001$
SES: $F = 8.9$, $df = 1$; $p \leq 0.01$

Table A39.
Use of Respondents' Parental Leave as an Alternative Childcare Arrangement:
Percentage Distributions by Country (N=400)

	France %	Italy %	Denmark %	Ireland %	All Countries %
Never	94.9	82.7	97.4	88.1	90.4
Rarely	0.0	5.1	0.0	5.0	2.7
Sometimes	2.0	7.1	1.3	5.0	4.0
Often	3.0	4.1	1.3	1.0	2.4
Always	0.0	1.0	0.0	1.0	0.5
Total	**100.0**	**100.0**	**100.0**	**100.0**	**100.0**

Table A40.
Use of Respondents' Parental Leave as an Alternative Childcare Arrangement:
Mean Scores by Country and Sector (N=400)

	France	Italy	Denmark	Ireland	Total
Public	1.2	1.5	1.1	1.3	**1.3**
Private	1.0	1.2	1.1	1.1	**1.1**
Total	**1.1**	**1.3**	**1.1**	**1.2**	**1.2**

(1 = never, 5 = always)
Country: $F = 2.90$, $df = 3$; $p \leq 0.05$
Sector: $F = 9.73$, $df = 1$; $p \leq 0.005$

Table A41.
Use of Partners' Parental Leave as an Alternative Childcare Arrangement:
Percentage Distributions by Country (N=400)

	France %	Italy %	Denmark %	Ireland %	All Countries %
Never	95.9	89.8	98.7	85.9	92.0
Rarely	2.0	1.0	0.0	6.1	2.7
Sometimes	0.0	5.1	0.0	6.1	2.9
Often	2.0	4.1	1.3	0.0	1.9
Always	0.0	0.0	0.0	2.0	0.5
Total	**100.0**	**100.0**	**100.0**	**100.0**	**100.0**

Table A42.
Use of Partners' Parental Leave as an Alternative Childcare Arrangement:
Mean Scores by Sex and SES (N=400)

	Male	Female
Low SES	1.1	1.1
High SES	1.4	1.0
Total	**1.3**	**1.1**

Sex: $F = 10.71$, $df = 1$; $p < 0.001$
Sex x SES: $F = 4.79$, $df = 1$; $p < 0.05$

Table A43.
Use of Partners' Parental Leave as an Alternative Childcare Arrangement: Mean Scores by Sector and Country (N=400)

	France	Italy	Denmark	Ireland	Total
Public	1.1	1.4	1.1	1.4	1.2
Private	1.1	1.1	1.0	1.2	1.1
Total	**1.1**	**1.2**	**1.0**	**1.3**	**1.2**

(1 = never, 5 = always)
Country: $F = 3.39$, $df = 3$; $p<0.05$
Sector: $F = 6.08$, $df = 1$; $p<0.05$

Table A44.
Use of Respondents' Informal Arrangements with Employer as an Alternative Childcare Arrangement: Percentage Distributions by Country (N=400)

	France %	Italy %	Denmark %	Ireland %	All Countries %
Never	62.6	72.2	43.9	46.5	56.2
Rarely	13.1	10.3	18.4	24.2	16.5
Sometimes	15.2	12.4	32.7	22.2	20.5
Often	7.1	2.1	2.0	5.1	4.3
Always	2.0	3.1	3.1	2.0	2.5
Total	**100.0**	**100.0**	**100.0**	**100.0**	**100.0**

Table A45.
Use of Respondents' Informal Arrangements with Employer as an Alternative Childcare Arrangement: Mean Scores by Country and SES (N=400)

	France	Italy	Denmark	Ireland
Low SES	2.0	1.5	1.8	1.7
High SES	1.5	1.6	2.2	2.2
Total	**1.7**	**1.5**	**2.0**	**1.9**

(1 = never, 5 = always)
Country: $F = 3.42$, $df = 3$; $p \leq 0.05$
Country x SES: $F = 4.55$, $df = 3$; $p \leq 0.005$

Table A46.
Use of Respondents' Informal Arrangements with Employer as an Alternative Childcare Arrangement: Mean Scores by Country, SES, Sector and Sex (N=400)

			France	Italy	Denmark	Ireland
Low SES	Public	M	1.8	1.2	1.6	1.9
		F	1.6	1.4	1.9	1.6
	Private	M	2.0	2.2	2.0	1.3
		F	2.4	1.2	1.6	2.0
High SES	Public	M	1.4	1.9	1.9	2.2
		F	1.9	1.2	1.8	2.2
	Private	M	1.3	1.3	2.6	2.2
		F	1.4	1.5	2.6	2.2

(1 = never, 5 = always)
Country x Sex x SES x Sector: $F = 4.13$, $df = 3$; $p \leq 0.01$

Table A47.
Use of Partners' Informal Arrangements with Employer as an Alternative Childcare Arrangement: Percentage Distributions by Country: (N=400)

	France %	Italy %	Denmark %	Ireland %	All Countries %
Never	60.2	68.7	51.5	58.0	59.7
Rarely	16.3	13.1	14.1	15.0	14.7
Sometimes	15.3	10.1	26.3	17.0	17.2
Often	4.1	4.0	1.0	7.0	4.1
Always	4.1	4.0	7.1	3.0	4.3
Total	**100.0**	**100.0**	**100.0**	**100.0**	**100.0**

Table A48.
Alternative Childcare Arrangement—Other Relative Percentage Distributions by Country (N=400)

	France %	Italy %	Denmark %	Ireland %	All Countries %
Never	15.5	19.6	19.8	45.9	25.2
Rarely	22.7	13.4	19.8	11.2	16.8
Sometimes	18.6	25.8	45.5	27.6	29.5
Often	35.1	32.0	8.9	12.2	21.9
Always	8.2	9.3	5.9	3.1	6.6
Total	**100.0**	**100.0**	**100.0**	**100.0**	**100.0**

Table A49.
Alternative Childcare Arrangements—Neighbour/Babysitter
Percentage Distributions by Country (N=400)

	France %	Italy %	Denmark %	Ireland %	All Countries %
Never	45.5	78.7	71.7	88.3	70.7
Rarely	14.1	7.4	13.1	4.3	9.8
Sometimes	19.2	7.4	12.1	5.3	11.1
Often	19.2	5.3	1.0	1.1	6.7
Always	2.0	1.1	2.0	1.1	1.6
Total	100.0	100.0	100.0	100.0	100.0

CHAPTER 8: 4. TIME PREFERENCES

Table A50.
How Much Time Respondents Would Like to Spend with their Family:
Percentage Distributions by Country (N=400)

	France %	Italy %	Denmark %	Ireland %	All Countries %
Much less time	0.0	0.0	0.0	0.0	0.0
Somewhat less time	2.0	.0	1.0	1.0	1.0
About the same	19.0	28.0	21.0	26.7	23.6
More time	53.0	54.0	53.0	48.5	52.4
Much more time	26.0	18.0	25.0	23.8	23.1
Total	100.0	100.0	100.0	100.0	100.0

Table A51.
How Much Time Respondents Would Like their Partner to Spend with their Family:
Percentage Distributions by Country (N=400)

	France %	Italy %	Denmark %	Ireland %	All countries %
Much less time	0.0	0.0	0.0	1.0	0.3
Somewhat less time	2.0	2.0	2.0	3.0	2.3
About the same	26.3	32.0	28.0	31.3	29.3
More time	52.5	50.0	50.0	45.5	49.6
Much more time	19.2	16.0	20.0	19.2	18.5
Total	**100.0**	**100.0**	**100.0**	**100.0**	**100.0**

Table A52.
How Much Personal Time Respondents Would Like to Have:
Percentage Distributions by Country (N=400)

	France %	**Italy %**	**Denmark %**	**Ireland %**	**All Countries %**
Much less time	0.0	0.0	0.0	0.0	0.0
Somewhat less time	1.0	0.0	2.0	0.0	0.7
About the same	7.0	28.0	36.0	24.0	23.7
More time	76.0	55.0	48.0	57.0	59.1
Much more time	16.0	17.0	14.0	19.0	16.5
Total	**100.0**	**100.0**	**100.0**	**100.0**	**100.0**

CHAPTER 9: 1. WORK PLACE DEMOGRAPHICS

Table A53.

Mean Number of Hours Partner Works per Week:
Mean Scores by Country and Sex (N=400)

	France	Italy	Denmark	Ireland
Male	36.2	34.4	36.3	32.5
Female	42.4	43.1	40.1	42.4

Table A54.

Whether or Not Respondent Normally Works Typical Hours:
Percentage Distributions by Country (N=400)

	France %	Italy %	Denmark %	Ireland %	All Countries %
No	32.3	40.0	30.0	20.0	30.6
Yes	67.7	60.0	70.0	80.0	69.4
Total	100.0	100.0	100.0	100.0	100.0

CHAPTER 9: 2. CHANGES IN WORK FOLLOWING THE BIRTH OF THE YOUNGEST CHILD

Table A55.

Whether Partners of Respondents Modified Their Working Time:
Percentage Distributions by Country and Sex (N=400)

	France %		Italy %		Denmark %		Ireland %		All Countries %	
	M	F	M	F	M	F	M	F	M	F
No	52.0	88.0	50.0	84.0	60.0	82.0	52.0	86.0	53.5	84.9
Yes	48.0	12.0	50.0	16.0	40.0	18.0	48.0	14.0	46.5	15.1
Total	100.0	100.0	100.0	100.0	100.0	100.0	100.0	100.0	100.0	100.0

Table A56.
When Respondents Altered their Working Time, Did They Increase or Decrease it? Percentage Distributions by Country and Sex (N=<400)

	France %		Italy %		Denmark %		Ireland %		All Countries %	
	M	F	M	F	M	F	M	F	M	F
Decreased	75.0	89.3	41.7	88.5	73.3	70.6	56.5	78.6	59.3	83.8
Stayed the same	25.0	7.1	58.3	3.8	6.7	11.8	26.1	17.9	29.6	10.1
Increased	0.0	3.6	0.0	7.7	20.0	17.6	17.4	3.6	11.1	6.1
Total	100.0	100.0	100.0	100.0	100.0	100.0	100.0	100.0	100.0	100.0

Table A57.
Percentage of Respondents and Partners Who Temporarily Interrupted their Working Activity: Percentage Distributions by Country and Sex (N=400)

	France %		Italy %		Denmark %		Ireland %		All Countries %	
	M	F	M	F	M	F	M	F	M	F
Respondents	0.0	20.8	8.0	38.0	62.5	92.0	16.0	46.0	21.2	49.7
Partners	12.0	2.0	38.0	2.0	71.1	62.5	46.0	6.0	41.0	17.3

CHAPTER 9: 3. POTENTIAL FOR FLEXIBILITY

Table A58.
How Much of the Workday is the Respondent Available for Their Child/ren Via Phone, Messages, Voicemail, etc.:
Percentage Distributions By Country and Sex (N=400)

	France %	Italy %	Denmark %	Ireland %	All Countries %		
					Male %	Female %	Total %
Not at all	8.0	4.0	0.0	1.0	3.5	3.0	3.3
Little of the day	23.0	7.0	0.0	4.0	7.0	9.5	8.3
Some of the day	43.0	5.0	0.0	3.0	12.5	13.0	12.8
Most of the day	18.0	11.0	12.0	17.8	18.0	11.0	14.5
All day	8.0	73.0	88.0	74.3	59.0	63.5	61.3
Total	100.0	100.0	100.0	100.0	100.0	100.0	100.0

Table A59.
Respondent's Ability to Keep in Contact with the Childminder/Crèche/Nursery/etc. During the Day for Child 1: Percentage Distributions by Country and Sex (N=400)

	France %	Italy %	Denmark %	Ireland %	All Countries %		
					Male %	Female %	Total %
Not at all	10.2	1.0	1.0	0.0	3.5	2.5	3.0
With difficulty	17.3	8.0	1.0	5.0	7.5	7.6	7.5
Easily	72.4	91.0	98.0	95.0	89.0	89.9	89.4
Total	100.0	100.0	100.0	100.0	100.0	100.0	100.0

Table A60.
Respondent's Ability to Keep in Contact with the Childminder/Crèche/Nursery/etc. During the Day for Child 2: Percentage Distributions by Country and Sex (N=400)

	France %	Italy %	Denmark %	Ireland %	All Countries %		
					Male %	Female %	Total %
N/A	5.1	0.0	0.0	1.7	2.1	0.9	1.5
Not at all	12.8	0.0	0.0	0.0	2.1	2.8	2.5
With difficulty	20.5	6.4	0.0	10.3	8.5	7.5	8.0
Easily	61.5	93.6	100.0	87.9	87.2	88.8	88.1
Total	100.0	100.0	100.0	100.0	100.0	100.0	100.0

Table A61.
Reasons for Difficulties in Contacting Youngest Child: Percentage Distributions by Country (N=400)

	France %	Italy %	Denmark %	Ireland %	All Countries %
Distance/transport	20.8	12.5	0.0	0.0	15.8
Access to telephone	20.8	62.5	100.0	40.0	34.2
Permission of employer	8.3	12.5	0.0	20.0	10.5
Other	50.0	12.5	0.0	40.0	39.5
Total	100.0	100.0	100.0	100.0	100.0

Table A62.
Respondent's Ability to Get Away from Work to Visit Child's Childminding Facility/Creche/Nursery/etc. for Child 1: Percentage Distributions by Country and Sex (N=400)

	France %	Italy %	Denmark %	Ireland %	All Countries %		
					Male %	Female %	Total %
Not at all	16.7	4.0	3.0	2.0	6.0	6.6	6.3
With difficulty	53.1	26.0	18.0	23.0	31.0	28.6	29.8
Easily	30.2	70.0	79.0	75.0	63.0	64.8	63.9
Total	**100.0**	**100.0**	**100.0**	**100.0**	**100.0**	**100.0**	**100.0**

Table A63.
Respondent's Ability to Get Away from Work to Visit Child's Childminding Facility/Creche/Nursery/etc. for Child 2: Percentage Distributions by Country and Sex (N=400)

	France %	Italy %	Denmark %	Ireland %	All Countries %		
					Male %	Female %	Total %
N/A	2.4	0.0	1.7	1.5	2.1	0.9	1.4
Not at all	19.0	6.5	1.7	1.5	6.3	6.0	6.1
With difficulty	40.5	26.1	15.3	16.7	22.9	23.1	23.0
Easily	38.1	67.4	81.4	80.3	68.8	70.1	69.5
Total	**100.0**	**100.0**	**100.0**	**100.0**	**100.0**	**100.0**	**100.0**

Table A64.
Reasons for Difficulties in Leaving Work to Visit Child:
Percentage Distributions by Country (N=400)

	France %	Italy %	Denmark %	Ireland %	All Countries %
Employer wouldn't allow	22.3	3.3	5.1	3.4	12.6
Employer might allow but with disapproval	23.6	22.6	21.4	26.6	23.6
Couldn't leave work	47.8	41.4	63.2	35.0	46.1
Distance/ transportation problems	31.0	26.7	9.7	37.3	28.4
Other	8.0	9.7	16.2	10.8	9.9

CHAPTER 10: 1. RECONCILING WORK AND FAMILY LIFE

Table A65
Ease *vs.* Difficulty in Combining Work and Family Life:
Percentage Distributions by Country and Sex (N=400)

	France %		Italy %		Denmark %		Ireland %		All Countries %		
	M	F	M	F	M	F	M	F	M	F	Total
Very easy	0.0	2.1	2.0	2.0	12.0	2.0	6.0	6.0	5.0	3.1	4.0
Easy	6.0	6.4	6.0	6.0	24.0	32.0	26.0	22.0	15.5	16.3	15.9
Somewhat easy	48.0	48.9	58.0	20.0	32.0	44.0	24.0	20.0	40.5	33.2	36.9
Somewhat difficult	34.0	29.8	30.0	50.0	26.0	18.0	26.0	30.0	29.0	32.1	30.6
Difficult	10.0	6.4	2.0	16.0	6.0	2.0	12.0	12.0	7.5	9.2	8.3
Very difficult	2.0	6.4	2.0	6.0	0.0	2.0	6.0	10.0	2.5	6.1	4.3
Total	100.0	100.0	100.0	100.0	100.0	100.0	100.0	100.0	100.0	100.0	100.0

Table A66
Do the Hours you Work Create Problems in your Childcare Arrangements?
Percentage Distributions by Country and Sex (N=400)

	France %		Italy %		Denmark %		Ireland %		All Countries %		
	M	F	M	F	M	F	M	F	M	F	Total
Not at all	14.3	24.0	26.0	26.0	42.9	47.9	40.0	56.0	31.0	38.1	34.5
Not very much	30.6	42.0	44.0	46.0	28.6	22.9	36.0	28.0	34.5	35.0	34.8
Yes to some extent	42.9	30.0	28.0	22.0	20.4	20.8	20.0	14.0	27.5	21.8	24.7
Yes a great deal	12.2	4.0	2.0	6.0	8.2	8.3	4.0	2.0	7.0	5.1	6.0
Total	100.0	100.0	100.0	100.0	100.0	100.0	100.0	100.0	100.0	100.0	100.0

CHAPTER 10: 2. WELL-BEING

Table A67

Satisfaction with Present State of Health:
Percentage Distribution by Country and Sex (N = 400)

	France %		Italy %		Denmark %		Ireland %		All Countries %		
	M	F	M	F	M	F	M	F	M	F	Total
Very Dissatisfied	0.0	0.0	0.0	0.0	0.0	0.0	0.0	2.0	0.0	0.5	0.3
Dissatisfied	4.1	4.2	2.0	8.0	2.0	4.0	7.8	4.0	4.0	5.0	4.5
Somewhat Dissatisfied	8.2	16.7	14.0	4.0	6.1	0.0	17.6	4.0	11.0	6.0	8.5
Somewhat Satisfied	32.7	20.8	28.0	34.0	12.2	14.0	17.6	14.0	23.0	20.1	21.6
Satisfied	34.7	45.8	40.0	38.0	44.9	50.0	35.3	42.0	39.0	44.2	41.6
Very Satisfied	20.4	12.5	16.0	16.0	34.7	32.0	21.6	34.0	23.0	24.1	23.6
Total	100.0	100.0	100.0	100.0	100.0	100.0	100.0	100.0	100.0	100.0	100.0

Table A68

Satisfaction with Present Work:
Percentage Distributions by Country and Sex (N= 400)

	France %		Italy %		Denmark %		Ireland %		All Countries %		
	M	F	M	F	M	F	M	F	M	F	Total
Very Dissatisfied	0.0	2.0	4.0	4.0	0.0	2.0	4.0	0.0	2.0	2.0	2.0
Dissatisfied	6.1	12.2	2.0	4.0	2.0	0.0	4.0	4.1	3.5	5.0	4.3
Somewhat Dissatisfied	16.3	14.3	8.0	4.0	4.0	12.0	14.0	4.1	10.5	8.5	9.5
Somewhat Satisfied	34.7	26.5	44.0	34.0	20.0	14.0	30.0	28.6	31.5	25.6	28.6
Satisfied	36.7	36.7	26.0	38.0	40.0	48.0	26.0	32.7	32.5	38.7	35.6
Very Satisfied	6.1	8.2	16.0	16.0	34.0	24.0	22.0	30.6	20.0	20.1	20.1
Total	100.0	100.0	100.0	100.0	100.0	100.0	100.0	100.0	100.0	100.0	100.0

Table A69

Satisfaction with Family Life:
Percentage Distributions by Country and Sex (N=400)

	France %		Italy %		Denmark %		Ireland %		All Countries %		
	M	F	M	F	M	F	M	F	M	F	Total
Very Dissatisfied	0.0	0.0	0.0	2.0	0.0	0.0	0.0	0.0	0.0	0.5	0.3
Dissatisfied	0.0	0.0	0.0	0.0	0.0	2.0	0.0	0.0	0.0	0.5	0.3
Somewhat Dissatisfied	6.0	10.0	4.0	0.0	2.0	0.0	8.0	4.1	5.0	3.5	4.3
Somewhat Satisfied	22.0	22.0	16.0	20.0	12.0	16.0	10.0	18.4	15.0	19.1	17.0
Satisfied	52.0	42.0	36.0	46.0	48.0	44.0	36.0	34.7	42.5	41.7	42.1
Very Satisfied	20.0	26.0	44.0	32.0	38.0	38.0	46.0	42.9	37.5	34.7	36.1
Total	100.0	100.0	100.0	100.0	100.0	100.0	100.0	100.0	100.0	100.0	100.0

Table A70

Satisfaction with Relationship with Partner:
Percentage Distributions by Country and Sex (N=400)

	France %		Italy %		Denmark %		Ireland %		All Countries %		
	M	F	M	F	M	F	M	F	M	F	Total
Very Dissatisfied	0.0	2.1	0.0	4.0	0.0	0.0	0.0	0.0	0.0	1.5	O.8
Dissatisfied	0.0	2.1	2.0	2.0	0.0	0.0	0.0	0.0	O.5	1.0	O.8
Somewhat Dissatisfied	4.1	10.6	2.0	8.0	4.0	0.0	4.0	5.9	3.5	5.6	4.5
Somewhat Satisfied	20.4	17.0	20.0	24.0	8.0	22.0	8.0	9.8	14.4	18.3	16.3
Satisfied	42.9	44.7	28.0	26.0	44.0	30.0	36.0	23.5	37.3	31.0	34.2
Very Satisfied	32.7	23.4	48.0	36.0	44.0	48.0	52.0	60.8	44.3	42.6	43.5
Total	100.0	100.0	100.0	100.0	100.0	100.0	100.0	100.0	100.0	100.0	100.0

Table A71

Satisfaction with Life in General:
Percentage Distributions by Country and Sex (N=400)

	France %		Italy %		Denmark %		Ireland %		All Countries %		
	M	F	M	F	M	F	M	F	M	F	Total
Very dissatisfied	0.0	2.0	0.0	0.0	0.0	0.0	0.0	0.0	0.0	0.5	0.3
Dissatisfied	0.0	2.0	2.0	2.0	0.0	0.0	0.0	0.0	0.5	1.0	0.8
Somewhat dissatisfied	2.0	6.0	2.0	0.0	0.0	0.0	10.0	6.0	3.5	3.0	3.3
Somewhat satisfied	44.0	24.0	30.0	22.0	16.0	4.0	16.0	10.0	26.1	15.1	20.6
Satisfied	44.0	52.0	44.0	48.0	42.0	44.0	44.0	42.0	44.2	46.2	45.2
Very satisfied	10.0	14.0	22.0	28.0	42.0	52.0	30.0	42.0	25.6	34.2	29.9
Total	100.0	100.0	100.0	100.0	100.0	100.0	100.0	100.0	100.0	100.0	100.0

APPENDIX B
QUESTIONNAIRE

Country
France | 1
Italy | 2
Denmark | 3
Ireland | 4

Subject I.D.

QUESTIONNAIRE

**FATHERS AND MOTHERS:
DILEMMAS OF THE WORK-LIFE BALANCE**

A Collaborative Study by:

Centre for Gender and Women's Studies,
Trinity College, Dublin

Dipartimento di Scienze Umane e Sociali,
Universita di Trento

Centre National de la Recherche Scientifique (CNRS),
Caisse Nationale des Allocations Familiales (CNAF)

Institute of Political Science, University of Copenhagen

[With support from the European Commission and the Irish Dept. of Justice, Equality and Law Reform]

September 2001

DEMOGRAPHICS

1. **Sex:**

Male	Female
1	2

2. **How old are you? Age (in years):**

3. **Are you married or co-habiting with your partner?**

Married	Co-habiting
1	2

4. **What is the highest level of education you have attained?**

Primary	1
Secondary (Inter. Cert.)	2
Secondary (Leaving Cert.)	3
University Degree	4
Postgraduate Degree	5

5. **What is the highest level of education your partner has attained?**

Primary	1
Secondary (Inter. Cert.)	2
Secondary (Leaving Cert.)	3
University Degree	4
Postgraduate Degree	5

6. **Please describe your occupation**

SES
1-8

7. **Please describe your partner's occupation**

SES
1-8

8. What, precisely is the activity of the establishment where you work?_____

9. What, precisely is the activity of the establishment where your partner works?__

10. **Do you work in the public or private sector?**

Public	Private
1	2

11. **Does your partner work in the public or private sector?**

Public	Private
1	2

12. **Is your immediate supervisor (boss):**

Male	Female
1	2

13. **How long does it take, on average, for you to get to work? (In minutes)**

14. **How long does it take, on average, for your partner to get to work? (In minutes)**

15. **What mode of transport do you usually use?**

Car	1
Train (DART, Metro)	2
Bus	3
Bicycle	4
Motorcycle	5
Walking	6
Other	7
_____	
Not applicable (work at home)	8

16. **How many hours on average do you work per week? (In hours)**

17. **How many hours on average does your partner work per week? (in hours)**

18. **Do you normally work typical hours (within the range 9am - 5:30pm)?**

Yes	No
2	1

YOU AND YOUR CHILDREN

19. How many children do you have?

20. What are their ages?

Child 1 (must be under 6 years of age)

Child 2 (must be 12 years old or under. If older - ignore and answer future questions for Child 1 only)

21. Did the birth of your youngest child ("Child 1") cause any significant changes for you, in relation to: (tick one for each)

a. The way you organised your day

None	A little	A fair amount	Very much
1	2	3	4

b. Your life habits

None	A little	A fair amount	Very much
1	2	3	4

c. Your professional tasks

None	A little	A fair amount	Very much
1	2	3	4

d. The amount of domestic chores

None	A little	A fair amount	Very much
1	2	3	4

e. Your friendships	None	A little	A fair amount	Very much
	1	2	3	4

f. Your free time	None	A little	A fair amount	Very much
	1	2	3	4

g. Your relationship with your partner	None	A little	A fair amount	Very much
	1	2	3	4

22. How did it change?

Very negatively	Negatively	Somewhat negatively	Somewhat positively	Positively	Very positively
1	2	3	4	5	6

23. Did you modify your working time after the birth of your youngest child (Child 1)?

Yes	No
2	1

24. If yes, did you decrease or increase your working time?

Decreased	Stayed the same	Increased
1	2	3

25. **Did the birth of your child oblige you to temporarily interrupt your activity (except for the period of paid maternity leave)?**

Yes	No
2	1

26. **Did your partner modify his/her working time after the birth of your youngest child (Child 1)?**

Yes	No
2	1

27. **If yes, did your partner decrease or increase his/her working time?**

Decreased	Stayed the same	Increased
1	2	3

28. **Did the birth of your child oblige your partner to temporarily interrupt his/her activity (except for the period of paid maternity leave)?**

Yes	No
2	1

29. **Please indicate which person usually carries out the following activities during the week (tick only one):**

General Household Management and Tasks

a. Shopping for food

Me	My partner	Both of us	Other
1	2	3	4

b. Preparing meals

Me	My partner	Both of us	Other
1	2	3	4

c. Washing up.

Me	My partner	Both of us	Other
1	2	3	4

d. Managing/ organising/ planning family tasks/ home-life	Me	My partner	Both of us	Other
	1	2	3	4

e. Washing/ironing clothes	Me	My partner	Both of us	Other
	1	2	3	4

f. Cleaning	Me	My partner	Both of us	Other
	1	2	3	4

g. Taking the children to creche, childminder, school etc	Me	My partner	Both of us	Other
	1	2	3	4

h. Playing with the child/ren.	Me	My partner	Both of us	Other
	1	2	3	4

i. Feeding the child/ren	Me	My partner	Both of us	Other
	1	2	3	4

j. Changing nappies/ dressing child/ren.	Me	My partner	Both of us	Other
	1	2	3	4

k.	Bathing the child/ren	Me	My partner	Both of us	Other
		1	2	3	4

l.	Picking up the child/ren when s/he cries at night	Me	My partner	Both of us	Other
		1	2	3	4

30. **Would you like to spend more time, less time or the same amount of time with your family?**

    Much more time... 5
    More time.. 4
    About the same... 3
    Somewhat less time....................................... 2
    Much less time... 1

31. **Would you like your partner to spend more time, less time or the same amount of time with your family?**

    Much more time... 5
    More time.. 4
    About the same... 3
    Somewhat less time....................................... 2
    Much less time... 1

32. **Would you like to have more personal time, less personal time or about the same amount of personal time?**

    Much more time... 5
    More time.. 4
    About the same... 3
    Somewhat less time....................................... 2
    Much less time... 1

CHILDCARE ARRANGEMENTS

I would now like to ask you some questions about your childcare arrangements.

33. **Who takes care of your youngest child (Child 1) when you are at work, most often, next most often and third most often? (tick one only in each of the 3 columns). SHOW CARD 1**

		Most	Next most	3rd most
a.	Self..	3	2	1
b.	Partner...	3	2	1
c.	Grandparent.................................	3	2	1
d.	Other relative..............................	3	2	1
e.	Workplace creche/childcare centre/nursery	3	2	1
f.	Other Creche/childcare centre/ nursery......	3	2	1
g.	School..	3	2	1
h.	Childminder (registered).............	3	2	1
i.	Childminder (unregistered)/babysitter/neighbou	3	2	1
j.	Other..	3	2	1
k.	N/A..	3	2	1

34. **Total hours that youngest child (Child 1) is in care (other than by parents):**

a. per day on average

b. per week on average

COMPLETE ONLY IF SECOND YOUNGEST CHILD IS 12 YEARS OR YOUNGER

35. Who takes care of your second youngest child (Child 2) when you are at work, most often, next most often and third most often? (tick one only in each of the 3 columns) SHOW CARD 1

		1 Most	2 Next most	3 3rd most
a.	Self...	3	2	1
b.	Partner...	3	2	1
c.	Grandparent.....................................	3	2	1
d.	Other relative...................................	3	2	1
e.	Workplace Creche/childcare centre/nursery	3	2	1
f.	Other Creche/childcare centre/ nursery......	3	2	1
g.	School..	3	2	1
h.	Childminder (registered)................	3	2	1

i.	Childminder (unregistered)/babysitter/neighbou	3	2	1
j.	Other..	3	2	1
k.	N.A...	3	2	1

36. **For Child 2 (only if child is not yet at school and goes to a childcare centre, creche, nursery or childminder: please give total hours in care:**

a. per day on average

b. per week on average

37. **When your childcare arrangements become unavailable (e.g., during holidays or when child-minder is ill), who usually cares for the child/ren? Please tick one for each item. INTERVIEWER MAY REFER TO CARD 2 IF NECESSARY**

	Never	Rarely	Some times	Often	Always
Respondent does					
a. by using own sick leave...............................	1	2	3	4	5
b. by using own annual leave (holiday)...........	1	2	3	4	5
c. by using flexi-time......................................	1	2	3	4	5

		1	2	3	4	5
d.	by using parental leave..................................					
e.	Informal arrangement between employer and self...					

Spouse/Partner does

		1	2	3	4	5
f.	by using sick leave..					
g.	by using annual leave (holiday)....................					
h.	by using flexi-time..					
i.	by using parental leave.................................					
j.	Informal arrangement between employer and partner...					
k.	**Other relative does**...............................					
l.	**Neighbour/ babysitter does**......................					

38. **If one of your child/ren is usually cared for by a childcare centre/ creche, what are the reasons for having chosen this option?**

Both parents work..	1
To relieve grandparents from their burden of care................	2
To stimulate the child, to favour her/his independence or socialization...	3
For the high level of professional skills of crèche personnel	4
Other...	5
N/A...	6

39. **If one of your child/ren is not usually cared for by a childcare centre/ creche, what are the reasons for not having chosen this option?**

High cost of creche...	1
Parents are generally unfavourable to crèche......................	2
It is better for a child to be cared by a relative...................	3
The child has some problems in adapting to crèche...........	4
Shortage of childcare places..	5
Child too young..	6
Schedule doesn't suit...	7
I am favourable to a creche, but only for part-time............	8
Other (please specify)_____	9
N/A..	10

40. **What is the total cost (excluding transport and incidentals), if any, per week of your childcare arrangements? (write 0 if no cost)**

    Irish £ [   ]   Euros [   ]

41. **Overall, how satisfied are you with your childcare arrangements?**

Very dissatisfied	Dissatisfied	Somewhat dissatisfied	Somewhat satisfied	Satisfied	Very satisfied
1	2	3	4	5	6

42. **If you are not satisfied, why not?**

It is too expensive...	1
It is not easily accessible..	2
I don't have enough confidence in the personnel who care for my child	3
I don't feel comfortable about it..	4
The hours are too rigid...	5
I have several modes of childcare and it is too complicated	6
I would prefer another mode of care..................................	7
Other (please specify)..	8

THE WORKPLACE

I would now like to ask you some questions about your working life

43. **Is it acceptable that one may leave earlier and/or arrive later due to problems regarding children?**

a. Among you and your colleagues

Very unacceptable	Unacceptable	Somewhat unacceptable	Somewhat acceptable	Acceptable	Very acceptable
1	2	3	4	5	6

b. By your managers

Very unacceptable	Unacceptable	Somewhat unacceptable	Somewhat acceptable	Acceptable	Very acceptable
1	2	3	4	5	6

44. **Is it acceptable that one may bring a child to work (for an hour) due to problems regarding childcare?**

a. Among you and your colleagues

Very unacceptable	Unacceptable	Somewhat unacceptable	Somewhat acceptable	Acceptable	Very acceptable
1	2	3	4	5	6

b. By your managers

Very unacceptable	Unacceptable	Somewhat unacceptable	Somewhat acceptable	Acceptable	Very acceptable
1	2	3	4	5	6

45. **How well do you think the following people take into account the fact that you have responsibility for a child/ren?**

a. Your colleagues

Not at all well	Not too well	So-so	Well	Very Well
1	2	3	4	5

b. Your immediate supervisor

Not at all well	Not too well	So-so	Well	Very Well
1	2	3	4	5

c. Your employer

Not at all well	Not too well	So-so	Well	Very Well
1	2	3	4	5

46. **I am now going to ask you if you can do the following things at work.**

a. Is it acceptable for you to run private errands such as shopping, go to a bank or a post office during work?

Yes	No	N/A
3	1	2

b. Do you have the possibility of owing work time?

Yes	No	N/A
3	1	2

c. Do you have a **formal** agreement of flexible working time?

Yes	No	N/A
3	1	2

d.	Do you have an **informal** agreement of flexible working time?	Yes	No	N/A
		3	1	2
e.	Is it possible for you to swap shifts/working time with co-workers?	Yes	No	N/A
		3	1	2
f.	Is it acceptable for you to make phone calls to doctors, handymen, call home, etc. during work?	Yes	No	N/A
		3	1	2

47. To what extent do you agree that in your workplace...

a. Many employees are resentful when men take extended leaves to care for newborn or adopted children.

DISAGREE				AGREE		
Strong	Moderate	Slight		Slight	Moderate	Strong
1	2	3	4	5	6	7

b. Many employees are resentful when women take extended leaves to care for newborn or adopted children.

DISAGREE				AGREE		
Strong	Moderate	Slight		Slight	Moderate	Strong
1	2	3	4	5	6	7

c. Men who participate in available work-family programmes (e.g. job-sharing, part-time work) are viewed as less serious about their career than those who do not participate in these programmes.

DISAGREE				AGREE		
Strong	Moderate	Slight	Slight	Moderate	Strong
1	2	3	4	5	6	7

d. Women who participate in available work-family programmes (e.g. job-sharing, part-time work) are viewed as less serious about their career than those who do not participate in these programmes.

DISAGREE				AGREE		
Strong	Moderate	Slight	Slight	Moderate	Strong
1	2	3	4	5	6	7

e. To get ahead employees are expected to work over and above the normal hours, whether at the workplace or at home.

DISAGREE				AGREE		
Strong	Moderate	Slight	Slight	Moderate	Strong
1	2	3	4	5	6	7

f. To be viewed favourably by top management, employees must constantly put their jobs ahead of their families or personal lives.

DISAGREE				AGREE		
Strong	Moderate	Slight	Slight	Moderate	Strong
1	2	3	4	5	6	7

48. The actual use of the possibilities for flexibility regarding children

a. Do you ever leave your job earlier or arrive late due to problems regarding childcare?...

Yes	No
2	1

b. Do you ever bring a child to work on occasion due to problems with childcare?...

Yes	No
2	1

c. Do you run private errands such as shopping, go to a bank or a post office during work?..

Yes	No
2	1

d. Do you make phone calls to doctors, handymen, call home etc. during work?..

Yes	No
2	1

49. How much of the workday are you normally available for your child/ren via phone messages, etc.?

All day		5
Most of the day		4
Some of the day		3
Very little of the day		2
Not at all		1

50. Can you keep in contact with the childminder/ babysitter, school or facility during the day by telephone or otherwise?

	a. Child 1 Youngest	b. Child 2 Next Youngest
Easily..	3	3
With difficulty...............................	2	2
Not at all.....................................	1	1
N/A...		0

51. **If "with difficulty" or not at all, what are the difficulties?**

	a. Child 1	b. Child 2
Distance/transport....................................	1	1
Lack of access to telephone......................	2	2
Permission of employer not forthcoming	3	3
Other (please specify)_____	4	4

N/A.. | | 5

52. **If the need arose, could you get away from work to visit your child's childminding facility?**

	a. Child 1	b. Child 2
Easily..	3	3
With difficulty..	2	2
Not at all...	1	1
N/A..		0

53. **If "with difficulty" or impossible, why?**

Employer wouldn't allow..	1
Employer might allow but with disapproval.........	2
Couldn't leave work...	3
Distance/ transportation problems........................	4
Other (please specify)_____	5

54. **What would be your ideal working schedule (with no change in your salary)?**
    (interviewee looks, interviewer ticks)

Longer day, fewer days a week............................	1
Shorter days..	2
Flexible hours..	3
More holiday time...	4
Stay the same..	5
Other (please specify)_____	6

_____

COMBINING WORK AND FAMILY LIFE

I would now like to ask you about how you reconcile your work with your family life.

55. How easy/difficult is it for you to combine your job and family life?

Very Easy	EASY	Somewhat easy	Somewhat difficult	Difficult	Very difficult
1	2	3	4	5	6

56. Do the hours you work create problems in your childcare arrangements?

Yes a great deal.......... 4
Yes to some extent...... 3
Not very much............ 2
Not at all.................... 1

57. What strategies do you use in order to reconcile work and family life?

		Not at all	To some extent	A great deal
a.	Better family management	1	2	3
b.	Higher level of partner's involvement	1	2	3
c.	Stronger support from the family network	1	2	3
d.	More flexibility of working schedules	1	2	3

e.	More flexibility of the working environment	Not at all	To some extent	A great deal
		1	2	3

f.	Other	Not at all	To some extent	A great deal
		1	2	3

INTRO. TO NEXT SET OF QUESTIONS
A number of policies have been devised to help working parents, although some of them would have relevance for all workers. Please tell me for each policy firstly whether or not it is available to you personally in your workplace, secondly whether or not you have used it, and lastly please indicate your attitude to the policy in general (whether it exists in your workplace or not).
INTERVIEWER MAY REFER TO CARD 3 IF NECESSARY

58. Paid maternity leave: Is it available in your workplace? If yes, have you used it? What is your attitude towards it?

a. Available?			b. Used?			c. Attitude		
Yes	No	Don't know	Yes	No	N/A	Not favour	Somewhat favour	Strongly favour
3	1	2	3	1	2	1	2	3

59. Unpaid maternity leave: Is it available in your workplace? If yes, have you used it? What is your attitude towards it?

a. Available?			b. Used?			c. Attitude		
Yes	No	Don't know	Yes	No	N/A	Not favour	Somewhat favour	Strongly favour
3	1	2	3	1	2	1	2	3

60. **Paid Paternity leave (for childbirth):** Is it available in your workplace? If yes, have you used it? What is your attitude towards it?

a. Available?			b. Used?			c. Attitude		
Yes	No	Don't know	Yes	No	N/A	Not favour	Somewhat favour	Strongly favour
3	1	2	3	1	2	1	2	3

61. **Unpaid Paternity leave (for childbirth):** Is it available in your workplace? If yes, have you used it? What is your attitude towards it?

a. Available?			b. Used?			c. Attitude		
Yes	No	Don't know	Yes	No	N/A	Not favour	Somewhat favour	Strongly favour
3	1	2	3	1	2	1	2	3

62. **Part-time working:** Is it available in your workplace? If yes, have you used it? What is your attitude towards it?

a. Available?			b. Used?			c. Attitude		
Yes	No	Don't know	Yes	No	N/A	Not favour	Somewhat favour	Strongly favour
3	1	2	3	1	2	1	2	3

63. **Job-sharing:** Is it available in your workplace? If yes, have you used it? What is your attitude towards it?

a. Available?			b. Used?			c. Attitude		
Yes	No	Don't know	Yes	No	N/A	Not favour	Somewhat favour	Strongly favour
3	1	2	3	1	2	1	2	3

64. **Flexible hours (Flexi-time):** Is it available in your workplace? If yes, have you used it? What is your attitude towards it?

a. Available?			b. Used?			c. Attitude		
Yes	No	Don't know	Yes	No	N/A	Not favour	Somewhat favour	Strongly favour
3	1	2	3	1	2	1	2	3

65. **Career breaks:** Is it available in your workplace? If yes, have you used it? What is your attitude towards it?

a. Available?			b. Used?			c. Attitude		
Yes	No	Don't know	Yes	No	N/A	Not favour	Somewhat favour	Strongly favour
3	1	2	3	1	2	1	2	3

66. **Term-time working (taking unpaid leave during school summer holidays):** Is it available in your workplace? If yes, have you used it? What is your attitude towards it?

a. Available?			b. Used?			c. Attitude		
Yes	No	Don't know	Yes	No	N/A	Not favour	Somewhat favour	Strongly favour
3	1	2	3	1	2	1	2	3

67. **Personalised (flexible) working hours:** Is it available in your workplace? If yes, have you used it? What is your attitude towards it?

a. Available?			b. Used?			c. Attitude		
Yes	No	Don't know	Yes	No	N/A	Not favour	Somewhat favour	Strongly favour
3	1	2	3	1	2	1	2	3

68. **Emergency/ Special leave:** Is it available in your workplace? If yes, have you used it? What is your attitude towards it?

a. Available?			b. Used?			c. Attitude		
Yes	No	Don't know	Yes	No	N/A	Not favour	Somewhat favour	Strongly favour
3	1	2	3	1	2	1	2	3

69. **Working from home (tele-working):** Is it available in your workplace? If yes, have you used it? What is your attitude towards it?

a. Available?			b. Used?			c. Attitude		
Yes	No	Don't know	Yes	No	N/A	Not favour	Somewhat favour	Strongly favour
3	1	2	3	1	2	1	2	3

70. **Is paid parental leave available in your or your partner's workplace?**

Mine only	Partners only	Both	Neither	Don't Know
1	2	3	4	5

71. **Is unpaid parental leave available in your or your partner's workplace?**

Mine only	Partners only	Both	Neither	Don't Know
1	2	3	4	5

72. **Have you or your partner used either paid or unpaid parental leave?**

a. Self: Paid leave

Yes	No
2	1

b. Self: Unpaid leave

Yes	No
2	1

c. Partner: Paid leave

Yes	No
2	1

d. Partner: Unpaid leave

Yes	No
2	1

73. **IF YES: For how long (in weeks) have you used it?**

a. Self: Paid leave   b. Self: Unpaid leave

c. Partner: Paid leave   d. Partner: Unpaid leave

74. **IF NO to paid leave:**

a. Why not? _____

_____

	Yes	No
b. Would you have taken it if it were paid more?	2	1

	Yes	No
c. Would your partner have taken it if it were paid more?	2	1

75. **IF NO to unpaid leave:**

a. Why not? _____

_____

	Yes	No
b. Would you have taken it if it was paid?	2	1

	Yes	No
c. Would your partner have taken it if it was paid?	2	1

76. **What is your attitude to paid parental leave in general?**

Not favour	Somewhat favour	Strongly favour
1	2	3

77. **What is your attitude to unpaid parental leave in general?**

Not favour	Somewhat favour	Strongly favour
1	2	3

WELL-BEING

(Let respondent tick)

78. How satisfied are you on the whole with your present state of health?

Very dissatisfied	Dissatisfied	Somewhat dissatisfied	Somewhat satisfied	Satisfied	Very satisfied
1	2	3	4	5	6

79. How satisfied are you, all in all, with your present work?

Very dissatisfied	Dissatisfied	Somewhat dissatisfied	Somewhat satisfied	Satisfied	Very satisfied
1	2	3	4	5	6

80. How satisfied are you, all in all, with your family life?

Very dissatisfied	Dissatisfied	Somewhat dissatisfied	Somewhat satisfied	Satisfied	Very satisfied
1	2	3	4	5	6

81. Overall, how satisfied are you with your relationship with your spouse/partner?

Very dissatisfied	Dissatisfied	Somewhat dissatisfied	Somewhat satisfied	Satisfied	Very satisfied
1	2	3	4	5	6

82. Overall, how satisfied are you with your life in general?

Very dissatisfied	Dissatisfied	Somewhat dissatisfied	Somewhat satisfied	Satisfied	Very satisfied
1	2	3	4	5	6

Thank you very much for your co-operation

REFERENCES

Addis, E. (1997) "Il tempo delle donne tra produzione e riproduzione." In: E. Addis (Ed.) *Economia e differenza di genere*. Bologna: Clueb.

Allain, L. & Sédillot, B. (1999) "L'effet de l'allocation parentale d'éducation sur l'activité des femmes." In: Majnoni d'Intignano, B. (Ed.), *Egalité entre femmes et hommes: aspects économiques*, Rapport du Conseil d'Analyse Economique, Paris, La Documentation Française.

Andersen, D. & Hestbæk, A. D. (1999) *Ansvar og værdier. En undersøgelse i børnefamilier*. København: Socialforskningsinstituttet.

Andersen, D. Appeldorn, A. & Weise, H. (1996) *Orlov: Evaluering af orlovsordningerne*. Kobenhavn: Socialforskningsinstitutet.

Anxo, D., Flood, L. & Kocoglu, Y. (2000) *Allocation du temps et partage des tâches en France et en Suède,* Research report. Paris: Ministry of Employment and Solidarity.

Arona, M. (1997) "Valutare la soddisfazione dei genitori rispetto al nido." *Bambini*, Aprile.

Aryee, S. Luc, V. & Stone, R. (1998) "Family-Responsive Variables and Retention-Relevant Outcomes Among Employed Parents", *Human Relations*, 51 (1) pp. 73-87.

Ascoli, U. & Pavolini, E. (2001) "Le politiche sociali della regione Emilia-Romagna". In: U. Ascoli, M. Barbagli, F. Cassentino, and G. Ecchia (Eds.) *Le politiche sociali in Emilia-Romagna*. Torino: Rosenberg & Sellier.

Badolato, G. (1993) *Identità paterna e relazione di coppia*. Milano: Giuffrè.

Balbo, L. (Ed.) (1991) *Tempi di vita. Studi e proposte per cambiarli*. Milano: Feltrinelli.

Balbo, L., May, M., & Micheli, G. (1990) *Vincoli e strategie nella vita quotidiana.* Milano: Angeli.

Barbagli, M., & Saraceno, C. (Eds.) (1997) *Lo stato delle famiglie in Italia*. Bologna: Il Mulino.

REFERENCES

Barrère-Maurisson, M.A., Minni, C. & Rivier, S. (2001) "Le partage des temps pour les hommes et les femmes, ou comment conjuguer travail rémunéré, non rémunéré et non-travail", DARES, *Premières synthèses*, n°11.

Barrère-Maurisson, M.A., Marchand, O. & Rivier, S. (2000) "Temps professionnel, temps parental. La charge parentale: un travail à mi-temps", DARES, *Premières synthèses*, n°20.

Barry, U. (1998) "Women, Equality and Public Policy." In: S. Healy and B. Reynolds (Eds.) *Social Policy in Ireland: Principles, Practice and Problems*. Dublin: Oak Tree Press.

Bassi, A., Casotti, G. & Sbordone, F. (2000) (Eds.) *Tempi di vita e tempi di lavoro. Donne e impresa sociale nel nuovo welfare*. Milano: Angeli.

Becchi, E., Bondioli, A. & Ferrari, M. (1999) "ISQUEN (Indicatori e Scala di valutazione della Qualità del Nido)" In: L. Cipollone (a cura di) *Strumenti e indicatori per valutare il nido*, Bergamo, Junior.

Belloni, C. (1984) *Il tempo delle città*. Milano: Angeli.

Belloni, C. (1995a) "Che cos'è il tempo libero?" *Sociologia del lavoro*, 56, pp.17-32.

Belloni, C. (1995b) "Il tempo quotidiano in Italia. La struttura del tempo quotidiano tra normazione sociale e scelte soggettive." *Polis*, 9(3), pp. 401-21.

Belloni, C. (1996) "Madri e padri, due tempi due organizzazioni." *Inchiesta*, 111, pp. 35-43.

Bergamaschi, M., Chiesi, A., De Filippi, F. & Sogni, G. (1993) *Orari di lavoro come strategia. Politiche aziendali e comportamenti di genere*. Milano: Angeli.

Bergamaschi, M., Omodei Zorini, E. & Schweizer, K. (1995) *Un benessere insopportabile. Identità femminile tra lavoro produttivo e lavoro di cura*. Milano: Angeli.

Bernardi, M.P. & Mancini, M.G. (1994) "Una donna a tempo pieno." In: C. Cipolla (Ed.) *La differenza come compatibilità*. Milano: Angeli.

Bertozzi, L. (1999) *Il lavoro di che genere?* Flessible, project of Assessorato alle politiche sociali e pari opportunità, Municipality of Forlì, Forlì

Bestetti, G. (1996) "Nascere come genitori: le parole delle madri e dei padri." In: C. Corinna (Ed.) *Percorsi di genere tra natura e cultura*. Milano: Unicopoli.

Bettio, F. & Villa, P. (1998) "A Mediterranean perspective on the breakdown of the relationship between participation and fertility," *Cambridge Journal of Economics*, 22,(2), pp. 137-171.

Bianchi, M. (2000) *Conciliabilità tra famiglia, lavoro di cura e lavoro retribuito in particolare per le donne in base a dati e documentazioni a livello europeo*. Research Report. Bolzano: Provincia Autonoma di Bolzano.

REFERENCES

Bielenski, H., Bosch, G. & Wagner, A. (2002) *Working time preferences in sixteen European countries.* Dublin: European Foundation for the Improvement of Living and Working Conditions.

Bielenski, H. & Kauppinen, T. (1999) "Working Time Needs of Europeans." Paper presented at the conference: *Working Time in Europe – Towards a European Working Time Policy*, Helsinki.

Bimbi, F. (1990) "Molteplicità dei tempi sociali; tempo quotidiano, esperienze di maternità e di paternità." In: F. Bimbi, and G. Castellano (Eds.) *Madri e padri.* Milano: Angeli.

Bimbi, F. (1991a) "Voci: differenza/parità, doppia presenza, l'economia del dono". In: L. Balbo (Ed.) *Tempi di vita. Studi e proposte per cambiarli.* Milano: Feltrinelli.

Bimbi, F. (1991b) "Madri e padri: relazioni asimmetriche e forme dell'intimità nel caso italiano," *Critica Sociologica*, 97-98, pp.1-14.

Bimbi, F. (1992) "Tre generazioni di donne. La trasformazione dei modelli d'identità femminile in Italia." In: S. Ulivieri (Ed.) *Educazione e ruolo femminile: la condizione delle donne in Italia dal dopoguerra ad oggi.* Firenze: La Nuova Italia.

Bimbi, F. (1993a) *Il genere e l'età: percorsi di formazione dell'identità.* Milano: Angeli.

Bimbi, F. (1993b) "Tradizione e trasmissione tra generazioni di donne." In: A. Carbonaro, and C. Facchini (Eds.) *Biografie e costruzione dell'identità.* Milano: Angeli.

Bimbi, F. (1995) "Metafore di genere tra lavoro non pagato e lavoro pagato," *Polis*, 9(3), pp. 379-400.

Bimbi, F. (1996) "Differenze di genere nelle decisioni di procreazione," *Inchiesta*, 111, pp.15-23.

Bimbi, F., & Castellano, G. (Eds.) (1990) *Madri e Padri.* Milano: Angeli.

Bonke, J. (1995) *Arbejde, tid og køn - i udvalgte lande.* København: Socialforskningsinstituttet.

Bonke, J. & Meilbak, N. T. (1999) *Danskere på fuldtid - deres faktiske og ønskede arbejdstid.* Servicerapport. København: SFI-Survey

Bowen, G. L. (1998) "Corporate supports for the lives of employees: A conceptual model for program planning and evaluation", *Family Relations*, 37, pp. 183-188.

Bozzao, P. (2001) "La protezione sociale della famiglia," *Lavoro e Diritto*, 15(1), pp. 55-96.

Bozzi, G., & Cristiani, C. (1996) "Cento padri a Milano: una ricerca sull'interazione precoce padre neonato." In: C. Corinna (Ed.) *Percorsi di genere tra natura e cultura.* Milano: Unicopoli.

Brousse, C. (1999) "La répartition du travail domestique entre conjoints : permanences et évolution de 1986 à 1999." In: *France, Portrait Social.* Paris: INSEE.

REFERENCES

Bué J., (2002) "Temps partiel des femmes: entre choix et contraintes," *Premières synthèses*, Dares, n° 08.2.

Burchell, B., & Fagan, C. (2002) "Gender and the intensification of work: Evidence from the 2000 European Working Conditions Survey." Paper presented at the *Work Intensification Conference*, Paris, November, pp 21-22.

Calafà, L. (2001) "La prestazione di lavoro tra assenze e (dis)equilibri familiari," *Lavoro e Diritto*, 15(1), pp. 143-161.

Calafà, L., and Gottardi, D. (1999) "Maternità, paternità e lavoro, recenti linee di ineludibili riforme," *Diritto del Mercato del Lavoro*, 12(3), pp. 431-446.

Cappellini, G. (1999) "Il part-time come strumento di politica dell'occupazione e del lavoro: analisi economica ed evidenza empirica," *Quaderni di economia del lavoro*. Special issue on: "Gestione del tempo di lavoro e lavoro femminile", 64, pp. 57-119.

Carlsen, S. (1994) "Mænds brug af fædre- og forældreorlov." In: Jørgen Elm Larsen & Søren Carlsen (Eds.) *Den svære balance. Om sammenhængen mellem arbejdsliv og familieliv set i et ligestillingsperspektiv*. Ligestillingsrådet.

Castelain-Meunier, C. (1998) *La paternité, Que-sais-je ?*, Paris, PUF.

Cazzaniga, P. (1999) "Azioni positive nelle aziende in favore della conciliazione. Un'esperienza del gruppo elettrolux-Zanussi." Paper presented at the conference on *Le famiglie interrogano le politiche sociali*. Bologna, 29-31 March.

CBI (1994) *Sickness Absence in Industry*. London: CBI/PERCOM.

Censis (1984) *La condizione dell'infanzia tra famiglia e istituzioni*. Roma: Ministero dell'Interno, Direzione Generale dei Servizi Civili.

Christenson, K. & Staines, G. L. (1990) "Flexi-time: A Viable Solution to Work-Family Conflict?" *Journal of Family Issues*, 11, pp. 455-476.

Clarke, H. (1999) *Growing up in the Context of Different Gender-Role Attitudes: A Comparison of Irish and Swedish Girls' Attitudes towards Men and Women's Work and Family Roles*. Unpublished MPhil thesis, Centre for Gender and Womens Studies, Trinity College, University of Dublin.

Commission on the Family (1998) *Strengthening Families for Life. Final Report of the Commission on the Family to the Minister for Social, Community and Family Affairs*. Dublin: Stationery Office.

Cooper, C. L. & Williams, S. (1994) *Creating Healthy Work Organizations*, Chichester: John Wiley and Sons.

Cooperativa Sociale Koine (2000) *Servizi all'infanzia e nuove imprese in uno scenario interculturale*. Firenze: atti del convegno, 23/2/2000. www.progettoarcobaleno.it

REFERENCES

CREDOC (1998) "Accueil des jeunes enfants, conciliation vie professionnelle – vie familiale et opinions sur les prestations familiales," *Collection des rapports* n°191, Paris.

CREDOC (2001) *Opinions sur la politique des prestations familiales et sur les CAF.* Research report for CNAF, Paris.

Crowley, N. (2002) "Opening of Conference" In: M. Fine-Davis, H. Clarke, and M. Berry (Eds.) *Fathers and Mothers: Dilemmas of the Work-Life Balance - Conference Proceedings.* Dublin: Centre for Gender and Women's Studies, Trinity College, pp. 3-7.

CSO (1999-2001) *Quarterly National Household Survey,* Dublin: Central Statistics Office.

CSO (2000) *Quarterly National Household Survey: Travel to Work, 1st Quarter 2000.* Dublin: Central Statistics Office.

CSO (2001) *Quarterly National Household Survey: Length and Pattern of Working Time, 2nd Quarter 2001.* Dublin: Central Statistics Office.

CSO (2002) *Quarterly National Household Survey, 1st Quarter 2002.* Dublin: Central Statistics Office.

CSO (2003) *Quarterly National Household Survey: Childcare, 4th Quarter 2002.* Dublin: Central Statistics Office.

CSO Labour Force Surveys (various). Dublin: Central Statistics Office

Csonka, A. (2000) *Ledelse og arbejde under forandring.* Københavns Universitet, Institut for Statskundskab. Ph.d-serien.

Damgaard, J. B. (1998) *Styring og effektivitet: Organisering af dansk børnepasning.* Institut for Statskundskab. Aarhus Universitet Ph.D.-serien.

Ligestillingsrådet & Danmarks Statistik (1999) Kvinder og Mænd.

Danmarks Statistik (2000a) Levevilkarsundersogelsen. Kobenhavn.

Danmarks Statistik (2000b) "Statistikbank" online, (www.dst.dk).

Danmarks Statistik (2002) *Børns Levevilkår* (Children's living conditions). Copenhagen: Danmarks Statistik.

Davis, E.E., Fine-Davis, M. & Meehan, G. (1982) "Demographic determinants of perceived well-being in eight European countries," *Social Indicators Research*, 10, pp. 341-358.

Davis, E. E. & Fine-Davis, M. (1991) "Social Indicators of Living Conditions in Ireland, with European Comparisons," *Social Indicators Research*, 25, (Whole Nos 2-4), pp. 103-365.

de Brito, I. (2003) Paper presented at Conference on Flexible and Innovative Ways to Facilitate Work-Life Balance and Social Inclusion, Centre for Gender and Women's Studies, Trinity College, Dublin, 23-24 January.

REFERENCES

De Simone, G. & Villa, P. (1998) *The care system and the employed population in Italy*. Bruxelles: European Commission, Network on "Gender and Employment", Equal Opportunities Unit, DG V.

Del Punta, R. (2000) "La nuova disciplina dei congedi parentali, familiari e formativi," *Rivista Italiana di Diritto del Lavoro*, 19(1), pp. 149-80.

Department of Education and Science (1999) *Ready to Learn - White Paper on Early Childhood Education*. Dublin: Stationery Office.

Department of Justice, Equality and Law Reform (2001) *Report of the Working Group on the Review and Improvement of the Maternity Protection Legislation*. Dublin: Stationery Office.

Dex, S. & Joshi, H. (1999) "Careers and motherhood: policies for compatibility," *Cambridge Journal of Economics*, 23, 641-659.

Di Vita, A. M. & Mancuso, R. (Eds.) (2000) *Oltre Proserpina: identità, rappresentazioni sociali e disagio nel ciclo di vita femminile*. Milano: Angeli.

Di Vita, A.M., Annino, M., Mancuso, R. and Marino, E. (2000) "Scelte professionali e identità di genere in un contesto palermitano. Un'indagine preliminare." In: A.M. Di Vita, and R. Mancuso (Eds.) *Oltre Proserpina: identità, rappresentazioni sociali e disagio nel ciclo di vita femminile*. Milano: Angeli.

Donati, P. (Ed.) (1997) *Uomo e donna in famiglia*. Milano: S.Paolo.

Drew, E., Emerek, R. & Mahon, E. (Eds.) (1998) *Women, Work and the Family in Europe*, London & New York: Routledge.

Drew, E., Humphreys, P. & Murphy, C. (2002) *Off the Treadmill: Achieving Work life Balance*. Dublin: National Framework Committee for the Development of Family Friendly Policies.

Dublin Transportation Office (2002) *Quality Bus Corridor Monitoring Survey*, November. Unpublished Annual Summary Report, Dublin Transportation Office.

Duclos, L. (2002) "Des politiques de la conciliation entre vie professionnelle, vie familiale et vie personnelle aux arrangements quotidiens dans la ville." Paper presented at the Conference, *Rencontres de la DIV*, Paris, 27 Juin.

Dutch Ministry of Social Affairs and Employment (2002) *Daily Routine Arrangements: Experiments in the Netherlands*. The Hague: Dutch Ministry of Social Affairs and Employment.

Ellingsæter, A. L. (1997) "Forældreskab og økonomisk forsørgelse: Fra mandsnorm til ligedeling". In: Jens Bonke (Ed.) *Dilemmaet arbejdsliv - familieliv i Norden*. København: Socialforskningsinstituttet.

REFERENCES

Emmott, M. & Hutchinson, S. (1998) "Employment flexiblity: Threat or promise?" In: P. Sparrow & M. Marchington (Eds.) *HRM: The New Agenda*. London: Pitman.

Equality Authority (1998) *About the Parental Leave Act 1988*. Dublin: Equality Authority.

Esping-Andersen, G. (1990) *The Three Worlds of Welfare Capitalism*. Cambridge: Polity.

Estrade, M. A., Méda, D. & Orain, R. (2001) "Les effets de la réduction du temps de travail sur les modes de vie: qu'en pensent les salaries un an après?" *Premières Synthèses*, DARES, n°21.

European Commission (1995) *Men as Carers: Towards a culture of Responsibility, Sharing and Reciprocity between Women and Men In the Care and Upbringing of Children*. Brussels: European Commission Equal Opportunities Unit.

European Commission Network on Childcare (1996) *A Review of Services for Young Children in the European Union*. Brussels: European Commission Directorate General V (Employment, Industrial Relations and Social Affairs) Equal Opportunities Unit.

European Commission (1997) *Reconciliation of work and family life for women and men and the quality of care services* (Report on Existing Research in the European Union). Brussels: European Commission.

Eurostat (2001) *The Social Situation in the European Union*. Luxembourg: Eursostat, European Commission.

Eurostat (2002) "La protection sociale en Europe," *Statistique en bref, Theme 3, No. 1*.

Evans, J. M. (2001) *Firms' Contribution to the Reconciliation Between Work and Family Life*, Occasional Papers, n°48, Paris: OECD.

Expert Working Group on Childcare (1999) *National Childcare Strategy - Report of the Partnership 2000 Expert Working Group on Childcare*. Dublin: The Stationery Office.

Fagnani, J. (1995) "L'allocation parentale d'éducation : effets pervers et ambiguités d'une prestation," *Droit Social*, n°3, pp. 287-295.

Fagnani, J. (1998a) "Recent changes in family policy in France: political trade-offs and economic constraints." In: E. Drew, R. Emerek & E. Mahon (Eds.) *Women, Work and the Family in Europe*. London, New-York: Routledge, pp. 58-65.

Fagnani, J. (1998b) "Helping mothers to combine paid and unpaid work - or fighting unemployment? The ambiguities of French family policy," *Community, Work and Family*, 1(3), pp. 297-312.

Fagnani J. (2000) *Un travail et des enfants. Petits arbitrages et grands dilemmas*. Bayard Ed., Paris.

REFERENCES

Fagnani, J. (2002a) "Why do French women have more children than German women? Family policies and attitudes towards childcare outside the home," *Community, Work and Family*, 5(1), pp. 103-119.

Fagnani, J. (2002b) "The French Experience." In: M. Fine-Davis, H. Clarke & M. Berry (Eds.) *Fathers and Mothers: Dilemmas of the Work-Life Balance – Conference Proceedings.* Dublin: Centre for Gender and Women's Studies, Trinity College, pp. 15-22.

Fagnani, J. & Letablier, M. T. (2000) *Enquete sur la conciliation de la vie familiale et de la vie professionnelle.* Paris: Caisse Nationale des Allocations Familiales.

Fagnani, J. & Letablier, M. T. (2003a) "La réduction du temps de travail a t-elle amélioré la vie quotidienne des parents de jeunes enfants?" *Premières Synthèses*, DARES, n°1-2.

Fagnani J. & Letablier M. T. (2003b) "Qui s'occupe des enfants pendant que les parents travaillent?" *Recherches et Prévisions, n°72.*

Fahey, T. & Fitzgerald, J. (1997) In *Medium Term Report.* Dublin: Economic and Social Research Institute.

Fenet F., Leprince F. & Périer L. (2001) *Les modes d'accueil des jeunes enfants, concilier vie familiale, vie professionnelle et vie sociale.* Actualités sociales hebdomadaires, n°187/189.

Fermanian J. D. (1999) "Le temps de travail des cadres," *INSEE Première*, n°671.

Fermanian, J. D. & Lagarde, P. (1998) "Les horaires de travail dans le couple," *Economie et Statistique,* n°321 – 322.

Ferrari, M. (1994) "Rilevare l'indice complessivo della qualità: una rassegna di ricerche nei nidi." In: M. Ferrari (Ed.) *La valutazione nei contesti prescolari: strumenti e realtà.* Bergamo: Edizioni Junior.

Ferrucci, F. (1998) "Gli orientamenti delle politiche familiari in Italia alla fine degli anni '90." *Sociologia e Politiche Sociali*, special issue on "Famiglia e Politiche di Welfare," 1(3), pp. 47-78.

Filippi, V. (1997) *Donne, lavoro, famiglia. Il caso di "Insieme Si Può, una cooperativa del nord-est.* Milano: Angeli.

Fine-Davis, M. (1977) *Attitudes towards the Status of Women: Implications for Equal Employment Opportunity.* Report to the Department of Labour, Dublin.

Fine-Davis, M. (1983a) *Women and Work in Ireland: A Social-Psychological Perspective.* Dublin: Council for the Status of Women.

Fine-Davis, M. (1983b) "Mothers' Attitudes toward Child Care and Employment: A Nationwide Survey." In: *Working Party on Child Care Facilities for Working Parents, Report to the Minister for Labour.* Dublin: Stationery Office, pp. 73 - 168.

REFERENCES

Fine-Davis, M. (1983c) "A society in transition: Structure and determinants of attitudes toward the role and status of women in Ireland." *Psychology of Women Quarterly*, 8(2), pp. 113-132.

Fine-Davis, M. (1985) *Women, Work and Well-Being in the European Community: Nationwide Results for 8 Countries* [V/55/85-EN]. Brussels: Commission of the European Communities.

Fine-Davis, M. (1988a) "Changing Attitudes to the Role of Women in Ireland: 1975-1986, Vol. I: 'Attitudes toward the Role and Status of Women, 1975-1986'". In: *First Report of the Second Joint Oireachtas [Parliamentary] Committee on Women's Rights* (Pl. 5609) Dublin: The Stationery Office, May.

Fine-Davis, M. (1988b) "Changing Attitudes to the Role of Women in Ireland: 1975-1986, Vol. III: 'Attitudes towards Moral Issues in Relation to Voting Behaviour in Recent Referenda, 1975-1986'". In: Third *Report of the Second Joint Oireachtas [Parliamentary] Committee on Women's Rights* (Pl. 5796) Dublin: The Stationery Office, July.

Fine-Davis, M. (1988c) "Changing Attitudes to the Role of Women in Ireland: 1975-1986, Vol. II: 'Issues Related to Equal Employment Opportunity'". In: *Second Report of the Second Joint Oireachtas [Parliamentary] Committee on Women's Rights* (Pl. 5673) Dublin: The Stationery Office, June.

Fine-Davis, M. (1989a) "Attitudes toward the role and status of women as part of a larger belief system." *Political Psychology*, 10 (2), 287-308.

Fine-Davis, M. (1989b) *The Economic and Social Benefits of Childcare in the Workplace*. Dublin: Irish Congress of Trade Unions.

Fine-Davis, M. (1994) *Changing Attitudes to the Role of Women*. Paper presented at European Research Workshop on Families, Labour Markets and Gender Roles, European Foundation for the Improvement of Living and Working Conditions, Shankill, Co. Dublin, 7-9 September.

Fine-Davis, M. (2001) *Childcare in Ireland: Policy Options and Recommendations*. Unpublished paper. Centre for Gender and Women's Studies, Trinity College, Dublin.

Fine-Davis, M. (2003) "The evolving childcare policy debate in Ireland: An overview." Submitted to *Administration*.

Fine-Davis, M. (2003, in press) "Balancing Work and Family in Ireland: Social Attitudes and Evolving Policy Debates." *Proceedings of Conference on Private and Professional Spheres: Towards a Recomposition of Roles and Actions*. (Belgian Presidency of the EU, Gembloux, November 8-9, 2001). Service des Etudes et de la Statistique, Walloon Region Ministry, De Boeck Université Publishers.

REFERENCES

Fine-Davis, M. & Clarke, H. (2002) "Ireland and Cross-National Comparisons" In: M. Fine-Davis, H. Clarke & M. Berry (Eds.) *Fathers and Mothers: Dilemmas of the Work-Life Balance – Conference Proceedings.* Dublin: Centre for Gender and Women's Studies, Trinity College, pp. 51-69.

Fine-Davis, M., Davis, E.E. & Bolger, N. (1981) *The quality of working life in the European Community: Multivariate analyses of the Irish data.* Final Report to the Statistical Office of the European Communities, Luxembourg. Dublin: Deparment of Psychology, Trinity College Dublin and Economic and Social Research Institute.

Fisher, H. (2000) *Investing in People: Family-Friendly Work Arrangements in Small and Medium-Sized Enterprises*, Dublin: Equality Authority.

Galinsky, E. & Stein, P. J. (1990) "The impact of human resource policies: Balancing work and family life." *Journal of Family Issues*, 11, pp. 368-383.

Gallou, R., & Simon, M. O. (1999) *Le devenir des sortants de l'allocation parentale d'éducation de rang deux*, Paris, Research report, CREDOC - CNAF.

Ganster, D. C. & Schaubroeck, J. (1991) "Work Stress and Employee Health," *Journal of Management*, 17, pp. 65-271.

Ghedini, P. (1995) "La qualità come strategia". *Bambini.* Giugno.

Gheido, M. R. & Casotti, A. (2000) "Permessi e congedi per gravi motivi," *Diritto e Pratica del Lavoro.* Special issue on "Congedi parentali e formativi. Astensione facoltativa, tutela del lavoratore padre, permessi per gravi motivi familiari," 11 (5).

Ginatempo, N. (1994) *Donne al confine: identità e corsi di vita femminili nelle città del sud.* Milano: Angeli.

Giovannini, D. (1998) "Are fathers changing? Comparing some different images on sharing of childcare and domestic work." In: E. Drew, R. Emerek, & E. Mahon (Eds.) *Women, Work and the Family in Europe.* London, New York: Routledge, pp. 191-199.

Giovannini, D. (2002) "The Italian Experience." In: M. Fine-Davis, H. Clarke & M. Berry (Eds.) *Fathers and Mothers: Dilemmas of the Work-Life Balance – Conference Proceedings.* Dublin: Centre for Gender and Women's Studies, Trinity College, pp. 23-38.

Giovannini, D., Goriup. E. & Cerrato, J. (in press) "La imagen de la paternidad en los progenitores: Un estudio sobre la interdependencia entre procesos representacionales y prácticas comportamentales." In: J. Cerrato & A. Palmonari (Eds.) *Representaciones Sociales: Perspectivas Teóricas y Aproximaciones.*

Giovannini, D. & Molinari, L. (1994) "Fathers' and Mothers' Involvement in Childcare as a Factor of Intersubjective Relationships." Paper presented at the Conference, *Social Practices and Symbolic Mediations*, Neuchatel, March.

Giovannini, D. & Ventimiglia, C. (Eds.) (1994) *Paternità e politiche per l'infanzia: Essere padri oggi* (Fatherhood and childcare policies: Being a father today). Unpublished report of research. Regione Emilia Romagna: Assessorato alla Formazione Professionale, Lavoro, Scuola e Università, Bologna.

Glass, J. & Fujimoto, T. (1995) "Employer Characteristics and the Provision of Family Responsive Policies," *Work and Occupations*, 22(4) pp. 380-411.

Glass, J. & Riley, L. (1998) "Family Responsive Policies and Employee Retention Following Childbirth," *Social Forces*, 76(4), pp. 1401-1435.

Glaude, M. (1999) "L'égalité entre femmes et hommes : où en sommes-nous." In: B. Majnoni d'Intignano (Ed.), *Egalité entre femmes et hommes : aspects économiques*. Rapport du Conseil d'Analyse Economique, Paris, La Documentation Française.

Goff, S. J., Mount, M. K. & Jamison, R. L. (1992) "Employer supported childcare, work/family conflict and absenteeism: A field study," *Personnel Psychology*, 43, pp. 793-809.

Goodbody Economic Consultants (1998) *The Economics of Childcare in Ireland*. Dublin: Goodbody Economic Consultants.

Goriup, E. (2001) *Rappresentazioni sociali della paternità e coppie genitoriali: una ricerca empirica nella zona di Cividale del Friuli*. Tesi di laurea, Università degli Studi di Trento (manoscritto non pubblicato).

Gottardi, D. (1999) "I congedi parentali nell'ordinamento Italiano." *Lavoro e Diritto*, 13(3), pp. 497-527.

Grecchi, A. (Ed.) (1999) *Competitività aziendale e pari opportunità. Casi di "buone pratiche"*. Roma: Presidenza del Consiglio dei Ministri, Commissione Nazionale per la parità e le Pari Opportunità tra Uomo e Donna.

Grover, Sl. L. & Crooker, K. J. (1995) "Who appreciates family-responsive human resource policies: The impact of family-friendly policies on the organizational attachment of parents and non-parents," *Personnel Psychology*, 48, pp. 271-288.

Haas, L. (1993) "Changing Gender Roles in Sweden." In J. C. Hood (Ed.) *Men, Work and Family*, CA: Sage Publications.

Hall, D. T. & Parker, V. A. (1993) "The Role of Workplace Flexibility in Managing Diversity", *Organizational Dynamics*, 21, pp. 5-18.

Hall, J. & Jones, D.C. (1950) "The social grading of occupations," *British Journal of Sociology*, 1, 31-55.

Hantrais L. & Letablier M.T. (1996) *Familles, travail et politiques familiales en Europe*. Paris: PUF.

Hantrais, L. (Ed.) (2000) *Gendered policies in Europe*. London: Macmillan Press.

REFERENCES

Hestbæk, A. D. (1995) *Forældreskab i 90'erne.* København: Socialforskningsinstituttet.

Hillage, J. & Simkin, C. (1992*) Family Friendly Working: New Hope or Old Hype.* IMS Report 224. Brighton: Institute of Manpower Studies.

Højgaard, L. (1990) *Vil Kvinder Lede?* Kobenhavn: Ligestillingsradet.

Højgaard, L. (1996a) "Work and Family - Life's Inseparable Pair." In: J. E. Larsen & S. Carlsen (Eds.) *The Equality Dilemma, Reconciling working life and family-life, viewed in an equality perspective.* The Danish Equal Status Council.

Højgaard, L. (1996b) *Kon og lon- En analyse af virksomhedskultur og lonforskelle mellem kvinder og mand i fire pivate virksomheder.* Kobenhavn: Samsundslitteratur.

Højgaard, L. (1997) "Working Fathers - Caught in the Web of the Symbolic Order of Gender," *Acta Sociologica,* 40.

Højgaard, L. (1998) "Workplace Culture, Family-supportive Policies and Gender Differences." In: E. Drew, R. Emerek & E. Mahon (Eds.) *Women, Work and the Family in Europe.* London & New York: Routledge, pp. 140-149.

Højgaard, L. (2002) "The Danish Experience." In: M. Fine-Davis, H. Clarke & M. Berry (Eds.) *Fathers and Mothers: Dilemmas of the Work-Life Balance – Conference Proceedings.* Dublin: Centre for Gender and Women's Studies, Trinity College, pp. 39-49.

Holt, H. (1994) *Forældre på arbejdspladsen - en analyse af tilpasningsmulighederne mellem arbejdsliv og familieliv i kvinde- og mandefag.* København: Socialforskningsinstituttet.

Holt, H. (1998) *En kortlægning af danske virksomheders sociale ansvar.* København: Socialforskningsinstituttet.

Holt, H. & Thaulow, I. (1996b) "Strategies to make more responsive to the needs of families." In H. Holt and I. Thaulow (eds.) *Reconciling Work and Family-life. An International Perspective on the Role of Companies.* København, Socialforskningsinstituttet.

Humphreys, P. C., Fleming, S. & O'Donnell, O. (2000) Balan*cing Work and Family Life*. Institute of Public Administration, Dublin.

Hutchinson, B. (1969) *Social status and inter-generational social mobility in Dublin.* Paper No. 48. Dublin: The Economic and Social Research Institute.

Inglehart, R. & Rabier, J. R. (1985) "If you're unhappy, this must be Belgium". *Public Opinion,* April/May, pp. 10-15.

Ingrosso, M. (1988) *Stelle di mare e fiocchi di neve. Le famiglie di fronte all'evento nido.* Firenze: La Nuova Italia.

REFERENCES

Irer (Istituto Regionale di Ricerca della Lombardia) (1998) "Conciliazione tra vita professionale e vita familiare, risorse e vincoli delle famiglie e sostegno istituzionale." *Quaderni Regionali di Ricerca*, n°25.

Irish Constitution (1937) *Bunreacht na hEireann - Constitution of Ireland.* Dublin: Stationery Office.

Irish Times, "Childcare here costs working parents more", 17 May 2001, p. 3.

Irish Times/ MRBI Poll (1997) In: G. Kennedy, "77% say limited abortion rights should be provided", *The Irish Times*, 11 Dec 1997, p. 1.

Istat (1993) *Indagine multiscopo sulle famiglie. Anni 1987-91.* Roma: Istat.

Kluwer, E. S., Heessink, J. A. M. & Van de Vliert, E. (1996) "Marital Conflict About the Division of Household Labor and Paid Work", *Journal of Marriage and the Family*, 58 (Nov), pp. 958-969.

Langford, S. (1999) "The Childcare Challenge." *Proceedings of the SIPTU National Women's Forum - 1999 - The Legal, Social and Economic Position of Women on the Verge of a new Century and Millennium.* Dublin: Equality Unit, SIPTU, pp. 66 - 73.

Lanquetin, M.T., Laufer, J., & Letablier, M. T. (2000) "From equality to reconciliation in France?" In: L. Hantrais (Ed.) *Gendered Policies in Europe*, London: Macmillan.

Lansdowne Market Research Poll (2001) In: K. Holland, "Irish should not have to travel for abortion - poll", *Irish Times*, 1 June 2001, p. 5.

Latta, M. & O'Conghaile, W. (2000) *Aspirations, Restrictions and Choices – Combining Life and Work in the EU.* European Foundation for the Improvement of Living and Working Conditions in Dublin, Dublin.

Laufer, J. (1998) "Les femmes cadres entre le pouvoir et le temps?" *Revue Française des Affaires Sociales*, 3.

Leccardi, C. (1994) "Ricomporre il tempo: le donne, il tempo, il lavoro," *Sociologia del lavoro,* 56, pp. 148-55.

Le Nove (1990) *Mappatura degli orari dei servizi di Modena città: primo rapporto della ricerca "Le donne nella città: tempi, bisogni, servizi".* Cooperative LeNove – Modena: Comune di Modena.

Lewis, J. (Ed.) (1998) *Gender, Social Care and Welfare State Restructuring in Europe.* Aldershot: Ashgate.

Lewis, S. & Cooper, C. L. (1995) "Balancing the Work/Home Interface: A European Perspective," *Human Resource Management Review*, 5(4), pp. 289-305.

Lurol, M., & Pélisse, J., (2001) "35 heures : les disparités entre hommes et femmes," *Quatre pages,* Bulletin du Centre d'Etudes de l'Emploi.

REFERENCES

Mahon, E. (1998) "Changing Gender Roles, State, Work and Family Lives". In: E. Drew, R. Emerek & E. Mahon (Eds.) *Women, Work and the Family in Europe.* London & New York: Routledge.

Mantovani (1999) "Misure di sostegno alla conciliazione dei ruoli nelle aziende e nelle organizzazioni." Paper presented at the conference on *Le famiglie interrogano le politiche sociali.* Bologna, 29-31 March.

Martin, J. (1998) "Politique familiale et travail des femmes mariées en France. Perspective historique: 1942 – 1982," *Population*, n°6.

Maruani, M. (2000) *Travail et emploi des femmes.* Coll. Repères, La Découverte, Paris.

Mauri, L., and Billari, F.C. (Eds) (1999) *Generazioni di donne a confronto.* Milano: Angeli.

McKeown, K., Ferguson, H. & Romney, D. (1998) "Fathers: Irish experience in an international context - an abstract of a report to the Commission on the Family." In: *Strengthening Families for Life. Final Report of the Commission on the Family to the Minister for Social, Community and Family Affairs.* Dublin: Stationery Office, pp. 404-454.

Méda, D. (2001) *Le temps des femmes. Pour un nouveau partage des rôles,* Flammarion, Paris.

Méda, D. & Orain R. (2002) "Transformations du travail et du hors travail: le jugement des salariés," *Travail et Emploi,* n°90, pp. 23-38.

Melchiorre, V. (Ed.) (1992) *Maschio-femmina: nuovi padri e nuove madri.* Milano: San Paolo.

Menniti, A. (1993) *Fatti e opinioni sulle politiche familiari.* Working Paper, Irp.

Menniti, A., and S. Terracina (1994) *Conciliare lavoro, famiglia ed aspirazioni di vita. Cosa pensano gli italiani.* Working Paper. Roma: IRP.

Merelli, M. (1989) *Quasi adulte. Percorsi e modelli di donna nella transizione dei vent'anni.* Milano: Angeli.

Merllié, D. & Paoli, P. (2000) *Third European Survey on Working Conditions.* Luxembourg, Office for Official Publications of the European Communities.

Meurs, D., Ponthieux, S. (2000) "Une mesure de la discrimination, dans l'écart de salaire entre hommes et femmes," *Economie et Statistique,* 337-338, pp. 135- 152.

Mol, D. (2002) "Innovations in the Netherlands." In: M. Fine-Davis, H. Clarke & M. Berry (Eds.) *Fathers and Mothers: Dilemmas of the Work-Life Balance Conference Proceedings.* Dublin: Centre for Gender and Women's Studies, Trinity College, pp. 87-101.

REFERENCES

Molinari, L. (1991) "Identità sociali e conflitto di ruoli: principi organizzatori di rappresentazioni sociali dello sviluppo infantile," *Giornale Italiano di Psicologia*, 18(1), pp. 97-118.

Molinari, L. (1994) "Motherhood, Fatherhood and Sharing of Childcare." Paper presented at the International Congress: *Changes in Family Patterns in Western Countries*, Bologna, (Italy), 6-8 October.

Molinari, L. (1996) Ritratti di famiglia nelle esperienze delle madri. In: C. Ventimiglia (Ed.) *Paternità in controluce*. Milano: Angeli.

Musatti, T. (1992) *La giornata del mio bambino: madri, lavoro e cura dei più piccoli nella vita quotidiana*. Bologna: Il Mulino.

Musatti, T. & D'Amico R. (1996) "Nonne e nipotini: lavoro di cura e solidarietà intergenerazionale," *Rassegna Italiana di Sociologia*, 37(4), pp. 559-84.

National Development Plan (2001) ICTU Statement in National Framework Committee for Family Friendly Policies: - "An Introduction to Family Friendly Working Arrangements" Programme for Prosperity and Fairness, *National Development Plan*. Dublin: Stationery Office.

National Framework Committee for the Development of Family-Friendly Policies (2001) *Case Studies*, www.familyfriendly.ie

Nava, P. (1996) "Il figlio unico. Modelli di doppia presenza e strategie di decisione delle coppie," *Inchiesta*, 111, pp. 5-15.

NCJW Center for the Child (1988) *Employer Supports for Child Care*, New York: National Council of Jewish Women.

Nebenfuhr, E. (1998) "Determinants of Preferences Regarding the Reconciliation of Work and the Family and Requests to Policy Makers," In: R. Palomba & H Moors (Eds.) *Population, Family and Welfare: A Comparative Survey of European Attitudes: Vol II*. Oxford: Clarendon Press, pp. 143-162.

Neyrand, G. (1999) "Savoirs et normes socials en matière de petite enfance," *Recherches et Prévisions*, n° 57 – 58, pp. 3 –16.

Nordio, S., Piazza, G., & Stefanini, P. (1983) *Diventare padri. La famiglia, i suoi simboli, il pediatra*. Milano: Angeli.

Department of Education and Science (1999) *"Ready to Learn" - White Paper on Early Childhood Education*. Dublin: The Stationery Office.

O'Donoghue, J., T. D. (1999) "National Childcare Infrastructure," Speech by Minister for Justice, Equality and Law Reform, Government Press Centre, Dublin, 3 December.

REFERENCES

O'Donoghue, J., T. D. (2001) Speech by Minister for Justice, Equality and Law Reform at the launch of: *The Report of the Working Group on the Review and Improvement of the Maternity Protection Legislation; the Review of the Parental Leave Act, 1998; and a Research Project identifying the Key Issues concerning the Reconciliation Of Work And Family Roles*, 28 February.

OECD (2001) "Balancing Work and Family Life: Helping Parents into Paid Employment." *Employment Outlook,* Chp. 4, pp. 129-166.

Ondina Greco, E.M. (2000) "Il sostegno della rete primaria nell'accudimento dei bambini piccoli," *Politiche Sociali e Servizi*, 2, pp.283-99.

Palomba, R. (1991) "Gli Italiani e le opinioni sulla natalità e le politiche demografiche." In: A. Golini (Ed.) *Famiglia, figli e società in Europa*. Torino: Fondazione Giovanni Agnelli.

Palomba, R. (1997) "I tempi in famiglia." In: M. Barbagli & C. Saraceno (Eds.). *Lo stato delle famiglie in Italia*. Bologna: Il Mulino.

Palomba, R. (Ed.) (1987) *Vita di coppia e figli. Le opinioni degli italiani degli anni Ottanta*. Firenze: La nuova Italia.

Palomba, R. & Sabbadini, L. L. (1994) *Tempi diversi. L'uso del tempo di uomini e donne nell'Italia di oggi*. Commissione Nazionale per le pari opportunità tra uoma e donna – ISTAT, Roma.

Pattaro, S. (2000) *Scelte individuali e vincoli sociali: la distribuzione del tempo di lavoro tra famiglia e mercato nelle coppie danesi e italiane*. Università degli Studi di Trento, tesi di laurea (manoscritto non pubblicato).

Pélisse, J. (2002) *From negotiation to implemention. A study of the reduction of working time in France*, Document n°17, Centre d'Etudes de l'Emploi.

Piazza, M. (1993) "Il tempo per sé: un anello forte nella costruzione del soggetto." In: A. Carbonaro & C. Facchini (Eds.) *Biografie e costruzione dell'identità*. Milano: Angeli.

Piazza, M. (1999) (Ed.) *La presenza femminile nel Comune di Reggio Emilia. Soggettività e comportamenti organizzativi*. Reggio Emilia: Comune di Reggio Emilia, Comitato Pari Opportunità.

Piazza, M., Ponzellini, A. M., Provenzano, E., Tempia, A. (1999) *Riprogettare il tempo. Manuale per la progettazione degli orari di lavoro*. Roma: Edizioni Lavoro.

Pierson, P. (2001) *The New Politics of the Welfare State*. Oxford: Oxford University Press.

Pleck, J. H. (1998) "Work-Family Policies in the United States." In: R. Palomba & H. Moors (Eds.) *Population, Family and Welfare: A Comparative Survey of European Attitudes: Vol II*. Oxford: Clarendon Press.

Rauti, I. (1998) "Reti di sostegno: tipologie auspicabili." Paper presented at the conference on "Ragioniamo di maternita," Rome, 28 May. In: Commissione Nazionale per la Parità e le Pari Opportunità tra Uomo e Donna, Presidenza del Consiglio dei Ministri. *Ragioniamo di maternità. Maternità, paternità e Riforma del Welfare.* Roma: Commissione Nazionale per la Parità e le Pari Opportunità tra Uomo e Donna, Presidenza del Consiglio dei Ministri.

Report on the National Forum for Early Childhood Education (1998) Dublin: The Stationery Office.

Riva, S. (1999) "Conciliare lavoro e vita familiare: vincolo o vantaggio competitivo?" Paper presented at the conference on *Le famiglie interrogano le politiche sociali*. Bologna, 29-31 March.

Romito, P. & Saurel Cubizzolles, M.J. (1997) "I costi della maternità nella vita delle donne." *Polis*, 11(1), pp. 67-88.

Rossi, G. (1999) "Studiare la famiglia come intreccio tra i sessi e le generazioni: implicazioni sociologiche". In: D. Bramanti (Ed.) *Coniugalità e genitorialità. I legami familiari nella società complessa*. Milano: Vita e Pensiero.

Sabbadini L.L. & Palomba R. (1994) *Tempi diversi*. Roma: Commissione Nazionale Parità, Presidenza del Consiglio dei Ministri.

Sabbadini, L.L. (2001) *Modelli di formazione e organizzazione della famiglia*. Roma: Istat (versione provvisoria).

Saitta, L. (1996) "I datori di lavoro e la paternità." In: C. Ventimiglia, *Paternità in controluce*. Milano: Angeli.

Saraceno, C. (1987) *Pluralità e mutamento: riflessioni sull'identità al femminile*. Milano: Angeli.

Saraceno, C. (1993a) "Elementi per un'analisi delle trasformazioni di genere nella società contemporanea e delle loro conseguenze sociali," *Rassegna Italiana di Sociologia*, 34, pp. 19-57.

Saraceno, C. (1993b) "Continuità e discontinuità nella riproduzione sociale." In: A. Carbonaro & C. Facchini (Eds.) *Biografia e costruzione dell'identità*. Milano: Angeli.

Saraceno, C. (1996) "Il costo dei figli: un diverso riconoscimento per madri e padri," *Inchiesta*, 111, pp. 23-33.

Saraceno, C. (1998) *Mutamenti della famiglia e politiche sociali in Italia*. Bologna, Il Mulino.

Saraceno, C. (2001) "Politiche del lavoro e politiche della famiglia: un'alleanza lunga e problematica," *Lavoro e Diritto*, 15(1), pp. 37-54.

Saraceno, C. & S. Piccone Stella (Eds.) (1996) *Genere, la costruzione sociale del maschile e del femminile*. Bologna: Il Mulino.

REFERENCES

Scabini, E., and P. Donati (Eds.) (1991) *Identità adulte e relazioni familiari, Studi interdisciplinari sulla famiglia*. Milano: Vita e pensiero.

Scabini, E. & Regalia, C. (1999) "Benessere psichico, qualità dei legami e transizioni familiari." In: P. Donati (Ed.) *Famiglia e società del benessere*. Milano: San Paolo.

Scarazzati, L. (1994) "Nel segno della differenza. Tendenze e prospettive nelle concezioni femminili del lavoro." In: C. Cipolla (Ed.) *La differenza come compatibilità*. Milano: Angeli.

Scisci, A. (1999) "La donna tra famiglia e lavoro: il caso Italiano," *Studi di Sociologia*, 37 (2), pp. 235-54.

Second Commission on the Status of Women (1993) *Report to Government*. Dublin: The Stationery Office.

Second Commission on the Status of Women (1994) *First Progress Report of the Monitoring Committee on the Implementation of the Recommendations of the Second Commission on the Status of Women*, Dublin: Government Publication.

Second Commission on the Status of Women (1996) *Second Progress Report of the Monitoring Committee on the Implementation of the Recommendations of the Second Commission on the Status of Women*, Dublin: Government Publication.

Sexton, J. J. and Dillon, M. (1984) "Recent Changes in Irish Fertility." In: T. J. Baker, T. Callan, S. Scott & D. Madden (Eds.) *Quarterly Economic Commentary*. Dublin: The Economic and Social Research Institute.

Sgritta, G. (1988) *Famiglia, mercato e stato*. Milano: Angeli.

Shaver, S. & Bradshaw, J. (1995) "The Recognition of Wifely Labour by Welfare States," *Social Policy and Administration*, 29(1), pp. 10-25.

Shepard, E. M., Clifton, T. J. & Kruse, D. (1996) "Flexible Work Hours and Productivity: Some Evidence from the Pharmaceutical Industry," *Industrial Relations*, 35(1), pp. 123-139.

Shinn, M., O, B., Morris, A., Simko, P. (1987) "Child Care Patterns, Stress, and Job Behaviors Among Working Parents." Paper presented at the *Conference of the American Psychological Association*, New York.

Siebert, R. (1991) *E' femmina però è bella. Tre generazioni di donne al sud*. Torino: Rosenber&Sellier.

Staines, G.L. (1990) "Flexitime and the Conflict Between Work and Family Life." Paper presented at the conference of the *American Psychological Association, Boston*.

Thaulow, I. & Holt, H. (1996) *Erfaringer fra et udviklingsprojekt om familievenlige arbejdspladser*. København: Socialforskningsinstituttet.

REFERENCES

Thompson, C. A., Thomas, C. C. & Maier, M. (1992) "Work-family conflict: Reassessing corporate policies and initiatives." In: U. Sekaran and F. T. L. Leong (Eds.) *Womanpower: Managing in times of demographic turbulence.* Newbury Park, CA: Sage Publications, pp. 59-84.

Trifiletti, R. (1996) "La politica dell'infanzia in Italia: lo spazio del discorso politico e la ricostruzione storica." In: R. Trafiletti and P. Turi, *Tutela del bambino e famiglia "invisibile". L'analisi di una politica sociale in Toscana.* Milano: Angeli.

Trifiletti, R., and Turi, P. (1996) *Tutela del bambino e famiglia invisibile.* Milano: Angeli.

Van de Walle, I. (1997) Le congé parental: stratégies des employeurs et des salariées, *Recherches et Prévisions,* n°49, pp. 19-29.

Ventimiglia, C. (1994) *Di padre in padre. Essere, sentirsi, diventare padri.* Milano: Angeli.

Ventimiglia, C. (1996) *Paternità in controluce.* Milano: Angeli.

Ventimiglia, C. (1999) "Mamme in regia, papà in panchina." *Famiglia Oggi.* 11, pp. 18-25.

Vilde, M. (1999) "Le misure adottate dalla Provincia di Milano per facilitare la conciliazione della vita professionale e familiare del personale." Paper presented at the conference on *Le famiglie interrogano le politiche sociali.* Bologna, 29-31 March.

Villa, P. (2002) "Family and Work can be made compatible? The European experience". National and European Meeting: *Which "kind" of reconciliation? Family, Labour and Gender: balances and imbalances,* Turin, August 28-29.

Wagner, D. L. & Neal, M. B. (1994) "Caregiving and Work: Consequences, Correlates and Workplace Responses", *Educational Gerontology,* 20, pp. 645-663.

Whelan, C.T. & Fahey, T. (1994) "Marriage and the Family." In: C. T. Whelan (Ed.) *Values and Social Change in Ireland.* Dublin: Gill and Macmillan, pp. 45-81.

Winett, R. A. & Neale, M. S. (1980) "Results of Experimental Study on Flexitime and Family Life," *Monthly Labour Review,* 103 (Nov.), pp. 29-323.

Working Group on Childcare Facilities for Working Parents (1994) *Report to the Minister for Equality and Law Reform.* Dublin: Stationery Office.

Working Party on Child Care Facilities for Working Parents (1983) *Report to the Minister for Labour.* Dublin: Stationery Office.

Working Party on Women's Affairs and Family Law Reform (1985) *Irish Women: Agenda for Practical Action.* Dublin: Stationery Office.

Yeates, P. (2001) "Childcare costs have more than doubled since 1998" *The Irish Times,* 6 August, p. 7.

REFERENCES

Zanatta, A. L. (1999) "Il coinvolgimento dei padri nella cura dei figli," *Polis,* 13 (3), pp. 469-84.

Zanuso, L. (1986) "Donne, lavoro e generazioni." *Politiche del lavoro*, 1, pp. 130-54.

Zanuso, L. (1987) "Gli studi sulla doppia presenza: dal conflitto alla norma." In: M.C. Marcuzzo, & A. Rossi-Doria (Eds.). *La ricerca delle donne. Studi femministi in Italia.* Torino: Rosenberg & Sellier.

AUTHOR INDEX

Addis, E. 34, 35, 321
Allain, L. 14, 321
Andersen, D. 43, 47, 48, 321
Annino, M. 37, 326
Anxo, D. 18, 321
Appeldorn, A. 47, 321
Arona, M. 35, 321
Aryee, S. 240, 321
Ascoli, U. 35, 321

Badolato, G. 38, 87, 225, 245, 321
Balbo, L. 32, 34, 35, 225, 244, 321
Barbagli, M. 36, 321, 336
Barrère-Maurisson, M. A. 18, 322
Barry, U. 69, 322
Bassi, A. 31, 322
Becchi, E. 31, 322
Belloni, C. 32–34, 244, 322
Bergamaschi, M. 30, 31, 322
Bernardi, M. P. 34, 225, 322
Bertozzi, L. 30, 322
Bestetti, G. 38, 322
Bettio, F. 78, 322
Bianchi, M. 30, 322
Bielenski, H. 1, 129, 184, 323
Billari, F.C. 36, 334
Bimbi, F. 32–34, 36–39, 86–88, 90, 220, 223–225, 244, 245, 323
Bolger, N. 330
Bondioli, A. 322
Bonke, J. 41–43, 323, 326
Bosch, G. 323
Bowen, G. L. 241, 323
Bozzao, P. 25, 27, 323
Bozzi, G. 38, 323
Bradshaw, J. 9, 337
Brousse, C. 18, 323
Burchell, B. 3, 4, 324

Calafà, L. 25, 324
Cappellini, G. 35, 324

Carlsen, S. 47, 48, 50, 51, 324, 332
Casotti, A. 25, 31, 322, 330
Castelain-Meunier, C. 17, 224, 324
Castellano, G. 32–34, 38, 86–88, 90, 223–225, 245, 323
Cazzaniga, P. 30, 324
CBI 243, 324
Censis 35, 324
Cerrato, J. 330
Chiesi, A. 31, 322
Christenson, K. 240, 324
Clarke, H. xiii, 324, 325, 328, 330, 332, 334
Clifton, T. J. 242, 338
Commission on the Family 58, 59, 63, 65, 324, 334
Cooper, C. L. 243, 324, 334
Cooperativa Sociale Koine 31, 324
CREDOC 13–15, 325
Cristiani, C. 38, 323
Crooker, K. J. 243, 331
Crowley, N. 242, 243, 325
CSO 58, 64, 123, 134, 135, 175, 229, 232, 325
Csonka, A. 41, 42, 52, 53, 86, 235, 325

D'Amico, R. 35, 337
Damgaard, J. B. 45, 325
Danmarks Statistik 41, 44, 45, 47, 78, 219, 220, 325
Davis, E. E. 91, 196, 325, 330
de Brito, I. 244, 325
De Filippi, F. 31, 322
De Simone, G. 23, 25, 326
Del Punta, R. 25, 326
Department of Education and Science 59, 63, 66, 326, 335
Department of Justice, Equality and Law Reform ix, xiii, 56, 326
Dex, S. 234, 326
Di Vita, A. M. 36, 37, 90, 326
Dillon, M. 69, 338
Donati, P. 36, 326, 338

AUTHOR INDEX

Drew, E. 62, 86, 242, 326, 327, 330, 332, 334
Dublin Transportation Office 134, 326
Dutch Ministry of Social Affairs and Employment 129, 244, 326

Ellingsæter, A. L. 53, 54, 326
Emerek, R. 326, 327, 330, 332, 334
Emmott, M. 242, 244, 327
Equality Authority 57, 60, 168, 327, 330
Esping-Andersen, G. vii, 2, 327
Estrade, M. A. 20, 327
European Commission ix, xii, xiii, 1, 291, 326, 327
European Commission Network on Childcare 57, 81, 327
Eurostat xi, 2, 17, 76, 78, 79, 94, 135, 222, 224, 229, 327
Evans, J. M. 16, 327
Expert Working Group on Childcare 57, 58, 63, 66, 121, 327

Fagan, C. 3, 4, 324
Fagnani, J. ix, xi, 4, 9, 13, 17, 20, 79, 91, 219, 225, 227, 229, 327, 328
Fahey, T. 64, 71, 328, 339
Ferguson, H. 334
Fermanian, J. D. 17, 18, 328
Ferrari, M. 31, 322, 328
Ferrucci, F. 24, 328
Filippi, V. 31, 328
Fine-Davis, M. xi, 4, 59, 62, 64, 65, 69, 70–72, 87, 91, 92, 121, 196, 220, 227, 232, 242, 325, 328–330, 332, 334
Fisher, H. 59, 60, 330
Fitzgerald, J. 64, 328
Fleming, S. 332
Flood, L. 321
Fujimoto, T. 331

Galinsky, E. 241, 330
Gallou, R. 13, 330
Ganster, D. C. 243, 330
Ghedini, P. 31, 330
Gheido, M. R. 25, 330
Ginatempo, N. 36, 37, 330
Giovannini, D. ix, xii, 4, 5, 32–34, 38, 39, 87, 90, 97, 103, 224, 225, 245, 330, 331
Glass, J. 240, 331
Glaude, M. 9, 331
Goff, S. J. 243, 331
Goodbody Economic Consultants 63–65, 121, 331
Goriup, E. ix, 34, 330, 331
Gottardi, D. 25, 324, 331
Grecchi, A. 29, 331
Grover, S. L. 243, 331

Haas, L. 91, 103, 331
Hall, D. T. 243, 331
Hall, J. 90, 94, 331
Hantrais, L. 16, 331, 333
Heessink, J. A. M. 333
Hestbæk, A. D. 43, 321, 332
Hillage, J. 243, 332
Højgaard, L. ix, xiii, 4, 44, 49–51, 87, 90, 147, 195, 237, 332
Holt, H. 43, 44, 46, 47, 50–52, 86, 90, 141, 147, 332, 338
Humphreys, P. 242, 326, 322
Hutchinson, B. 90, 94, 332
Hutchinson, S. 242, 244, 327

Inglehart, R. 196, 332
Ingrosso, M. 31, 35, 90, 332
Irer (Istituto Regionale di Ricerca della Lombardia) 32–35, 37, 223, 333
Irish Constitution 68, 69, 333
Irish Times 68, 71, 333, 339
Istat 32, 333, 336, 337

Jamison, R. L. 331
Jones, D. C. 90, 94, 331
Joshi, H. 234, 326

Kauppinen, T. 1, 184, 323
Kocoglu, Y. 321
Kruse, D. 242, 338

Lagarde, P. 18, 328
Langford, S. 65, 68, 333
Lanquetin, M. T. 15, 333
Lansdowne Market Research 71, 333

AUTHOR INDEX

Latta, M. 183, 234, 333
Laufer, J. 18, 333
Le Nove 32,. 244, 333
Leccardi, C. 34, 333
Leprince, F. 328
Letablier, M. T. xii, 16, 20, 91, 227, 328, 331, 333
Lewis, J. 3, 333
Lewis, S. 243, 333
LigestillingsrÅdet 41, 44, 45, 219, 324, 325, 332
Luc, V. 321
Lurol, M. 243, 333

Mahon, E. 59, 326, 327, 330, 332, 334
Maier, M. 241, 339
Mancini, M. G. 34, 225, 322
Mancuso, R. 36, 37, 326
Mantovani 30, 334
Marchand, O. 322
Marino, E. 326
Martin, J. 9, 334
Maruani, M. 9, 334
Mauri, L. 36, 334
May, M. 321
McKeown, K. 73, 88, 245, 334
Méda, D. 21, 327, 334
Meehan, G. 325
Meilbak, N. T. 42, 43, 323, 325
Melchiorre, V. 36, 334
Menniti, A. 33, 35, 334
Merllié, D. 3, 334
Meurs, D. 9, 334
Micheli, G. 321
Minni, C. 322
Mol, D. 244, 334
Molinari, L. 5, 33, 38, 39, 330, 335
Morris, A. 338
Mount, M. K. 331
MRBI 71, 333
Murphy, C. 326
Musatti, T. 35, 90, 335

National Development Plan ix, 59, 335
National Framework Committee for the Development of Family-Friendly Policies 57, 59, 61, 86, 326, 335

Nava, P. 33, 37, 335
NCJW Center for the Child 242, 335
Neal, M. B. 243, 339
Neale, M. S. 240, 339
Nebenfuhr, E. 226, 232, 335
Neyrand, G. 17, 224, 335
Nordio, S. 38, 335

O'Conghaile, W. 183, 234, 333
O'Donnell, O. 332
O'Donoghue, J. 56–58, 335, 336
OECD 57, 58, 76, 77, 220, 327, 336
Omodei Zorini, E. 30, 322
Ondina Greco, E. M. 35, 336
Orain, R. 327, 334

Palomba, R. 32–34, 37, 88, 223, 225, 335–337
Paoli, P. 3, 334
Parker, V. A. 243, 331
Pattaro, S. ix, 32, 33, 88, 223, 336
Pavolini, E. 35, 321
Pélisse, J. 243, 333, 336
Périer, L. 328
Piazza, G. 335
Piazza, M. 28, 34, 336
Piccone, S. 337
Pierson, P. 2, 3, 220, 336
Pleck, J. H. 240, 336
Ponthieux, S. 9, 334
Ponzellini, A. M. 336
Provenzano, E. 336

Rabier, J. R. 196, 332
Rauti, I. 24, 337
Regalia, C. 35, 338
Report on the National Forum for Early Childhood Education 57, 63, 66, 121, 337
Riley, L. 240, 331
Riva, S. 30, 337
Rivier, S. 322
Romito, P. 37, 337
Romney, D. 334
Rossi, G. 34, 35, 337

Terracina, S. 33, 334

Sabbadini, L. L. 32–35, 88, 223, 225, 336, 337

Saitta, L. 33, 223, 337
Saraceno, C. 23–25, 36, 37, 321, 336, 337
Saurel Cubizzolles, M. J. 37, 337
Sbordone, F. 31, 322
Scabini, E. 35, 36, 338
Scarazzati, L. 37, 338
Schaubroeck, J. 243, 330
Schweizer, K. 30, 322
Scisci, A. 33–35, 86, 87, 338
Second Commission on the Status of Women 62, 63, 338
Sédillot, B. 14, 321
Sexton, J. J. 69, 338
Sgritta, G. 35, 338
Shaver, S. 9, 338
Shepard, E. M. 242, 338
Shinn, M. O. B. 239, 338
Siebert, R. 36, 338
Simkin, C. 243, 332
Simko, P. 338
Simon, M. O. 13, 239, 338
Sogni, G. 31, 322
Staines, G. L. 240, 324, 338
Stefanini, P. 335
Stein, P. J. 241, 330
Stone, R. 321

Tempia, A. 336
Thaulow, I 44, 332, 338
Thomas, C. C. 241, 339

Thompson, C. A. 241, 339
Trifiletti, R. 23, 24, 35, 339
Turi, P. 35, 339

Van de Vliert, E. 333
Van de Walle, I. 16, 339
Ventimiglia, C. 32–34, 38, 87, 88, 90, 97, 103, 223–225, 245, 331, 335, 337, 339
Vilde, M. 30, 339
Villa, P. 23, 25, 75, 76, 78, 79, 322, 326, 339

Wagner, A. 323
Wagner, D. L. 243, 339
Weise, H. 47, 321
Whelan, C.T. 71, 339
Williams, S. 243, 324
Winett, R. A. 240, 339
Working Group on Childcare Facilities for Working Parents 63, 339
Working Party on Child Care Facilities for Working Parents xi, 62, 63, 65, 71, 328, 339
Working Party on Women's Affairs and Family Law Reform 63, 339

Yeates, P. 68, 339

Zanatta, A. L. 33, 90, 103, 223, 340
Zanuso, L. 36, 37, 340

SUBJECT INDEX

Annual leave 56, 72, 124, 125, 127–129, 227, 228, 265–267, 302, 303
Attitudes:
    acceptance of workers' family responsibilities 147, 230
    attitudes towards childcare 3, 14, 47, 119
    attitudes towards parental leave 168
    attitudes of colleagues 7, 133, 147, 149, 228
    attitudes of employers 7, 16, 19, 21, 47, 133, 146, 147, 149, 150, 186, 188, 190, 191, 206–209, 220, 224, 228, 230, 231, 240, 244, 307
    gender role attitudes xi, 6, 17, 36, 69, 70, 71, 73, 88, 157
    people availing of family-friendly policies 150, 233
    perceived work pressure 158, 234
    perceived attitudes in the workplace 205–208
    workplace attitudes 48, 146, 160, 205, 209, 215, 230, 235, 243

Care-day 47
Care-work 23, 30, 32
Child sick day 85, 124, 125
    child's first sick day 47, 85
    leave for caring of a sick child 26, 85
Childbirth 37, 44, 72, 220, 240, 315
    child-delivery 44
    effects of the birth of the youngest child 6, 97–103, 133, 138–140, 223, 228, 251, 277
    significant changes, caused by 91, 97, 295
Childcare
    alternative arrangements 124, 227
    cost of childcare 58, 91, 122, 123, 226
    hours youngest child is in care 119, 120, 257
    public provision 3, 9, 57, 81, 87, 195, 219, 220, 226, 227, 236, 237
    reasons for choosing childcare options 121
    satisfaction with childcare 3, 7, 91, 123, 202–204, 239, 263
Childcare arrangements
    asilo nido 24
    babysitter 118, 121, 128, 129, 145, 255, 256, 258–260, 275, 300, 302, 303, 310
    childcare centre 16, 71, 89, 119, 121, 122, 181, 261, 262, 300–302, 304
    childminder 10, 11, 14, 15, 19, 45, 65, 118, 119, 145, 181, 226, 229, 255, 256, 258–260, 279, 280, 298, 300–302, 310
    crèche 10, 15, 19, 24, 31, 35, 36, 58, 72, 81, 86, 110, 111, 117, 118, 120–122, 124, 224, 226, 227, 255, 256, 258, 259, 261, 262, 279–281, 298, 300–302, 304
    crèches familiales 10
    crèches collectives 10
    day-care v, 10, 24, 41, 44–47, 52, 81, 195, 226, 237
    day-care facilities on site 44
    day-care institutions 41, 45, 46, 52
    école maternelle 10, 11, 117, 118, 120, 226, 256, 258
    grandparents 15, 35, 117–122, 124, 181, 226, 227, 255, 256, 258–261, 300, 301, 304
    haltes-garderies 10
    individual-demand services 24
    informal arrangements 124, 127–129, 228, 272–274, 303
    informal networks 35, 81
    kindergarten 24, 35, 45, 81
    neighbour 118, 121, 128, 129, 255, 256, 258–260, 275, 300, 302, 303
    nursery 10, 11, 45, 117, 118, 120, 226, 255, 256, 258, 259, 279–281, 300–302
    private childcare services 35
    registered childminders 10, 11, 14, 15, 45, 118, 226, 255, 258, 259, 300, 301
    scuola maternal 24

SUBJECT INDEX

unregistered childminders 15, 117, 118, 121, 255, 256, 258, 259, 300, 302
work crèche 118, 255, 258, 259
workplace childcare 67, 120, 242
Childcare leave – *see* Parental leave
Childcare providers 56
Childcare supply 65
Child-rearing practices 37
Combining work and family life 6–8, 20, 91–93, 158, 179–181, 185–191, 196, 212–215, 229, 230, 234, 236–238, 241, 244, 283, 313
Commuting 4, 7, 34, 91, 133, 134, 185–191, 197–201, 225, 228, 229, 236, 238, 244
Compulsory leave – *see* Statutory leave

Daily life management 32
   child-rearing practices – *see* Child rearing practices
   family management 33, 313
   interchangeability 33
   negotiation processes 20, 33, 34
   parental costs (of reproduction choices) 37
Day-care – *see* Childcare arrangements
Domestic and childcare activities 103, 114–116, 130
   division of labour within the household 6, 32, 103
   domestic activities 73, 104, 108, 115, 116, 245
   HELPINDEX 7, 116, 117, 186, 188, 190, 191, 202, 203
   how much help respondents receive 116, 117
   who usually [does] . . . 91, 103–116, 302
Domestic help 8, 180, 202–204, 239
Double burden 1, 33, 34, 36, 37, 39, 86, 219

Early childhood education 57, 63, 66, 67, 121
Educational childcare 65, 66, 121
Employers' motives for implementing family-friendly policies
   advantages of family-friendly working policies 242
   optimising female resources 29
Employment policy – *see* State policy

Employment rates 75, 76, 78
   female employment rate 76, 78
   female participation 2, 17, 41, 53, 64, 79, 219
   labour force participation rate 2, 220

Family friendly
   family friendly opportunities 51
   public support for family-friendly policies 71
   family friendly working arrangements – *see* Flexible Working
   family friendly workplace policies – *see* Flexible working
Family policy – *see* State policy
Fathers vi, vii, xii, 1, 3–5, 9, 12, 17–20, 26, 31–33, 38, 42–44, 47–52, 56, 73, 80, 84, 86–88, 103, 114, 123–125, 131, 138, 164, 180, 209, 220, 223–227, 229, 232–235, 237–241, 243, 245
   masculinity – *see* Gender roles, masculinity
   new fathers 38, 87, 245
   paternal involvement in childcare 33, 34, 38, 86, 223
   playing-expressive element 38
Fathers on leave – *see* Paternity leave
Femininity 49, 51, 87
Fertility rate 2, 44, 78, 79, 219
   total fertility rate 79, 219
Flexibility
   actual flexibility 7, 8, 92, 133, 140–144, 179, 211–214, 228, 230, 239
   flexible working – *see* Flexible working
   flexi-jobs 52
   potential flexibility 92, 141, 142, 211–214, 239
   potential for contact 144
   pragmatic flexibility 43
   time flexibility 53
Flexible working xi, 1, 3, 4, 6, 19, 27–29, 34, 55, 59, 60, 62, 86, 87, 142, 166, 173, 219, 230–232, 242–245, 307, 308, 316
   annualizzazione degli orari 29
   career breaks 60, 62, 92, 173, 231, 243, 316

SUBJECT INDEX

contratti di solidarietà 27, 28, 86
de-standardisation of labour-relations 27
e-working 60
family-friendliness of the workplace 8, 52, 176, 177, 179, 196, 210–214, 231, 237, 239
family friendly working arrangements 55, 59, 61, 236, 242
family friendly workplace policies 7, 55, 60, 133, 231, 240
flexible hours 20, 60, 72, 92, 172, 173, 182, 183, 231, 312, 316
informal agreements 43, 141, 142, 308
job-sharing 7, 27, 29, 55, 60–62, 86, 92, 133, 154–157, 171, 172, 210, 228, 231, 233, 234, 241, 243, 244, 309, 315
lavoro mobile 28
mobile work 28
part-time working 7, 14, 27, 29, 35, 53, 55, 60, 62, 77, 92, 133, 154–157, 170, 171, 184, 210, 228, 231, 232, 234, 243, 309, 315
personalised working hours 174, 175
shift work 29, 140–142, 308
tele-working 28, 55, 60–62, 86, 92, 175, 176, 242, 317
term-time working 55, 60, 173, 174, 231, 316
working time-schedules – *see* Working hours
year-based working schedules 29
Force majeur 57, 81, 85, 124, 227

Gender gap
  in employment rate 75, 76
  in hours and professional life 2
  in wages xiii, 42,
Gender issues / roles 5, 17, 36, 43, 55, 68–71, 73, 86–88, 220, 221, 235, 236
  asymmetry vi, 16, 18, 32–34, 39, 49, 86, 87, 224, 241
  attitudes towards gender roles xi, 6, 17, 36, 69, 70, 71, 73, 88, 157
  femininity – *see* Femininity
  gender asymmetries 32, 39, 87
  gender-based roles 36
  gendered division of labour 18, 20, 23, 24
  masculinity – *see* Masculinity
  re-distribution of care-work 32
  re-definition of gender and parental roles 39
  sharing equality 34
  symbolic order of gender 49, 50, 87
  traditional gender order 49
Gender segregation – vi, 41, 48, 235, 242

Horizontal and vertical segregation of women – *see* gender segregation

Implicit partner 23, 81

Labour force participation rate – *see* Employment rates
Leave of absence 29, 45, 46

Market-oriented work 37
Masculinity 49, 87
Maternity leave 11, 13–16, 24–26, 45, 55, 80, 82, 83, 92, 127
  Paid maternity leave 11, 12, 44–46, 55, 56, 83, 138, 140, 161–163, 165, 166, 176, 195, 223, 231, 237, 243, 297, 314
  Unpaid maternity leave 55, 56, 162, 163, 165, 166, 231, 314

National household surveys 58
National leave policies 161
Negotiation processes – *see* Daily life management
Normative-value model 34

Optional leave 25–27, 55, 80, 82, 84

Paid leave – *see* Statutory leave
Parental leave v, 4, 12–16, 23–27, 29, 33, 45, 47–49, 55, 57, 61, 72, 80, 82–84, 92, 124, 127–129, 166–170, 195, 220, 223, 227, 231, 232, 237, 243, 270–272, 303, 317, 319
  daily leave 26, 82
  sick child 26, 80, 81, 85, 124
  optional leave 25–27, 80, 84
  paid parental leave 166–170, 195, 220, 223, 231, 232, 237, 243, 317, 319

SUBJECT INDEX

unpaid parental leave 13, 166–170, 231, 317, 319
paternal involvement in childcare – *see* Fathers
Paternity Leave 12, 21, 24, 25, 27, 45, 47–50, 55, 57, 72, 80, 83, 84, 92, 138, 166, 243
   paid paternity leave 57, 61, 80, 83, 138, 163–166, 223, 231, 243, 315
   unpaid paternity leave 83, 164, 165, 166, 231, 315
Presenteeism 7, 243

Reconciliation xii, xiii, 1, 2, 5, 6, 9, 20, 28, 30–33, 36, 37
   combining work and family life; predictors of ease vs. difficulty 92, 93, 181, 185, 186, 188–190, 191, 196, 212–214, 236, 241, 244
   reconciliation policies 28
   optimising female resources – *see* Employers' motives for implementing family-friendly policies
   reconciling work and family; ease vs. difficulty 7, 53, 179–181, 215., 236, 283
Role strain – *see* Double burden

Sick leave 4, 72, 124, 125, 127, 129, 227, 228, 242, 243, 264, 265, 302, 303
Social indicators xi, 5, 179, 196, 221, 222, 236
State policies/Acts: Denmark
   government sponsored childcare provision 44
State policies/Acts: France
   Aide à la Famillle pour l'Emploi d'une Assistante Maternelle Agree (AFEAMA) 11, 224, 226
   Allocation de Garde d'Enfant a'Domicile (AGED) 11, 15
   Allocation Parentale d' Education (APE) – Child Rearing Benefit 13, 14, 18, 80
   Caisse d' Allocations Familiales (CAF) 10, 19
   Conge Parental d' Education (CPE) 12, 13, 16, 17, 84
   Contrat Enfance (CNAF) ix, xi, xii, 10

   Family allowance fund – *see* Caisse d'Allocations Familiales (CAF)
   Protection Maternelle et Infantile (PMI) 10
State policies/Acts: Ireland
   Anti-Discrimination (Pay) Act 69
   Child Benefit Allowance 67
   Employment Equality Act 1977 69
   Employment Equality Agency 69
   Equal Pay Act in 1975 70
   Force Majeur 57, 81, 85, 124, 227
   Maternity (Protection of Employees) Act of 1981 55
   Maternity Protection Act of 1994 55
   Parental Leave Act, 1998 57, 168
   Protection of Employees (Part-time Work) Act, 2001 60
State policies/Acts: Italy
   Act. No. 242/1902 26
   Act No. 1044/1971 24
   Act No. 1204/1971 25
   Act No. 891/1977 24, 25
   Act No. 903/1977 25
   Act No. 285/1997 24
   Act No. 493/1999 23
   Act No. 53/2000 23, 25–27
   Act No. 151/2001 ("Testo Unico") 23, 25, 26
   Act. No. 115/2003 25
   Contributi figurativi 27, 124
   Copertura Contributiva Ridotta 27, 85
   Law No. 53 – *see* Act. No. 53
   Law No. 626/1994 28
State policies: EU Directives
   EU Directive of 1992 56
   Directive 97/81/EC 60
State policy
   de-standardisation of labour-relations 27
   employment policy 17, 59
   family policy xii, 1, 2, 5, 9, 10, 12, 15, 17, 18, 23, 73, 80, 221, 240
   family protection to citizenship rights 27
   social responsibility 46, 52
   welfare state v, vii, 2, 3, 32, 44, 49, 54, 80, 220
Statutory Leave
   force majeur – *see* Force majeur
   maternity leave – *see* Maternity leave

SUBJECT INDEX

paid leave 45, 56, 80, 82, 84, 166, 168, 231, 232, 317, 318
parental leave – *see* Parental leave
paternity leave – *see* Paternity leave
sick leave – *see* Sick leave
unpaid leave 56, 57, 72, 166, 168, 227, 232, 316–318
Supervisor, sex of 91, 137, 138

Time
 commuting time 91, 134, 185–191, 197–201, 228, 229, 236, 238, 239, 244
 differentiated timing 34
 elasticity of daily working schedules 29
 hours at work – *see* Working hours
 ideal working schedule – *see* Working hours
 re-distribution of care-work – *see* Gender issues / roles
 time economies 32
 time preferences – *see* Time preferences
 time of towns 32, 244
 time-crossing 34, 225
 urban space-time relations 32, 244
 work-oriented time and family-oriented time 36
Time preferences 129, 275
 personal time 80, 91, 129, 131, 198–201, 224, 238, 276, 299
 time with the family 4, 20, 34, 87, 91, 129, 130, 198, 199, 223, 224–226, 245, 299
 time for oneself 32, 34, 223, 226

Unpaid leave – *see* Statutory leave

Welfare State – *see* State policy
Well-being 2, 3, 5, 87, 91–93, 179, 192, 195–218, 221, 228, 236–241, 244, 246, 285, 320
 Correlates of well-being 7, 8, 179, 196, 237
 Life satisfaction 7, 93, 194, 195, 199–204, 206–210, 212–218, 238–241
 Satisfaction with family life 7, 92, 93, 97, 179, 193–195, 197–204, 206–210, 212–218, 238, 239, 241, 287
 Satisfaction with health 7, 92, 93, 179, 192, 195, 198–204, 206–209, 211–218, 239, 241, 244
 Satisfaction with relationship with spouse/partner 7, 92, 93, 179, 194, 195, 198–209, 212–218, 288
 Satisfaction with work 7, 92, 93, 179, 192, 193, 195, 198–210, 212–218, 236
Work permit 29
Working hours 2, 3, 14, 17, 19, 20, 25–27, 42, 43, 55, 56, 58, 87, 92, 133, 135, 140, 141, 174, 175, 182, 195, 215, 229, 231, 236–238, 241, 244, 316
 hours worked per week 13, 14, 19, 29, 42, 61, 86, 135–137, 183, 185–191, 197–201, 226, 229, 236, 238, 277, 294, 312
 ideal working schedule 179, 182, 183, 236, 312
 working time schedule 27, 29, 240
Workplace culture xiii, 7, 16, 42, 50–52, 133, 228, 144, 160, 185, 195, 230, 235–237, 240, 241

Social Indicators Research Series

1. V. Møller (ed.): *Quality of Life in South Africa.* 1997   ISBN 0-7923-4797-8
2. G. Baechler: *Violence Through Environmental Discrimination.* Causes, Rwanda Arena, and Conflict Model. 1999   ISBN 0-7923-5495-8
3. P. Bowles and L.T. Woods (eds.): *Japan after the Economic Miracle.* In Search of New Directories. 1999   ISBN 0-7923-6031-1
4. E. Diener and D.R. Rahtz (eds.): *Advances in Quality of Life Theory and Research.* Volume I. 1999   ISBN 0-7923-6060-5
5. Kwong-leung Tang (ed.): *Social Development in Asia.* 2000   ISBN 0-7923-6256-X
6. M.M. Beyerlein (ed.): *Work Teams: Past, Present and Future.* 2000   ISBN 0-7923-6699-9
7. A. Ben-Arieh, N.H. Kaufman, A.B. Andrews, R. Goerge, B.J. Lee, J.L. Aber (eds.): *Measuring and Monitoring Children's Well-Being.* 2001   ISBN 0-7923-6789-8
8. M.J. Sirgy: *Handbook of Quality-of-Life Research. An Ethical Marketing Perspective.* 2001   ISBN 1-4020-0172-X
9. G. Preyer and M. Bös (eds.): *Borderlines in a Globalized World.* New Perspectives in a Sociology of the World-System. 2002   ISBN 1-4020-0515-6
10. V. Nikolic-Ristanovic: *Social Change, Gender and Violence: Post-communist and war affected societies.* 2002   ISBN 1-4020-0726-4
11. M.R. Hagerty, J. Vogel and V. Møller: *Assessing Quality of Life and Living Conditions to Guide National Policy.* 2002   ISBN 1-4020-0727-2
12. M.J. Sirgy: *The Psychology of Quality of Life.* 2002   ISBN 1-4020-0800-7
13. S. McBride, L. Dobuzinskis, M. Griffin Cohen and J. Busumtwi-Sam (eds.): *Global Instability.* Uncertainty and new visions in political economy. 2002   ISBN 1-4020-0946-1
14. Doh. Chull Shin, C.P. Rutkowski and Chong-Min Park (eds.): *The Quality of Life in Korea.* Comparative and Dynamic Perspectives. 2003   ISBN 1-4020-0947-X
15. W. Glatzer: *Rich and Poor.* Disparities, Perceptions, Concomitants. 2002   ISBN 1-4020-1012-5
16. E. Gullone and R.A. Cummins (eds.): *The Universality of Subjective Wellbeing Indicators.* A Multi-disciplinary and Multi-national Perspective. 200?   ISBN 1-4020-1044-3
17. B.D. Zumbo (ed.): *Advances in Quality of Life Research 2001.* 2003   ISBN 1-4020-1100-8
18. J. Vogel, T. Theorell, S. Svalifors, H.-H. Noll and B. Christoph (eds.): *European Welfare Production. Institutional Configurates and Distributional Outcome.* 2003   ISBN 1-4020-1149-0
19. A.C. Michalos: *Essays on the Quality of Life.* 2003   ISBN 1-4020-1342-6
20. M. Joseph Sirgy, D. Rathz and A. Coskun Samli (eds.): *Advances in Quality-of-Life Theory and Research.* 2003   ISBN 1-4020-1474-0
21. M. Fine-Davis, J. Fagnani, D. Giovannini, L. Hojgaard and H. Clarke (eds.): *Fathers and Mothers: Dilemmas of the Work-Life Balance.* 2004   ISBN 1-4020-1807-X

KLUWER ACADEMIC PUBLISHERS – DORDRECHT / LONDON / BOSTON